WOMEN'S ISSUES

A LOOK AT MATERNAL HEALTH AND REPRODUCTIVE RIGHTS

WOMEN'S ISSUES

Additional books and e-books in this series can be found
on Nova's website under the Series tab.

WOMEN'S ISSUES

A LOOK AT MATERNAL HEALTH AND REPRODUCTIVE RIGHTS

LISA R. FLORES
EDITOR

snova
New York

Library of Congress Cataloging-in-Publication Data

ISBN: 978-1-53619-760-0

Published by Nova Science Publishers, Inc. † New York

CONTENTS

PREFACE

The United States is the most dangerous place in the developed world to deliver a baby. Each year, about 700 American women die and 50,000 women are severely injured due to complications related to childbirth. If you are a Black woman in the United States, it is even more dangerous to give birth.

Chapter 1 reports on ways to save mothers' lives. Chapter 2 and 3 examine how state and federal policies are impacting residents' access to comprehensive reproductive healthcare services, including abortion.

In: A Look at Maternal Health and Reproductive Rights ISBN: 978-1-53619-760-0
Editor: Lisa R. Flores

Chapter 1

IMPROVING MATERNAL HEALTH: LEGISLATION TO ADVANCE PREVENTION EFFORTS AND ACCESS TO CARE*

Committee on Energy and Commerce

Tuesday, September 10, 2019
House of Representatives,
Subcommittee on Health,
Committee on Energy and Commerce,
Washington, DC.

The subcommittee met, pursuant to call, at 10:01 a.m., in the John D. Dingell Room 2123, Rayburn House Office Building, Hon. Anna G. Eshoo (chairwoman of the subcommittee) presiding. Members present: Representatives Eshoo, Engel, Butterfield, Matsui, Castor, Sarbanes, Lujá n, Schrader, Kennedy, Cárdenas, Welch, Ruiz, Dingell, Kuster, Kelly, Barragán, Blunt Rochester, Rush, Pallone (ex officio), Burgess (subcommittee ranking member), Upton, Shimkus, Guthrie, Griffith, Bilirakis, Long, Bucshon, Brooks, Mullin, Hudson, Carter, Gianforte, and Walden (ex officio).

Also present: Representatives Schakowsky and Soto.

Staff present: Jacquelyn Bolen, Counsel; Jeffrey C. Carroll, Staff Director; Waverly Gordon, Deputy Chief Counsel; Tiffany Guarascio, Deputy Staff Director; Stephen Holland, Health Counsel; Zach Kahan, Outreach and Member Service Coordinator; Josh Krantz, Policy Analyst; Una Lee, Chief Health Counsel; Aisling McDonough, Policy Coordinator; Meghan Mullon, Staff Assistant; Joe Orlando, Staff Assistant; Kaitlyn Peel, Digital Director; Tim Robinson, Chief Counsel; Kimberlee

* This is an edited, reformatted and augmented version of Hearing before the Subcommittee on Health, of the Committee on Energy and Commerce, House of Representatives, One Hundred Sixteenth Congress, First Session, Publication No. Serial No. 116–58, dated September 10, 2019.

Trzeciak, Chief Health Advisor; Rick Van Buren, Health Counsel; Margaret Tucker Fogarty, Minority Staff Assistant; Caleb Graff, Minority Professional Staff Member, Health; Peter Kielty, Minority General Counsel; J. P. Paluskiewicz, Minority Chief Counsel, Health; Brannon Rains, Minority Legislative Clerk; Zack Roday, Minority Director of Communications; and Kristen Shatynski, Minority Professional Staff Member, Health.

Ms. ESHOO. The Subcommittee on Health will come to order.

Welcome back, everyone. I hope you had a productive August and that you have got some rest with your families, and we will roll up our sleeves and get back to work.

The Chair now recognizes herself for 5 minutes for an opening statement.

And the witnesses, please come to the table. And thank you each one for being here.

Opening Statement of Hon. Anna G. Eshoo, a Representative in Congress from the State of California

"The United States is the most dangerous place in the developed world to deliver a baby." That is a quote and the conclusion after major investigation by USA Today last year. Each year, about 700 American women die and 50,000 women are severely injured due to complications related to childbirth. If you are a Black woman in the United States, it is even more dangerous to give birth.

Black and American Indian and Alaska Native women are three to four times more likely to die from pregnancy-related causes. This is absolutely unacceptable. And what is more, it is preventable. The CDC estimates that more than 60 percent—more than 60 percent—of these deaths could be prevented.

Our witnesses will instruct us today that there is a clear way to save mothers' lives. We need to make sure that women have highquality care and coverage before, during, and after their pregnancy. And the four bills we are considering today do just that.[1]

Congresswoman Kelly's MOMMA's Act uses standardized data to inform healthcare professionals about the best practices and protocols to manage a mother's care in an emergency, such as when a mother hemorrhages after birth. This data-driven approach was spearheaded in my district at Stanford, California's Maternal Quality Care Collaborative, which has reduced severe health problems from pregnancy-related hemorrhages by 21 percent to date and has contributed to reducing the maternal mortality rate in California by a whopping 55 percent.

Representative Engel's Quality Care for Moms and Babies Act also works to improve maternal care through data by using care surveys, quality measures, and perinatal quality collaboratives.

---

[1] The legislation has been retained in committee files and also is available at https://docs.house.gov/Committee/Calendar/ByEvent.aspx?EventID=109919.

Both Congresswoman Kelly's legislation and Congresswoman Pressley's Healthy MOMMIES Act recognizes that to truly make progress, women must be able to get medical care when they need it.

Women are more likely to die of a pregnancy-related condition in the weeks following birth than during pregnancy or delivery, but many American mothers lack health insurance during that critical postpartum period. Every year, hundreds of thousands of mothers are kicked off Medicaid only 2 months after giving birth. The MOMMA'S Act and the Healthy MOMMIES Act extend Medicaid for a full year postpartum. These bills make sure the Medicaid safety net is there for women at one of the most vulnerable times in their lives, and this extension makes sense. That is why State legislatures in California, New Jersey, Texas, South Carolina, and Illinois are seriously considering measures to extend Medicaid for 1 year for eligible new mothers.

Finally, the Maternal CARE Act introduced by Congresswoman Alma Adams addresses the insidious way racism kills Black mothers. The bill funds implicit bias training programs for health professionals. As Nina Martin describes in her investigative series "Lost Mothers," African-American mothers repeatedly report being devalued and disrespected by medical providers who did not take their medical concerns seriously.

I will conclude as I began: The United States is the most dangerous place in the developed world to deliver a baby. Shame on us. I believe a high maternal death rate is a reflection of how much a society values women. As the first chairwoman of this subcommittee, I think it is time we reverse this by making a healthcare system that better cares for women.

[The prepared statement of Ms. Eshoo follows:]

PREPARED STATEMENT OF HON. ANNA G. ESHOO

"The U.S. is the most the dangerous place in the developed world to deliver a baby." This quote was the conclusion of a major investigation by *USA Today* last year.

Each year, about 700 American women die and 50,000 women are severely injured due to complications related to childbirth. If you're a black woman in the U.S., it is even more dangerous to give birth. Black women are three to four times more likely to die from childbirth than white women.

This is unacceptable, and what's more, it's preventable. The CDC estimates more than 60% of these deaths could be prevented.

Our witnesses will instruct us today that there is a clear way to save mothers' lives.

We need to make sure women have high quality care and coverage before, during, and after their pregnancy. The four bills we're considering today do just that.

Congresswoman Kelly's *MOMMA's Act* (H.R. 1897) uses standardized data to inform health care professionals about the best practices and protocols to manage a mother's care in an emergency, such as when a mother hemorrhages after birth.

This data-driven approach was spearheaded in my District. Stanford's California Maternal Quality Care Collaborative has reduced severe health problems from pregnancy-related hemorrhages by 21% and has contributed to reducing the maternal mortality rate in California by 55%.

Representative Engel's *Quality Care for Moms and Babies Act* (H.R. 1551) also works to improve maternal care through data by using care surveys, quality measures, and perinatal quality collaboratives.

Both Congresswoman Kelly's *MOMMA's Act* (H.R. 1897) and Congresswoman Pressley's *Healthy MOMMIES Act (*H.R. 2602) recognize that to truly make progress, women must be able to get medical care when they need it.

Women are more likely to die of a pregnancy-related condition in the weeks following birth than during pregnancy or delivery, but many American mothers lack health insurance during that critical postpartum period.

Every year, hundreds of thousands of mothers are kicked off Medicaid only two months after giving birth.

The *MOMMA's Act* and the *Healthy MOMMIES Act* extend Medicaid for a full year postpartum. These bills make sure the Medicaid safety net is there for women at one of the most vulnerable times in their lives.

This extension makes sense. That's why state legislatures in California, New Jersey, Texas, South Carolina, and Illinois are seriously considering measures to extend Medicaid for one year for eligible new mothers.

Finally, the *Maternal CARE Act* (H.R. 2902), introduced by Congresswoman Alma Adams, addresses the insidious way racism kills black mothers. The bill funds implicit bias training programs for health professionals.

As Nina Martin describes in her investigative series *Lost Mothers*, African-American mothers repeatedly report being devalued and disrespected by medical providers who did not take their medical concerns seriously.

I'll conclude as I began. The United States is the most dangerous place in the developed world to deliver a baby.

I believe a high maternal death rate is a reflection of how much a society values women. As the first Chairwoman of the Health Subcommittee, I think it's time we reverse this by making a health care system that better cares for women.

I yield the remainder of my time to Representative Engel, the author of H.R. 1551 the *Quality Care for Moms and Babies Act.*

Ms. ESHOO. I now would like to yield the remainder of my time to Representative Engel, the author of H.R. 1551, the Quality Care for Moms and Babies Act. Oh, he is not here. All right.

Well, the Chair will now recognize Dr. Burgess, the ranking member of our subcommittee, for 5 minutes for his opening statement.

OPENING STATEMENT OF HON. MICHAEL C. BURGESS, A REPRESENTATIVE IN CONGRESS FROM THE STATE OF TEXAS

Mr. BURGESS. Thank you, Chairwoman Eshoo. Thanks for the recognition.

And I certainly appreciate that our Health Subcommittee is revisiting the issue of maternal mortality. Certainly we addressed this last year when we held the hearing on Jaime Herrera Beutler's H.R. 1318, the Preventing Maternal Deaths Act, which was signed into law last December. And whether the people realize it or not—I don't know how many people do realize it—unusual for the House of Representatives to pass a stand-alone bill dealing with maternal mortality, but it did indeed happen in the last Congress.

And now we are here today to see if we can build on that success, build on that progress, utilize the data that is going to become available because of getting H.R. 1318 across the finish line.

By authorizing grants and allowing States to establish Maternal Mortality Review Committees, such as the one that Texas established back in 2013, States will be able to clearly identify the causes of maternal mortality and use that data to inform solutions. Given the robust bipartisan discussions that occurred last year, we do want to continue those robust bipartisan discussions. Unfortunately, today the bills that we have before us are all on the majority side. Our staffs have spent some time in preparation for this hearing. So it is unfortunate that that could not have been a little more expansive. Dr. Bucshon on this committee and Representative Andre´ Carson, a member of the majority, introduced a bipartisan bill, H.R. 4215, the Excellence in Maternal Health Act, along with a number of Energy and Commerce members, and I believe that a version of this language could become law and be signed by the President, and we should discuss the merits of such a policy at this hearing.

I think it is worthwhile to have a productive dialogue about the ideas put forth in all of the bills before us today, but there certainly are some questions about how implementation would occur and whether the bills would actually make a difference.

I in my former life did practice obstetrics and gynecology. Now as a Member of Congress, I want you know that addressing maternal mortality is one of my top priorities. And that is why I advocated, along with Representative Herrera Beutler last year, for the passage of H.R. 1318. Over the course of this year, I have been carefully looking at the right next step to build on the success we had last year. I have engaged with the Congressional Budget Office on several policy options related to Medicaid coverage of pregnancy, and I am committed to finding a way to address this issue, but we do need to be tactful and inclusive in this approach.

As we move through the discussion of these bills, I have some questions that I would like our witnesses to have in mind.

First, what is the Centers for Disease Control and Prevention already doing to aid States process data through Maternal Mortality Review Committees? And do these bills we have before us today, are they additive or are they simply duplicative of existing efforts?

Secondly, more than 40 percent of the births in the United States are covered by Medicaid. What tools do States need to address the unique needs of their own Medicaid populations?

Thirdly, some States are already submitting 1115 waivers to expand Medicaid coverage for 1 year postpartum without any intervening Federal legislation. How would these existing State efforts be impacted by a Federal law, and is there any danger of hampering State innovation?

Fourthly, how can we support hospitals' existing efforts to coordinate care and maintain access to physicians throughout the delivery?

Fifth, are any States employing innovative maternity care models in Medicaid that would be worthy of exploring at a demonstration at a Federal level?

And then, finally, what are the main barriers to women receiving pre- and postnatal care? And what are the best practices that can be deployed to address maternal mortality and severe morbidity, the so-called near misses that occur when someone actually survives but has a very untoward event?

Now, I do want to spend a moment and give a special thanks and a special Texas welcome to Dr. David Nelson, the chief of obstetrics at Parkland Hospital.

Chairwoman, you said, quoting from USA Today, that the United States is the most dangerous place in the world to have a baby. I would submit that Parkland Hospital is probably the safest place in the world to have a baby. It is because of the tremendous leadership, the clinical staff, and the dedicated staff of UT Southwestern and the residents and house officers and the nurses who all provide care to the medically indigent in Dallas County, Texas.

So, as a former Parkland resident, I am looking forward to hearing about the practices that your team employs to ensure safe delivery for both mothers and babies in Dallas, down in Texas.

And I yield back my time.

[The prepared statement of Mr. Burgess follows:]

PREPARED STATEMENT OF HON. MICHAEL C. BURGESS

Thank you, Chairwoman Eshoo. I appreciate that our Health Subcommittee is revisiting the issue of maternal mortality, one that we addressed last year when we held a hearing on Rep. Jaime Herrera Beutler's H.R. 1318, the Preventing Maternal Deaths Act, which President Trump signed into law in December. It was critical that we work in a bipartisan fashion to get H.R. 1318 across the finish line because stakeholders continued to tell us that there was a lack of data about why these maternal deaths were occurring, and that it is difficult to address problems that have yet to be clearly identified.

By authorizing grants allowing states to establish maternal mortality review committees, such as the one that Texas established in 2013, states will be able to clearly identify the causes of maternal mortality, eventually using that data to inform solutions.

Given the robust bipartisan discussions that occurred last year, I am frustrated that the Majority did not collaborate with us much in preparation of this hearing. For example, our staffs had spoken months ago about building upon language included in the bipartisan Senate HELP Committee's health care costs package to continue this Subcommittee's commitment to addressing the issue of maternal mortality. Unfortunately, you decided you did not want to move forward on this language together. In fact, you even tried to add a bill at the last minute on Friday afternoon and still refused to include the HELP language as introduced by Dr. Bucshon.

Dr. Bucshon and Rep. Andre Carson introduced a bipartisan bill, H.R. 4215, the Excellence in Maternal Health Act of 2019, along with me and a number of other Energy and Commerce Members. I believe that a version of this language could become law, and that we should discuss the merits of such a policy at this hearing. I think it is worthwhile to have a productive dialogue about the ideas put forth in the four bills before us today, but I have a lot of questions about how these policies would be implemented and if they would actually make a difference.

As an OB/GYN and a Member of Congress, addressing maternal mortality is one of my top priorities, which is why I advocated alongside Rep. Herrera Beutler last year for passage of H.R. 1318. Over the course of this year, I have been carefully looking for the right next step to build on the successes of H.R. 1318. I have engaged with CBO on several policy options related to Medicaid coverage of pregnancy, and I am committed to finding a way to address this issue, but we must be tactful in our approach. I do wish that this hearing had been planned in advance such that agencies that would be on the front lines of implementing the policies before us today.

As we move through our discussion of these bills, I have some questions that I would like our witnesses and other Members to have in mind.

1. What is the Center for Disease Control and Prevention already doing to aid states process data through maternal mortality review committees as a result of H.R. 1318, and do these other bills duplicate existing efforts?
2. More than 40 percent of births in the United States are covered by Medicaid. What tools do States need to address the unique needs within their own Medicaid populations?
3. States are already submitting 1115 waivers to expand Medicaid coverage to one-year post-partum without federal legislation. How would these existing state efforts be impacted by a federal law and would state innovation be hampered?
4. How can we support hospitals' existing efforts to coordinate care and maintain access to physicians throughout delivery?
5. Are any states employing innovative maternity care models in Medicaid that would be worthy exploring in a demonstration or at a federal level?

6. What are the main barriers to women receiving pre- and post- natal care, and what are best practices that can be deployed to address maternal morbidity and mortality?

I would like to give a special Texas welcome to Dr. David Nelson, the Chief of Obstetrics at Parkland Hospital. As a former Parkland resident, I look forward to hearing more about the practices he and his team employ to ensure safe delivery for both mothers and babies in Dallas.

Thank you, and I yield back.

Ms. ESHOO. The Chair thanks the ranking member for his comments. Let me just add something to them. The committee is hearing four bills today, and together they contain all of the provisions in the Senate health bill and Representative Bucshon's bill, but they also go beyond those provisions to include extending Medicaid coverage for post partum women. So I wanted to add that to the conversation.

The Chair is now pleased to recognize the chairman of the full committee, Mr. Pallone, for his 5 minutes for his opening statement.

OPENING STATEMENT OF HON. FRANK PALLONE, JR., A REPRESENTATIVE IN CONGRESS FROM THE STATE OF NEW JERSEY

Mr. PALLLONE. Thank you, Madam Chair.

Today, we are examining the often tragic reality of the maternal health system in our Nation and a number of policies that could dramatically improve health outcomes for new mothers and their children. Every year, about 700 women die here in the United States from a pregnancy-related condition, and thousands more face severe maternal morbidity. That is simply disgraceful. And when you compare these outcomes to other countries around the world, the United States is near the bottom. We are also the only industrialized country in the world with a rising maternal death rate.

In a nation as wealthy as ours, these statistics are simply shocking and inexcusable, but I am hopeful that we can begin to turn the tide to improve maternal health. The Centers for Disease Control and Prevention estimates that 60 percent of maternal deaths in the U.S. are preventable, and the legislation we are discussing today is a strong step forward.

Now, a number of the bills that we have today will strengthen prevention efforts that already exist, including policies that follow up on the Preventing Maternal Deaths Act, which was enacted last year. This new law improved data collection and helped to expand Maternal Mortality Review Committees to all 50 States. The legislation also authorizes and strengthens the Alliance for Innovation on Maternal Health and Safety, or the AIM program. This program helps physicians and health systems implement evidence-based practices that have been shown to improve patient outcomes when performed in a healthcare setting but have not yet been implemented nationwide.

Maternal mortality and morbidity are problems that affect women throughout our country, but especially in African-American and Native American communities, where women are three times as likely to die due to pregnancy-related conditions as White women. The bills also offer a number of proposals to reduce health disparities along racial, ethnic, and cultural lines.

We are also going to be looking at ways to improve health coverage for new mothers. According to the CDC, one-third of all pregnancy-related deaths occur between 1 week and 1 year post partum. And while Medicaid and the Children's Health Insurance Program cover more than half of all births in the U.S., coverage for some new mothers ends just 60 days after delivery. That is why I am glad we will be reviewing additional proposals to extend that coverage to 1 year after delivery, extending access to regular physician checkups and other health services that help women and their healthcare providers detect and treat health issues such as high blood pressure and heart disease, two of the most common causes of pregnancy-related deaths. It is my sincere hope to work with our Republican colleagues to enact a bipartisan proposal to extend this vital health coverage for new mothers.

Our witnesses today offer views from diverse backgrounds, and I am confident that their experiences and expertise will help us all learn more about the problems we are facing and the solutions that will make a real difference. I thank them all for being here.

And I also want to recognize the leadership of so many bipartisan Members of the House who testified on this important topic at our recent Member Day hearing, including several members of the Congressional Caucus on Maternity Care and the Black Maternal Health Caucus.

So I have a couple of minutes left. I would like to yield that to the woman from Chicago, Ms. Kelly, the author of the H.R. 1897, the MOMMA's Act.

PREPARED STATEMENT OF HON. FRANK PALLONE, JR.

Today we are examining the often-tragic reality of the maternal health system in our nation, and a number of policies that could dramatically improve health outcomes for new mothers and their children.

Every year, about 700 women die here in the United States from a pregnancy-related condition, and thousands more face severe maternal morbidity. That's simply disgraceful. And when you compare these outcomes to other countries around the world, the United States is near the bottom. We are also the only industrialized country in the world with a rising maternal death rate.

In a nation as wealthy as ours, these statistics are simply shocking and inexcusable, but I am hopeful that we can begin to turn the tide to improve maternal health. The Centers for Disease Control and Prevention (CDC) estimates that 60 percent of maternal deaths in the United States are preventable, and the legislation that we are discussing today is a strong step forward.

A number of the bills will strengthen prevention efforts that already exist, including policies that follow up on the Preventing Maternal Deaths Act, which was enacted last year. This new law improved data collection and helped to expand Maternal Mortality Review Committees to all fifty states. The legislation also authorizes and strengthens the Alliance for Innovation in Maternal Health and Safety, or the AIM program. This program helps physicians and health systems implement evidence-based practices that have been shown to improve patient outcomes when performed in a health care setting but have not yet been implemented nationwide.

Maternal mortality and morbidity are problems that affect women throughout our country, but especially in African American and Native American communities, where women are three times as likely to die due to pregnancy-related conditions as white women. The bills also offer a number of proposals to reduce health disparities along racial, ethnic, and cultural lines.

We are also going to be looking at ways to improve health coverage for new mothers. According to the CDC, one-third of all pregnancy-related deaths occur between one week and one year postpartum. While Medicaid and the Children's Health Insurance Program cover more than half of all births in the United States, coverage for some new mothers ends just 60 days after delivery. That is why I am glad we will be reviewing additional proposals to extend that coverage to one year after delivery. Extending access to regular physician check-ups and other health services could help women and their health care providers detect and treat health issues such as high blood pressure and heart disease, two of the most common causes of pregnancy-related death. It is my sincere hope to work with our Republican colleagues to enact a bipartisan proposal to extend this vital health care coverage for new mothers.

Our witnesses today offer views from diverse backgrounds and I am confident that their experiences and expertise will help all of us learn more about the problems we are facing and the solutions that will make a real difference. I thank them all for being here.

I also want to recognize the leadership of so many bipartisan members of the House who testified on this important topic at our recent Member Day hearing, including several members of the Congressional Caucus on Maternity Care and the Black Maternal Health Caucus.

I'd now like to yield the remainder of my time to Representative Kelly, the author of H.R. 1897, the MOMMA's Act.

Ms. KELLY. Thank you, Mr. Chair.

Chairman Pallone, Chairwoman Eshoo, and Ranking Member Burgess, thank you for allowing me to make this brief opening statement.

Like you, I am shocked by our Nation's growing maternal mortality crisis. While losing 700 to 900 new moms each year is devastating, this crisis, like too many others, takes a disproportionate toll on communities of color. Nationwide, Black mothers die three to four times the rate of White mothers. In my home State of

Illinois, that disparity climbs to six times. In the State of Washington, American Indian moms die eight times the rate of their White counterparts.

It is clear that race is playing a role in these deaths. That is why my proposal, the MOMMA's Act, which I will discuss in depth later, includes provisions to ensure cultural competency training to ensure all moms and families are listened to during their childbirth journey.

However, this provision will only take us so far. It is imperative that we continue investing in diversifying the provider pipeline. The racial disparities underlying the shocking maternal mortality statistics make an already tragic situation more tragic. However, these challenges are not insurmountable. Today's hearing and the commitment from this subcommittee give me great hope for a future where all mamas get the chance to be mamas. I thank the chairwoman for the time and appreciate your efforts in addressing the crisis.

I yield back.

Ms. ESHOO. We thank the gentlewoman for her work on her important legislation.

I now would like to recognize the ranking member of the full committee, my friend Mr. Walden, for his 5 minutes for an opening statement.

OPENING STATEMENT OF HON. GREG WALDEN, A REPRESENTATIVE IN CONGRESS FROM THE STATE OF OREGON

Mr. WALDEN. Thank you, Madam Chair. And thanks for having this very important hearing.

I appreciate all the witnesses who are here to share your stories and to comment on the legislation before us.

This critical issue of maternity morbidity and mortality, it is an issue that is quite literally a matter of life and death and for all women across the country. It is a difficult topic. It is one that is close to my heart.

Despite massive innovation in healthcare and advancements in technology, recent reports have indicated that the number of women dying due to pregnancy complications has increased in recent years. The effects of such a tragedy on any family are impossible to comprehend.

This hearing builds off the important work of our committee in the last Congress under the leadership of Dr. Burgess and the Health Subcommittee. Last year, as you have heard, the President signed into law H.R. 1318, the Preventing Maternal Deaths Act. This important law, led by Representative Jaime Herrera Beutler of Washington State and Diana DeGette of Colorado, seeks to improve data collection reporting around maternal mortality and develop systems at the local, State, and national levels in order to better understand the burden of maternal complications.

These efforts include identifying the reasons for disparity in maternal care, health risks that contribute to maternal mortality, and clinical practices that would improve health outcomes for moms and babies.

We have continued to lead the way this Congress as well—and on a bipartisan basis, I would add—sending letters earlier this year to six Health and Human Service agencies where we asked for the latest information on what they are doing to combat maternal mortality. I hope we finish the briefings requested in those letters very soon.

Unfortunately, I do have to say I am dismayed at the way that this legislative hearing today came together. For an issue that is absolutely bipartisan, I am just disappointed the majority would not allow consideration of Dr. Bucshon's bill, H.R. 4215, the Excellence in Maternal Health Act. It is a bipartisan bill. It is led by Dr. Bucshon. It serves as the House companion to the maternal mortality provisions in Senator Alexander and Senator Murray's bipartisan Senate legislation, Lowering Health Care Costs Act.

So I strongly support the bipartisan language in this bill as it demonstrates our commitment to further addressing maternal mortality, just as we did in a bipartisan way last Congress. The bill authorizes grants to identify, develop, and disseminate maternal health quality best practices, supports training at health profession schools to reduce and prevent discrimination and implicit biases, enhances Federal efforts to establish or support perinatal quality collaboratives, and authorizes grants for establishing and/or operating innovative evidence-informed programs that deliver integrated services to pregnant and post partum women.

The language in this bill passed the United States Senate Committee on Health, Education, Labor, and Pensions as part of Senator Alexander and Senator Murray's bipartisan package, and so I truly don't understand why we wouldn't have had that on the docket today for consideration as well. I just hope we will. I hope there will be another hearing where we can hear from Dr. Bucshon on his legislation.

Some of today's bills would expand Medicaid and CHIP coverage for pregnant and postpartum women from 60 days to 1 year. This is a significant policy change and one, of course, we need to carefully consider before we advance such a policy through the committee. Importantly, several States have already undertaken such initiatives. And we should gain a greater understanding about the State experiences, as that will be critical as we move forward.

Given the huge impact some of these bills will have on HHS, I would also note that HHS is not here before us today to discuss what they are already doing to address maternal mortality—we would benefit from hearing from them—nor to provide their thoughts on the incomplete list of bills before us today.

Given this absence, I call on the majority to schedule a second legislative hearing before moving to a markup. And I strongly urge the majority to include H.R. 4215 in such a hearing. It is a goodfaith, bipartisan bill with Senate support that deserves consider- ation in the House.

Despite my concerns about this process, I have no concerns about our distinguished witnesses today and our panel of experts. I want to thank you all again for being here today to talk about the bills before us, to share your stories and your expertise. I know we will learn much about the landscape of maternal mortality and care and what more we can do to improve the health outcomes in expectant and new mothers across the country. That is a goal we all share. So thank you for being here.

Madam Chair, with that, I yield back.

PREPARED STATEMENT OF HON. GREG WALDEN

The critical issue of maternal morbidity and mortality – an issue that is literally a matter of life and death for women all across the country – is a difficult topic, and one that is close to my heart.

Despite massive innovation in health care and advancements in technology, recent reports have indicated that the number of women dying due to pregnancy complications has increased in recent years. The effects of such a tragedy on any family are impossible to comprehend.

This hearing builds off the important work of our committee in the last Congress under the leadership of Dr. Burgess and the Health Subcommittee. Last year, the President signed into law H.R. 1318, the Preventing Maternal Deaths Act. This important law, led by Representatives Jaime Herrera Beutler (R-WA) and Diana DeGette (D-CO) seeks to improve data collection and reporting around maternal mortality, and develop systems at the local, state, and national level in order to better understand the burden of maternal complications. These efforts include identifying the reasons for disparities in maternal care, health risks that contribute to maternal mortality, and clinical practices that improve health outcomes for moms and babies.

We have continued to lead the way this Congress as well – and on a bipartisan basis, I might add – sending letters earlier this year to six HHS agencies asking for the latest information on what they are doing to combat maternal mortality. I hope that we finish the briefings requested in those letters soon.

Unfortunately, I'm dismayed at the way the majority handled our legislative process to get to this hearing. For an issue that is absolutely bipartisan, I'm disappointed that the majority would not allow consideration of H.R. 4215, the Excellence in Maternal Health Act, a bipartisan bill led by Dr. Bucshon that serves as the House companion to the maternal mortality provisions in Senator Alexander and Senator Murray's bipartisan Lowering Health Care Costs Act. I strongly support the bipartisan language in this bill as it demonstrates our commitment to further addressing maternal mortality. The bill authorizes grants to identify, develop, and disseminate maternal health quality best practices, supports training at health professions schools to reduce and prevent discrimination and implicit biases, enhances Federal efforts to establish or support perinatal quality collaboratives, and authorizes grants for establishing and/or operating innovative evidence-informed programs that deliver integrated services to pregnant and postpartum women. The language in this bill passed the U.S. Senate Committee on Health, Education, Labor and Pensions as a part of Senator Alexander and Senator Murray's bipartisan package. I truly don't understand why the majority refused to include H.R. 4215 in today's hearing.

Regarding the four bills that we ARE reviewing today, only one of the bills has a Republican cosponsor. I am also concerned that despite coming off of a six week district work period we didn't have witnesses agreed to until last Thursday and Members weren't able to review testimony until yesterday. Such a broken process is disrespectful of this important issue.

Some of today's bills would expand Medicaid and CHIP coverage for pregnant and postpartum women from 60 days to one year. This would be a significant policy change and one we need to carefully consider before we advance such a policy through the Committee. Importantly, several states have already undertaken such initiatives and understanding that state experience will be critical as we move forward.

Given the huge impact that some of these bills will have on HHS, I would also note that HHS is not here today to discuss what they have already been doing to address maternal mortality, nor to provide their thoughts on the incomplete list of bills before us today. Given this absence, I call on the majority to schedule a second legislative hearing before moving to a markup. And I strongly urge the majority to include H.R. 4215 in such a hearing. It's a good faith, bipartisan bill that deserves consideration, too.

Despite my concerns about this process, I have no concerns about our distinguished witnesses here today. I'd like thank our witnesses for being here and sharing your stories and expertise. I know we will learn much about the landscape of maternity care and what more we can do to improve the health outcomes in expectant or new mothers across the country.

Ms. ESHOO. The gentleman yields back.

It is always a pleasure to be joined by former Members of Congress, and this morning former Congressman Phil Gingrey is with us. So welcome, and thank you for being here.

I want to remind Members that, pursuant to committee rules, all Members' written opening statements will be made part of the record.

I now would like to introduce the witnesses for today's hearing, beginning with Ms. Wanda Irving, the mother of Shalon Irving. Thank you very much for being here. Your very moving piece in ProPublica—anyone that has read that, I think you are really not the same person after you read it. So thank you very much for being here today.

Dr. Patrice Harris is president of the Board of Trustees of the American Medical Association. Thank you to you for being here.

Dr. Elizabeth Howell, director of the Blavatnik Family Women's Health Research Institute at the Icahn School of Medicine at Mount Sinai, welcome to you and thank you.

Dr. David Nelson, assistant professor of obstetrics and gynecology at the University of Texas Southwestern Medical Center, thank you to you for being here.

And Ms. Usha Ranji, the associate director of women's health policy at the Kaiser Family Foundation, our thanks to you.

We are very grateful because this is—as the ranking member of the full committee said—this is a very important hearing. And we look forward to your testimony. So, at this time, the Chair will recognize each witness for 5 minutes to provide their opening statements. If you are not familiar with the light system, green obviously is go. When you see that the light has turned yellow, you will have 1 minutes remaining. And guess what? When it turns red, your time is up.

So I will begin by recognizing the very distinguish Ms. Wanda Irving for your 5 minutes of testimony.

You need to turn the mic on. That is it. And get close to it. We don't want to miss a word. We have some very energetic people outside of our hearing room. So get the microphone even closer so we don't miss a word. Thank you.

Statements of Wanda Irving, Mother of Dr. Shalon Irving; Patrice Harris, MD, President, Board of Trustees, American Medical Association; Elizabeth A. Howell, MD, Director, Blavatnik Family Women's Health Research Institute, Icahn School of Medicine at Mount Sinai; David Nelson, MD, Chief of Obstetrics, Parkland Health And Hospital System; and Usha Ranji, Associate Director, Women's Health Policy, Kaiser Family Foundation

Statement of Wanda Irving

Ms. IRVING. Good morning, Chairwoman Eshoo, Ranking Member Burgess, distinguished members of the committee. Thank you for the opportunity to address you.

New data released from the CDC demonstrates that pregnancy-related deaths for Black women with at least a college degree are five times higher than that of a White woman with similar education. Shalon MauRene Irving had a dual titled Ph.D. in sociology and gerontology and a master of science, both summa cum laude, from Purdue University and earned before the age of 25. By 26, she was a college professor at Hofstra University but decided, after watching her older brother who suffered numerous indignities during treatment for multiple sclerosis, that she wanted to work on the front lines fighting for health equity. She earned a master of public health from Johns Hopkins, also summa cum laude, and became certified as a health education specialist while being a weekend caregiver for her brother, who was then in a wheelchair.

She started her public health career as a Kellogg Fellow, working with pregnant women at Healthy Start in Baltimore. From there, she was hired as a consultant to the CDC, working on former First Lady Michelle Obama's Let's Move! Initiative. She went on to be accepted into the globally renowned Epidemic Intelligence Service and was quickly promoted to lieutenant commander.

As a well-respected epidemiologist at the CDC, she made major contributions to several scientific books written by colleagues and wrote various articles published in scientific and medical journals. She was dedicated and committed to racial equality and health equity. On her Twitter profile, Shalon said: "I see inequity wherever it exists, call it by name, and work hard to eliminate it. I vow to create a better Earth."

She believed in action over words and launched a consulting firm specializing in inclusivity training. This is the picture of Shalon Irving the professional, but she was so much more than that. She was my only daughter, born between two brothers that she idolized. Shalon was every mother's prayer and the one few of us are lucky enough to receive.

An unexpected pregnancy at 36 only added to the fullness of her life. She was so excited to become a mother. On January 3rd, Shalon underwent a planned c-section and gave birth to a beautiful baby girl she named Soleil Meena Daniele. Shalon thought Soleil was her greatest accomplishment. The 3 weeks that followed Soleil's birth should have been filled with joy and happiness, but it wasn't.

Instead, Shalon's general state of health steadily declined, while her blood pressure rose. She experienced leg swelling, decreased urine output, weight gains, and headaches. But despite repeated visits to her healthcare providers during this period, her complaints were not adequately addressed.

Shalon suffered cardiac arrest at home on the night of January 24th, 2017, 21 days after the birth of her daughter and just a few hours after her last trip to her health provider. My beautiful, vibrant, brilliant daughter was officially declared brain dead on Thursday, January 26th. Believe me, there is nothing more heartwrenching than seeing your child connected to life support. On January 28th, life support was removed. After reading her medical directive, the handwritten last line shattered my heart: "Mommy, I will fight hard, but if there is no hope, please let me go."

Shalon fought hard. She did what she was supposed to do. It was the medical profession that let her down. She was a 36-year-old woman of color who went to healthcare workers again and again in distress and was not properly treated. Imagine the many gerontology breakthroughs, epidemiology victories, and social advances that Shalon could have generated if only her medical providers had listened to her and addressed her cries for help.

Shalon's daughter, Soleil, is transitioning into a little girl. She is 31 months old now with a smile every bit as brilliant as her mother's. Soleil is fearless and determined like her mother. She constantly amazes me with her rapidly expanding vocabulary, her capacity for learning French, her athleticism as a gymnast, and her love for art and ballet. But there are no words in the English language to adequately portray the pain I feel when Soleil looks up at me and asks, "Where's my mommy,

Nona? Why can't I see her?" or cries, "I want my mommy" while clutching a picture of Shalon.

The loss of my daughter has earned me the right to demand the transformation of the healthcare system. I ask you—no, I implore you—to take three points from my words today. Not every maternal mortality is because of lack of insurance nor access to care, poverty, or lack of education. The dialogue needs to be reframed so it widens the lens to include the insured, those with access, and the educated.

Most pregnancy-related deaths can be prevented. According the latest CDC Morbidity and Mortality Weekly Report, further identification and evaluation of factors contributing to racial and ethnic disparities are crucial to inform and implement prevention strategies that will effectively reduce disparities in pregnancy-related mortality.

Quality of care plays a pivotal role in pregnancy-related deaths and associated racial disparities. It is imperative that more aggressive strategies to break down racial bias and prejudice be deployed now. Sending medical folks to cultural sensitivity or implicit bias training is not going to fix the problem without a redesign of medical school curricula. Post partum care must be redefined and optimized as well. Healthcare professionals must be accountable.

The reduction of preventable maternal death among Black women is a national disgrace and has become an urgent national priority. To paraphrase a line from Abraham Lincoln, it is the cause for which my daughter gave her last measure of devotion.

Thank you.

[The prepared statement of Ms. Irving follows:]

STATEMENT OF WANDA IRVING, HOUSE ENERGY & COMMERCE COMMITTEE, HEALTH SUBCOMMITTEE, HEARING ON IMPROVING MATERNAL HEALTH, SEPTEMBER 10, 2019

Chairwoman Eshoo, Ranking Member Burgess, Chairman Pallone, Ranking Member Walden, and Members of the Committee, thank you for the opportunity to sharing my story with such a prestigious group.

Lately, I've been called brave and courageous a lot. I'm not sure I agree. I am just a grieving mother, trying to move forward by putting one foot in front of the other and taking it one day at a time. What I want you to know as I tell Shalon's story is that I relive Shalon's death every time I share her story. It is painful, and yes – it would be easier not to do this, to sidestep this fresh pain a few times a month. But if my daughter had to leave me, I've got to find some meaning in her death, it must help someone else: save someone else's daughter or sister or wife. That's what my daughter would have wanted.

I am here today to put a face to what decades of research has shown—black women aren't being seen or heard when it comes to their health—especially during and after pregnancy. I want to share with you a remarkable woman, my daughter Dr. Shalon MauRene Irving, who became a maternal mortality statistic and to let you know what the aftermath of her preventable death has been like for her child and me.

Shalon was my only daughter, born between two brothers that she adored. She was an exceptional child. She loved to learn. She was generous, kind, passionate and a staunch champion for equity.

Shalon Grew into a Strong, Vibrant, Beautiful Woman

Shalon was fearless. She lived her truth each and every day. She never lost sight of who she was or what she wanted, and she never failed to answer the call when her expertise was needed. She was funny. Her smile was luminous and her melodic laughter touched your heart. She was readily accepting of everyone she met and fiercely loyal to her friends who told me Shalon had a way of making your day brighter and your load suddenly seem lighter.

Shalon Was Smart

She'd skipped two grades before high school and earned a bachelor's degree, a master's degree and a dual titled PhD in Sociology and Gerontology—the first student to do so at Purdue University—all Summa cum Laude. By the age of 25 she was a college professor at Hofstra University, but decided she wanted to be on the front line working to eliminate racial health injustices. So, she went on to acquire an MPH from Johns Hopkins University — also Summa Cum Laude— while being a weekend caretaker for the older brother she so adored, who was wheelchair bound as a result of multiple sclerosis—and began her career working to end health disparities. Shalon had an impressive career path that led to her work as a Lt. Commander in the prestigious Epidemic Intelligence Service of the U.S. Health Service, and a well-respected epidemiologist at the Centers for Disease Control and Prevention.

Shalon Was Well Travelled

Over the course of 10 years, we had vacationed extensively throughout the Caribbean and traveled to over 20 foreign countries on three continents. In fact, Shalon wanted to share her love of travel right away with her child. We had just made the final payments for a 2-week vacation to Dubai, which was to begin 5 days after Shalon died.

Shalon Was a Brilliant Writer and Published Author

She could take even the most complex scientific jargon and rewrite it so a seventh grader could understand it. She was an accomplished author—with major contributions to several scientific books written by colleagues, various published articles in medical journals, plus co-authored an introspective self-help book called *"Beautifully Bare and Undeniably You"* that was published posthumously in 2018.

Shalon Was the Epitome of a Modern-Day Renaissance Woman

She was always thinking, "what's next" for her. She owned her own home, was an avid gardener, a skilled photographer, and a talented chef and volunteered at several organizations to help young girls become the phenomenal women they were meant to be. Shalon had just launched a consulting firm, called Inclusivity Standard, LLC, to help first-generation college girls prepare for college and enable businesses and schools to embrace inclusivity to assist organizations in becoming more inclusive.

Shalon Was a Distinguished Scientist

She was a Lt. Commander in the globally recognized Epidemic Intelligence Service and a well-respected Epidemiologist at the Centers for Disease Control and Prevention in Atlanta, Georgia.

Most Importantly, Shalon Had a Passion for Ending All Health Disparities

She was dedicated and committed to racial equality and health equity. According to her Twitter profile, Shalon said, *"I see inequity wherever it exists, call it by name, and work hard to eliminate it. I vow to create a better earth."* Throughout her career, Shalon passionately advocated for a participatory approach to all research so that communities could immediately benefit from the research.

Yet, this vibrant, beautiful, intelligent woman fell victim to maternal mortality exemplifying that maternal mortality can happen to any woman giving birth.

According to the CDC over 700 women die every year from causes related to pregnancy and childbirth in the United States. Almost 70% of those deaths are preventable. What's worst, the CDC reports that black mothers in the U.S. die at three to four times the rate of white women, making it one of the widest of all racial disparities in women's health. Let me spell this out another way: a black woman is 22 percent more likely to die from heart disease than a white woman, 71 percent more likely to perish from cervical cancer, but 243 percent more likely to die from pregnancy- or childbirth-related causes than a white woman. Sure, some of it has to do with lack of insurance, no access to medical care, insufficient financial well-being. But, unfortunately, it also has to do with the appalling way black women are—or are not—attended to or listened to. Which was exactly the case for Shalon. She did not live in poverty. She was not uneducated. She was not complacent about her health. She had access to the kind of healthcare that should have saved her life, but she ended up a maternal mortality statistic. You tell me why.

Even though her pregnancy was unexpected, Shalon was overjoyed. She knew her pregnancy was high risk but, at that time, I did not know that she was among the country's most vulnerable pregnancy population. I never thought for a moment that as a black woman my daughter was three to four times more likely to die than a white woman from birth related complications, largely attributed to institutional racism and the stress that our bodies endure because of it.

Shalon did not take her pregnancy lightly. She did everything right. She rushed back from a deployment in Puerto Rico and immediately went to her GYN/OB doctor. She got tested for the Zika virus, which came back negative. She followed her OB's instructions to the letter. She never missed an OB appointment. Several months before she became pregnant, Shalon had discovered she had factor v leiden and took a pill daily to prevent any blood clots. But now that she was pregnant, her hematologist prescribed 2 painful shots into her stomach each day to keep her blood from clotting and protect her baby. Though her stomach resembled a black and blue pincushion, she never complained—not once. Shalon spent days creating a highly detailed birth plan with everything from who could be in the delivery room to the type of music and conversations that could go on in the delivery room. The plan included several tasks for me, starting with—sterilizing her hospital room, bed, chairs and bathroom with disinfectant. Shalon gave a lot of thought to preparing for her baby, but trusted that her doctors to look out for *her* in the days and weeks after her baby arrived.

On January 3, 2017 Shalon underwent a caesarean and gave birth to a beautiful baby girl she named Soleil Meena Daniele. In her journal entry on the morning of Soleil's birth, she wrote:

> Good morning! I am up and just sitting in my calming room meditating a bit before we leave for the hospital. I can't believe that the next time I sit in this room it will be as a mother with my beautiful little one. I barely slept (either out of excitement or nervousness), yet I'm not tired nor do I feel any nervousness now. I am prepared. I am surrounded by love (both present and virtual) and I am ready to meet this tiny human that I've been sharing space with for 37 weeks! It is inconceivable that someone so loving, so ready for motherhood, was cheated of the experience.

Though Soleil was delivered three weeks early, with some respiratory problems and suffered from colic, Shalon thought she was perfect—the fulfillment of a mother's dream. According to Shalon, Soleil was her greatest accomplishment.

However, that euphoria was short lived.

The 3 short weeks that followed Soleil's birth should have been filled with joy, happiness, and improving health. Instead, Shalon's general state of health steadily declined during this period. She suffered from elevated blood pressure. She experienced leg swelling. She had decreased urine output. She put on weight. She had headaches. Instead of improving over time, she felt increasingly worse and not her normal self. Shalon and I knew something was terribly wrong. Despite frequent visits to her health care providers during this period, her complaints were not adequately addressed and routinely dismissed with the dismissive words "it's to be expected; you just had a baby."

Shalon suffered an arrest at home on the night of January 24, 2017, 21 days after the birth of her daughter and just a few hours after returning home from yet another visit to her medical provider. 911 was called, and Shalon was transferred to a local hospital, where we learned that complications from hypertension had led to the cardiac arrest which deprived her brain of oxygen for a significant period of time.

My vibrant, brilliant, beautiful 36-year old daughter, with everything in the world to live for, was officially declared brain dead on Thursday, January 26th. There is nothing so heartwrenching as seeing your child unconscious, connected to instruments that can only say she is dying but cannot save her, unable to open her eyes to tell you she loves you one more time. Even with the dismal diagnosis, I could not let her go. Thursday evening, my cousin who was tasked with getting Shalon's papers in order found her medical directive and brought it to me at the hospital where I had kept a bedside vigil since my daughter was admitted. In the directive there was a paragraph Shalon had handwritten to me. The last line of that paragraph shattered my heart. She wrote: "*Mommy, I will fight hard, but if there is no hope, please let me go.*" But I couldn't. I just could not. My bedside vigil continued. It wasn't until Friday morning when I saw a single tear roll down Shalon's cheek, I knew my daughter was ready to go. I sat by her bedside again that night and cried. Then on Saturday morning, January 28, 2017, with both her father and me at her bedside, life support was removed. Fourteen minutes later, she was gone.

What infuriates me is that Shalon's death was a preventable tragedy. She was a 36-year-old woman of color who went to her health care workers again and again in distress – and she was not properly treated. Imagine the many gerontology breakthroughs, health miracles, epidemiology victories and social advancements that Shalon could have generated, if only her medical providers had listened to her and adequately addressed her cries for help. Even Shalon's many advantages — her B.A. in sociology, her two master's degrees, her dual titled Ph.D. in Sociology and Gerontology, her CHES certification, her work as an epidemiologist, her gold-plated insurance, and rock-solid support system — had not been enough to ensure Shalon's survival. Shalon deserved better. Soleil deserved to know her mother.

Shalon's death has been called "shameful." "Sad." "Senseless." "Tragic." One thing is certain in my mind: it was definitely a tragedy—a shameful, sad, senseless and preventable tragedy. IT SHOULD NOT HAVE HAPPENED. My granddaughter will grow up without her phenomenal mother by her side and the incredible influence Shalon would have had on Soleil's life.

Since my daughter's death, my life has been framed by unbearable pain and unrelenting sadness. At this point in my life, I did not expect to be raising my granddaughter. I wanted to be that indulgent grandmother on the sidelines, watching my daughter and granddaughter grow together. Instead, I am acutely aware that I will face the rest of my days without my daughter and my best friend. Her clothes still hang in her closets. Her shoe racks still display all her shoes. Everything is still organized exactly as she left it. Visitors must still remove their shoes before entering her home. The wind chimes she hung on her front porch still add a sense of peacefulness. Her house is still her house. For months after her death I convinced myself that she would be home after work. Day in day out, I looked forward to 4:30pm only to go into a grief spiral the later it got. I still catch myself hoping she will come through the door at 4:30pm. Nights are still the loneliest times of my day, and many a night I don't sleep at all. It is when the tears still come. Even with a very vocal 31month old in the house, it is surprising how quiet my life has become without my daughter. I miss our conversations. I miss her words of wisdom. I miss her insight, which was always right on point. I miss her smile. I miss her laughter. I miss her hugs. Most important, I miss her love. Depression is an ever-present companion now. Shalon loved the holidays. But holidays don't exist at her house now. It seems so wrong without Shalon. No Easter bunny. No 4th of July barbecues. No trick or treating. No Thanksgiving turkey and sweet potato pies. No Christmas trees. No Santa Claus. No joyous and merry holiday seasons. No New Year's Jamaican food extravaganzas prepared by Chef Shalon. I know at some point, for Soleil's sake I must recognize the holidays, especially now, thanks to her I Pad, she knows about Santa Claus and sings Jingle bells on a regular basis.

Soleil is transitioning from a toddler to a little girl. She is 31 months old now. I see Shalon in her daughter. Soleil's smile is every bit as brilliant as her mother's. I only wish Shalon were here raising Soleil and guiding her life. I never meant to be on the front lines, raising a spirited little one who is ramping up her energy and excitement for the world – She constantly amazes me with her rapidly expanding vocabulary, her capacity for learning French, her athleticism as a gymnast and her love for art and ballet.

Each morning Soleil and I say good morning to mommy's picture. I want her to know she had a truly remarkable mother who loved her dearly and would have done anything to be here raising her. But it is no easy task. There are no words in the English language to adequately portray what our life is like without my daughter—or the pain I feel when Soleil looks up at me and asks "Where is my Mommy, Nona? Why can't I see her?" Soleil has a favorite picture of her Mommy, which she hugs and tells me "I love Mommy." It brings tears to my eyes because Soleil should be hugging her Mommy. Shalon did not have to die. Shalon thought Doc McStuffins was a good role model for little girls. Soleil loves Doc McStuffins. She has a doctor's coat, a stethoscope, and a doctors bag filled with other doctor's instruments—ironically, the blood pressure cup is her favorite. She gives me regular check ups. Shalon would be so proud of her.

Assembling an extended family village for Soleil was very important to Shalon. She had some incredible friends who have tried to be there for me in everyway, for which I am eternally grateful. They have been there to celebrate each of Soleil's milestones. Shalon would definitely be thankful that her village stepped up and rallied around Soleil and me. What I have trouble explaining to them is that as much as they love Soleil and me, some days we must walk this difficult journey alone. I take it day by day. It is only my granddaughter's smile that motivates me to get up every morning, with the same goal each day—wake up, honor Shalon's legacy, take care of her daughter, as she would have wanted. This goal keeps me moving forward. That, and a letter Shalon wrote two years preceding her death, and left for me in the event of her death. Following is the last paragraph of that letter:

> Mommy, I am sorry that I have left you. On the particular day that I am writing this I have no idea how that may have occurred but know that I would never choose to leave you. It troubles me deeply that you are grieving. I know it seems impossible right now, but Mommy please do not let this break you. I want you to be happy and smile. I want you to know that my brothers and grandma are watching over me and that we are all watching over you. Mommy, please try not to cry. Use your energy instead to feel my love through time and space. Nothing can break the bond we have and you will forever be my mommy and I your baby girl! I love you for always! Lon

I have spent the last year trying to use my energy to feel her love by continuing her work. There is no mistaking the difference Dr. Shalon MauRene Irving made in this world. The difference her story continues to make every time I share it. Given the pain and turmoil I have experienced, I can never return to the ME that existed before losing my daughter. If I could go back in time and save my daughter, I would do anything. GIVE ANYTHING. If only I knew then what I know now. But, I take a small measure of comfort in knowing that Shalon's story has ignited a passion in some legislators, doctors and health care advocates to transform the health care system when it comes to lowering the maternal mortality rates and making changes to postpartum care protocol. To paraphrase a line from Abraham Lincoln's Gettysburg Address "it is the cause for which Shalon gave her last full measure of devotion." It is up to us the living to carry on. Babies deserve a lot of care and attention after birth, but I can't emphasize enough that mothers are equally as important. They deserve care and attention after birth as well as before giving birth. I know my daughter did. Shalon did not have to die.

Dr. Brian Yablon, an EIS colleague of Shalon and internist at Hennepin Healthcare said, "Shalon was a kind, thoughtful, and principled woman. As a sociologist, she brought a unique and much needed perspective to the science of epidemiology. She advised that we not get so caught up in the science that we forget the people behind the numbers. Her wisdom and moral compass were just two qualities that made Shalon an exceptional human being."

If Shalon were here today, she would also caution you not to get so caught up in the data, the maternal mortality statistics that you forget that behind every single number there is a face. The face of a woman who is loved. The face of a woman who had so much to offer the world. The face of a woman who will not get the opportunity to raise her beloved baby. If you take that face and multiple it, that one statistic not only includes the face of a woman who will be immeasurably mourned and forever missed but also the families left devastated by her death—the babies, the other children, the woman's mothers, like me, the fathers, the husbands, the friends, the colleagues. The domino effect of that one statistic is incomprehensible. So whenever you are tempted to think of maternal mortality statistics as just data or numbers, put Shalon's face in front of that number and remember my words. In closing, I ask you, no I implore you to take 3 points from my words today.

- One: Not every maternal mortality is because of lack of insurance, non-access to care, poverty or lack of education.
- Two: The majority of maternal deaths are preventable.
- Three: We must demand that postpartum care be redefined and optimized. We must hold health care professionals accountable for improving the quality of care and ensuring equity.

Sending folks to cultural sensitivity or implicit bias training is not going to fix the problem. We must demand the transformation of the health care systems in order to better respond to the needs and priorities of women, especially women of color. The reduction of preventable maternal deaths must become a national priority. It is for me. It was for Shalon. It should be for you too.

Thank you.

Mr. LONG. Madam Chair, Madam Chair, I don't know if I need to ask for a point of personal privilege or what, but I am going to say something.

I am a member of the Black Maternal Health Caucus, and I care deeply about this issue, and I think it is repugnant that we have to sit here and listen to whatever in the world is going on out there in the hall. These women deserve better. These women that passed away during and after childbirth. This is a very serious hearing, and that—whatever they are celebrating or complaining about out there in the hall, the Capitol Hill Police need to put a stop to it. If you could ask them to do it, I appreciate it.

I yield back.

Ms. ESHOO. I thank the gentleman.

Thank you, Ms. Irwin, for your—this is the first step to the promise that you are asking us to keep. Thank you for being here today.

Dr. Patrice Harris, you are recognized for your 5 minutes.

STATEMENT OF PATRICE HARRIS, MD

Dr. HARRIS. Good morning, Chairwoman Eshoo, Ranking Member Burgess, and committee members.

The American Medical Association commends you for holding today's legislative hearing. My name is Dr. Patrice Harris, and I am president of the AMA. I am a practicing child and adolescent psychiatrist from Atlanta, and I am adjunct faculty at the Emory University School of Medicine and the Morehouse School of Medicine. I thank you for the opportunity to testify.

The data on maternal mortality in the U.S. are deeply alarming. The U.S. is only one of three countries in the world where the rate of maternal deaths is rising. Moreover, there is a large disparity in maternal deaths. As you have heard, a recent CDC report found that Black women are three to four times and Native American/ Alaska Native women are two and a half times more likely to die from pregnancy-related causes as White women. And Black and Hispanic women are disproportionately affected by severe maternal morbidity, defined as life-threatening complications during or after childbirth. Most alarmingly, 60 percent of pregnancy-related deaths are preventable. This is simply unacceptable when we know these inequities and disparities are avoidable. Inequities and disparities do not have to exist, and we must collectively increase our efforts to close the gap.

What is causing these deaths? And why is the rate so much higher, particularly for Black and Native American women? Among the factors that play a role are as follows: Millions of women still lack insurance or have inadequate coverage prior to, during, and after pregnancy. There is increased closures of maternity units both in rural and urban communities and, thereby, reduced access to quality maternal care. There is a lack of appropriately trained interprofessional teams in best practices, and that also impacts quality of care. There are structural determinants of health, which include public policies, laws, and racism. And those impact the social determinants of health, which include education, employment, housing, and transportation. Discrimination, racism, implicit biases exacerbates stress, which negatively affects the body and can result in hypertension, heart disease, and gestational diabetes during pregnancy.

The evidence tells us that clinician and institutional biases can lead to missed warning signs—can and do lead, I must say, to missed warning signs and delayed diagnoses. Women of color are not being heard.

So how do we move forward? Regarding specific solutions, the AMA believes that ongoing surveillance and activities to promote appropriate screening, referral, and treatment are needed. I want to thank the House Energy and Commerce Committee for advancing H.R. 1318. We continue to support the expansion of State Maternal Mortality Review Committees and appreciate continued funding to support prevention efforts.

We also support the MOMMA's Act to improve data collection, spread that information from that data on effective interventions, and expand access to healthcare and social services for post partum women. And to ensure optimal health for women at risk for medical or mental health conditions leading to maternal death, addi- tional insurance coverage is required. And the AMA believes that Medicaid coverage should be extended to cover women 1 year post partum.

And, finally, let me highlight what the AMA is doing in this space internally in our own house. The medical community absolutely has a role to play here. The AMA recently hired Dr. Aletha Maybank as the AMA's first chief health equity officer, and she is initiating our new and explicit path to advanced health equity through the AMA Center for Health Equity and, although our Center for Health Equity is just getting up and running, there is great potential to partner with Congress to expand implicit bias training and other structural competency trainings in medical schools, residencies, and throughout the physician's career.

So it will take all of us working in partnership, and the AMA is committed to doing so, to build and continue on a path forward to more holistically and effectively improve maternal health and advance health equity.

Thank you.

[The prepared statement of Dr. Harris follows:]

Statement of the American Medical Association to the U.S. House of Representatives, Committee on Energy & Commerce, Subcommittee on Health, Re: Improving Maternal Health: Legislation to Advance Prevention Efforts and Access to Care, Presented by: Patrice Harris, MD, MA President AMA Board of Trustees, September 10, 2019

The American Medical Association (AMA) appreciates the opportunity to provide testimony to the U.S. House of Representatives Committee on Energy & Commerce, Subcommittee on Health, as part of the hearing entitled, "Improving Maternal Health: Legislation to Advance Prevention Efforts and Access to Care." The AMA commends the Committee for focusing on this critically important issue, which disproportionately affects Black women and Native American/Alaska Native women. The AMA also commends the many advocates who have paved the way for this issue to capture the attention of media, policy makers, and the health care sector. As the largest professional association for physicians and the umbrella organization for state and national specialty medical societies, the AMA is committed to working with other stakeholders to support efforts to reduce and prevent rising rates of maternal mortality and serious or near-fatal maternal morbidity.

The Problem: Rising Maternal Mortality and Morbidity in the U.S.

According to the Alliance for Innovation on Maternal Health (AIM), the U.S. is one of only three countries in the world—Sudan and Afghanistan being the others—where the rate of maternal deaths is on the rise. While maternal deaths are rare—approximately 700 occurring yearly out of 3.8 million births— an additional 50,000 women have serious maternal morbidity. Maternal mortality (pregnancy-related death) is defined as the death of a woman while pregnant or within one year of the end of a pregnancy— regardless of the outcome, duration, or site of the pregnancy—from any cause related to or aggravated by the pregnancy or its management, but not from accidental or incidental causes.[2] Severe maternal morbidity is a life-threatening complication during childbirth, which can include heavy bleeding, kidney failure, and stroke or heart attack during delivery. Experiencing severe maternal morbidity can have serious and life-long consequences for women and their families.

In a recent report by the Centers of Disease Control and Prevention (CDC)—which looked at pregnancy-related deaths from 2011 to 2015 and reviewed more detailed data from 2013 to 2017 provided by maternal mortality review committees in 13 states—there were significant disparities in the death rate for different racial, ethnic, and age groups.[3] Alarmingly, the CDC found that Black women were three to four times more likely (42.8 deaths for every 100,000 live births) than white women (13 deaths for every 100,000 live births) to die from a pregnancy-related cause; Native American and Alaska Native women were 2.5 times more likely (32.5 deaths for every 100,000 live births) to suffer a pregnancy-related death. Moreover, the rate differed by location, with the rate much higher in some states. The study also found that pregnancy-related deaths were occurring across a lengthy time span: more than 31 percent of deaths were during pregnancy; 36 percent occurred during delivery or in the week after birth; and 33 percent happened one week to one-year post-partum. Overall, heart disease and stroke were the leading cause of pregnancy-related deaths each year from 2011 to 2017, but the causes were different depending on when the deaths occurred. For example, obstetric emergencies such as hemorrhage (e.g., severe bleeding) and amniotic fluid embolisms caused most deaths at delivery; hemorrhage, high blood pressure, and infection were most common in the week after delivery; and cardiomyopathy (weakened heart muscle) caused most deaths one week to one year after delivery. Perhaps the most significant and troubling finding in the study is that the CDC estimates that 60 percent of all maternal deaths are preventable.

---

[2] https://www.cdc.gov/reproductivehealth/maternalinfanthealth/pregnancy-mortality-surveillance-system.htm.

[3] https://www.cdc.gov/mmwr/volumes/68/wr/mm6818e1.htm?s_cid=mm6818e1_w.

Health Equity and Social Determinants of Health

The AMA defines health equity as "optimal health for all" and recognizes the importance and urgency of advancing health equity and addressing SDOH to ensure that all people and communities reach their full health potential. The World Health Organization (WHO) defines health equity as the "absence of unfair and avoidable or remediable differences in health among social groups." This definition clarifies that inequities and disparities do not have to exist, but that inequities are produced; they do not just happen; the people who are negatively impacted by experiencing the injustice are not to blame; and there is something that we can actually do to close the gap.

Health disparities—i.e., differences in health outcomes—in maternal health are the result of conditions that are similar for other disparities that exist. These conditions are widely understood to be the SDOH. According to Healthy People 2020, the "social determinants of health are conditions in the environment in which people are born, live, learn, work, play, worship, and age that affect a wide range of health, functioning, and quality of life outcomes and risk." These social determinants include education, housing, wealth, income, and employment. We all experience conditions that socially determine our health or the SDOH. However, we do not all experience them equally.

The SDOH are impacted by larger and powerful systems that lead to discrimination, exploitation, marginalization, exclusion, and isolation. In this country, these historic and systemic realities are baked into structures, policies, and practices and produce, exacerbate, and perpetuate inequities among the SDOH, and therefore affect health itself. These larger, powerful systems of racism and gender oppression—also known as the root cause inequities—are upstream to the social determinants of health. They have shaped the social conditions in which women and families live, and they work to produce inequities across society in complex ways, especially for those marginalized at the intersection of race and gender, i.e., Black and Native American women.

Birth inequities arise at the intersection of discrimination by race and gender for Black and Native American women. We know that in some places across the country, Black women with at least a college degree had higher severe maternal morbidity rates than women of other races/ethnicities who never graduated high school. It is clear that racism and discrimination—at the provider, institutional, and societal levels—is an attributable etiology of the increased proportion of Black and Native American mothers inclusive of inequitable access to and quality of care, institutional racism, mistrust for health care institutions, and delayed response to medical emergencies by both medical providers and patients, and a culture of disrespect that can lead to mistrust for health care institutions. Stories from Black women also tell us about a culture of disrespect as well as realities of not being listened to or heard.

At the provider and institutional levels, there is a growing body of evidence demonstrating that implicit and explicit biases exist that negatively impact the quality of health care equity and patient safety and drive these inequities. This was described originally in an Institute of Medicine (now the National Academy of Medicine) report, more than 16 years ago.[4] The evidence shows that Blacks are more likely to receive poorer quality of care and less likely to receive the standard of care even when controlling for insurance status and income. This was linked with higher death rates for Blacks.

In addition, there has been a growing body of work examining the impact of structural racism on health in this country. In 2017, Dr. Zinzi Bailey et al. published a study in the *Lancet*, "Structural Racism and Health Inequities in the US: Evidence and Interventions," that explains structural racism to be the "totality of ways in which societies foster racial discrimination through mutually reinforcing systems of housing, education, employment, earnings, benefits, credit, media, health care, and criminal justice. These patterns and practices in turn reinforce discriminatory beliefs, values, and distribution of resources." And one key example of structural racism included how "residential segregation systemically shapes health care access, utilization, and quality at the neighborhood level, health-care system, and provider levels."

This spring, the *New England Journal of Medicine* published "Structural Racism—A 60-Year-Old Black Woman with Breast Cancer," exposing the impact of racism, not just race, on health outcomes. One of the authors, our Chicagoan colleague and partner from Rush Medical Center, Dr. David Ansell, says "we must be willing to identify the health impact of racism. The biological differences between groups are tiny, yet the gaps in outcomes are simply too wide to continue to see race as a disease risk factor when the root cause is racism."

While more research is needed on the relationship of discrimination and chronic stress of racism on maternal and infant health outcomes, there is evidence that experiences of discrimination and racism have a "weathering" effect on the body. Dr. Arline Geronimus, who coined the "weathering" hypothesis, explained that "Blacks experience early health deterioration as a consequence of the cumulative impact of repeated experience with social or economic adversity and political marginalization" over one's life course.[5] This physiologic pressure, also later described as allostatic load, can cause stress hormones, such as cortisol, and cause organ and cardiovascular, metabolic, and immune systems damage over time. In addition, chronic stress and trauma due to discrimination that occurs as early in-utero and early childhood, also known as adverse childhood experiences, have been associated with poor health outcomes and early death as an adult.

---

[4] Institute of Medicine. 2003. Unequal Treatment: Confronting Racial and Ethnic Disparities in Health Care. Washington, DC: The National Academies Press. https://doi.org/10.17226/10260.

[5] https://www.ncbi.nlm.nih.gov/pmc/articles/PMC1470581/.

SDOH Impact on Maternal Mortality and Morbidity

Insurance and Access to Quality Reproductive Health Care

Almost half of all U.S. births are to women with public insurance.[6] Public insurance has large coverage gaps for the low-income women who require it: in many states this coverage is not available prior to pregnancy, when women with medical conditions require it.[7] Insurance also terminates in the months following pregnancy when the vast majority of maternal deaths occur.[8] Medicaid coverage has improved maternal outcomes for low-income women.9 In addition, research has shown Medicaid expansion has made progress in increasing pre-pregnancy coverage rates.10 We strongly urge Congress to safeguard Medicaid funding so as to not exacerbate the problem of maternal mortality and morbidity in the U.S. Furthermore, in order to assure optimal health care for the women at risk for medical or mental health conditions leading to maternal death, we believe additional insurance coverage is required. As mentioned earlier, the CDC has found that about one-third or 33 percent of maternal deaths happened one week to one-year post-partum. Several states, including Texas, Illinois, New Jersey, South Carolina, and California, have proposed bills that would extend Medicaid coverage for a year postpartum, and federal legislation has also been proposed to extend Medicaid. It is critical that Congress works in a bipartisan manner to ensure Medicaid coverage for one-year post-partum.

Reduced Access to Quality Maternity Care

Safe maternity care requires access to hospitals with quality Obstetric units and access to appropriately trained medical teams led by obstetric physicians. Concurrent with the increased focus on maternal care delivery, hospitals with smaller maternity units have been closing. This trend in the U.S. is true for both urban and rural maternity units. Data from the American Hospital Association (AHA) reveals that 500,000 women deliver in rural hospitals each year. Women in rural hospitals are less likely to have Obstetric physicians provide care. According to data reported by HRSA, over 28 million reproductive-aged women (18-44) live in rural U.S. counties. Between 2004 and 2014, the percentage of rural counties that lacked hospital obstetrics units increased from 45 to 54 percent.[11] Medicaid expansion is credited with keeping many rural hospitals afloat. Research has shown that low volume maternity units have an increasing risk of closure of maternity units.[12] Hospitals with low volume maternity units are also more likely to share nursing staffing with other units and less likely to have trained emergency medicine physicians.

---

[6] https://www.cdc.gov/nchs/products/databriefs/db318.htm.

[7] https://www.macpac.gov/wp-content/uploads/2018/11/Pregnant-Women-and-Medicaid.pdf.

[8] Id.

[9] https://ccf.georgetown.edu/2019/05/09/medicaid-expansion-fills-gaps-in-maternal-health-coverage-leading-to-healthier-mothers-and-babies/.

[10] https://www.ncbi.nlm.nih.gov/pubmed/30156498.

[11] https://www.hrsa.gov/enews/past-issues/2017/march-16/rural-ob.html.

[12] https://onlinelibrary.wiley.com/doi/epdf/10.1111/1475-6773.12441.

Mental Health throughout the Pregnancy Spectrum

The CDC reports higher rates of depression in women of color, and lower rates of treatment.[13] Depression in pregnancy is associated with poor maternal outcomes including maternal death. With regards to postpartum depression, it is a mood disorder that can affect women after childbirth. Mothers with postpartum depression experience feelings of extreme sadness, anxiety, and exhaustion that may make it difficult for them to complete daily care activities for themselves or for others. Postpartum depression occurs in nearly 15 percent of births. It is important to note that postpartum depression does not have a single cause, but likely results from a combination of physical and emotional factors. Postpartum depression does not occur because of something a mother does or does not do. Without treatment, postpartum depression can last for months or years. In addition to affecting the mother's health, it can interfere with her ability to connect with and care for her baby and may cause the baby to have problems with sleeping, eating, and behavior as he or she grows.[14] The AMA believes that ongoing surveillance and activities to promote appropriate screening, referral, and treatment are needed to reduce depression and suicide among women before, during, and after pregnancy.

What the AMA Is Doing to Address Maternal Mortality and Morbidity

A commitment to health equity means we must address the SDOH and we must elevate and name the root causes of why health inequities exist and how they came to be—both in society and at the institutional level. The AMA demonstrates its commitment through addressing the social conditions that impact health, increasing health workforce diversity, advocating for equity in health care access, promoting equity in care, and ensuring equitable practices and processes in research and data collection. Although the AMA and physicians cannot control all factors that need to change to achieve health equity, the AMA views as its role to identify their importance and to urge and educate those who can have a direct role to act.

The AMA supports efforts designed to integrate training in social determinants of health and cultural competence across the undergraduate medical school curriculum to assure that medical students are prepared to provide patients with safe, high quality, and patient-centered care. In 2013, the AMA launched the "Accelerating Change in Medical Education" initiative. Today, the 37-member consortium, which represents almost one-fifth of allopathic and osteopathic medical schools, is delivering forward-thinking educational experiences to approximately 19,000 medical students—students who will provide care to a potential 33 million patients annually. One of the earliest innovations to come from the Consortium was the new and innovative curriculum on health systems science, which includes a chapter on the social determinants of health. Nearly all the 37 schools in the consortium are

---

[13] https://www.cdc.gov/mmwr/volumes/66/wr/mm6606a1.htm?s_cid=mm6606a1_w.
[14] https://www.nimh.nih.gov/health/publications/postpartum-depression-facts/index.shtml.

addressing the social determinants of health with a focus on ensuring that students recognize the impact of social determinants on health outcomes and are working with inter-professional colleagues to address them.

In 2019, the AMA announced its Reimaging Residency Initiative, designed to transform residency training to best address the workforce needs of our current and future health care system. Many of the applications to the graduate medical education initiative have included health systems science training in their proposals.

For practicing physicians, the AMA launched STEPSforward,™ an interactive practice transformation series offering innovative strategies that will allow physicians and their staff to thrive in the evolving health care environment by working smarter, not harder. This series includes a continuing medical education module on "Addressing Social Determinants of Health: Beyond the Clinic Walls." The interactive module helps physicians identify how to best understand the needs of their community, define a plan to begin addressing social determinants of health, and explains the tools available to screen patients and link them to resources.

The AMA also supports payment reform policy proposals that incentivize screening for social determinants of health and referral to community support systems. Last month, the AMA and UnitedHealthcare announced a new collaboration to better identify and address social determinants of health to improve access to care and patient outcomes. The goal is to standardize data collection, processing, and integration regarding critical social and environmental factors that contribute to patient well-being through the creation of nearly two dozen new ICD-10 codes related to SDOH. By combining traditional medical data with self-reported SDOH data, the codes trigger referrals to social and government services to address people's unique needs, connecting them directly to local and national resources in their communities.

On the policy side, specifically related to addressing maternal mortality and morbidity, the AMA supported legislation enacted into law last year, H.R. 1318 (P.L. 115-344), the "Preventing Maternal Deaths Act," that supports state maternal mortality review committees (MMRCs). MMRCs bring together local experts—ob-gyns, nurses, social workers, patient advocates, and other health care professionals—to review individual maternal deaths and recommend specific ways to prevent them in the future. We appreciate that Congress appropriated $50 million in Fiscal Year 2019 to support prevention efforts. MMRCs are a critical first step in efforts to make pregnancy safer for women.

In addition, the AMA is supporting legislation introduced in the 116th Congress, the "Mothers and Offspring Mortality and Morbidity Awareness (MOMMA's) Act" (H.R. 1897/S. 916), which would improve data collection, disseminate information on effective interventions, and expand access to health care and social services for postpartum women. The bill would enhance federal efforts to support states in collecting, standardizing, and sharing maternal mortality and morbidity data, and authorizes and expands existing federal grant programs dedicated to scaling best practices to improve maternity care. The MOMMA's Act would also authorize states to expand coverage under Medicaid, CHIP, and the Special Supplemental Nutrition

Program for Women, Infants, and Children (WIC) through a longer post-partum period for women. The bill would also ensure improved access to culturally-competent care training and workforce practices throughout the care delivery system. We understand that there are several other pieces of legislation that have been or will be introduced in the coming days/weeks and we offer our commitment to continue working with Congress to address this critical issue.

In addition, to improve health equity, the AMA's strategic and focused approach includes a multi-pronged, multi-year investment, strategic partnerships, and advocacy. Our goals are to champion health equity and promote greater diversity within the medical workforce. To date, our most recent and greatest demonstration of a commitment to health equity is creating a new role and hiring our first Chief Health Equity Officer, Aletha Maybank, MD, a pediatrician with extensive experience championing health equity who most recently worked in the New York City Public Health Department and was the founding director of the city's Center for Health Equity. In her new role, Dr. Maybank will launch the Center for Health Equity at the AMA, initiating our new and explicit path to advance health equity.

In response to advocacy by our Board and management arms of the organization, Dr. Maybank's role at the AMA as their first Chief Health Equity Officer is to embed health equity across the AMA so that health equity becomes part of the practice, process, action, innovation, and organizational performance and outcomes. The best measure of our long-term success and most desired outcome is meaningful, relevant, and impactful inclusion of health equity into the strategic and operational objectives of the AMA.

Providers' and Health Care Systems' Role in Maternal Morbidity and Mortality

Providers, hospitals, and health care systems play a critical role in ensuring that all mothers and families have healthy and safe experiences around the time of birth. We applaud the growing number of places and people that are making significant investments to meaningfully engage health care systems and providers to improve the quality and safety of care for women. This is being done by enhancing data tracking and analysis of maternal and pregnancy-related morbidity and mortality events in order to stop preventable complications; integrating structural competency, cultural sensitivity, and implicit bias training opportunities; and working with partners from different sectors and with patients to better inform system changes and improvements. Narratives from the lived experiences of Black women indicate there is a rupture of trust between Black women and the health care system that must also be addressed.

Medical education curriculum incorporates teaching and training on implicit and explicit biases, to provide tools and build skills to recognize and eliminate bias, and integrate structural competency education, which as described by Jonathan Metzel "is a framework for conceptualizing and addressing health-related social justice issues that emphasizes diagnostic recognition of economic and political conditions producing and racializing inequalities in health."[15] Although the AMA's Center for Health Equity is just getting up and running, there is great potential to enter this space and conduct an assessment of medical schools to find out which institutions offer and/or require implicit bias and other structural competency trainings. There also may be an opportunity to advance criteria on what needs to be included in the training as well as a list of organizations or individuals who could offer robust training in this area.

We encourage health care systems to work alongside other partners such as women, community-based organizations, public health systems, and insurers to identify and adopt standards for respectful care at birth. We note specifically programs similar to NYC's Maternal Hospital Quality Improvement Network and collaborative efforts with 38 hospitals and clinical providers and 100 community-based organizations fostering a sense of team work and shared–decision making to ensure respectful, safe, and quality care at the time of delivery and after. Also, key to NYC's model are enhancing meaningful community engagement and data quality and timeliness for collection and review as well as hospitals implementing Trauma and Resilience Informed Systems to provide a shared language and understanding of how stress and trauma affect individuals, institutions, and communities and provide tools for clinical setting and promote resilience within the workforce and patient population.

Conclusion

The scientific evidence shows that there are concrete actions that can be taken to reduce and prevent rising rates of maternal mortality and serious or near-fatal maternal morbidity in the United States. The AMA is committed to working with the Committee on legislation to support efforts to address this critically important issue.

Ms. ESHOO. Thank you, Dr. Harris.

We now will call on Dr. Elizabeth Howell, director of the Blavatnik Family Women's Health Research Institute at Mount Sinai. You have 5 minutes for your testimony. Welcome and thank you.

STATEMENT OF ELIZABETH A. HOWELL, MD

Dr. HOWELL. Chairwoman Eshoo, Ranking Member Burgess, Representative Engel of New York, and members of the Subcommittee on Health, thank you for inviting me to testify.

---

15 https://journals.lww.com/academicmedicine/Fulltext/2017/03000/Integrating_and_Assessing_Structural_Competency_in.30.aspx.

My name is Elizabeth Howell, and I am an obstetrician/gynecologist and a researcher. I serve as a professor in the Departments of Population Health Science and Policy and Obstetrics, Gynecology, and Reproductive Science. I also direct the Blavatnik Women's Family Health Research Institute at the Icahn School of Medicine at Mount Sinai.

So we are here today because the United States is in a maternal healthcare crisis. You have heard that every year in our country around 700 women die from pregnancy-related causes. Our maternal mortality rate is higher than all other high-income countries. And our numbers, as you have heard, are far worse for women of color. While leading causes of maternal death include heart conditions, high blood pressure, infections, blood clots, rates of maternal death from overdose and suicide are rapidly climbing. And opioid-related deaths have doubled over the last decade.

But a maternal death is just the tip of the iceberg. For every death, over a hundred women experience a life-threatening complication related to pregnancy and childbirth. Severe maternal morbidity impacts over 50,000 women every year in our Nation. Every hour, six new moms will have a tragic event like a stroke, a blood clot, or kidney failure. As you heard, the good news is that over half of these tragic events, actually 60 percent, are preventable if we improve the quality of care women receive before, during, and after pregnancy.

Quality of care includes women, no matter who they are and where they live, having access to doctors and nurses who are well-trained, prepared, and equipped with the right tools. It also means having systems in place that make it easy for women to receive evidence-based care. That means hospitals equipped with adequate resources, policies, and practices, staffing, and more. If we raised quality of care for pregnant women, we could lower the rates of these tragic events.

And quality of care differs for women of color. You have heard that Black women are three to four times and American Indian women are three times more likely to experience a pregnancy-related death than are White women. In New York City, Black women are 8 to 12 times more likely to experience a maternal death than are White women.

Although many want to think that income differences drive these disparities, it goes beyond class. A Black woman with a college education is nearly twice as likely to die as a White woman with less than a high school education, and she is nearly three times more likely to experience a severe maternal morbidity.

There is a growing recognition that social determinants of health, like racism and segregated housing, contribute to these disparities, and the powerful story you heard from Ms. Irving about her daughter highlights an additional underlying cause: quality of care, lack of standards, and post partum care. Her daughter was seen multiple times by clinicians after her delivery, but she still died.

Reasons for Black/White differences highlight the need to adequately resource programs that enhance quality of care. Research by our team and others has shown that, for a variety of reasons, Black women tend to deliver in a specific set of hospitals. And those hospitals have higher rates of severe maternal morbidity for both Black and White moms, regardless of patient risk factors. This is true overall in the United States, where about three-quarters of all Black women deliver in these hospitals but less than one-fifth of White women do.

In New York City, a woman's risk of having a life-threatening complication during her delivery in one hospital can be six times higher than in another hospital. Black and Latina mothers are more likely to deliver in hospitals with worse outcomes. In fact, differences in delivery hospital explain nearly one-half of the Black/White disparity in severe maternal morbidity in New York City.

But it does not have to be this way. We can come up with simple and effective ways to measure and improve quality of care for childbearing women, whether they are Black or White, rich or poor, rural or urban. I am pleased today to provide testimony in strong support of a number of elements discussed in the bills.

First, development of maternal health quality measures that are patient-centered and address disparities; authorization of the Alliance for Innovation in Maternal Health, the AIM program, which is a national partnership that works to reduce maternal mortality and morbidity by implementing standardized care practices across hospitals and health systems; extension of Medicaid for 12 months post partum to ensure access to needed care; development and expansion of State perinatal care quality collaboratives to improve quality of care for moms and infants; support for healthcare professional training to address implicit bias. I would expand this to include training on patient-centered communication, shared decisionmaking, and actions to address both implicit and explicit bias. And, last, I would echo efforts that are already started, but we need more to build a better infrastructure to support data collection and measurement.

I would like to end my testimony by saying that we have to value pregnant women from every community. We can and must do better. I thank you for this opportunity to provide testimony, and I look forward to your questions.

[The prepared statement of Dr. Howell follows:]

TESTIMONY OF ELIZABETH A. HOWELL, MD, MPP, PROFESSOR OF POPULATION HEALTH SCIENCE & POLICY AND OBSTETRICS, GYNECOLOGY, AND REPRODUCTIVE SCIENCE, DIRECTOR OF THE BLAVATNIK FAMILY WOMEN'S HEALTH RESEARCH INSTITUTE, ICAHN SCHOOL OF MEDICINE AT MOUNT SINAI, TO THE UNITED STATES HOUSE OF REPRESENTATIVES, COMMITTEE ON ENERGY AND COMMERCE, SUBCOMMITTEE ON HEALTH

Madam Chairman Eshoo, Ranking Member Burgess, Representative Engel of New York and Members of the Subcommittee on Health, thank you for inviting me to testify and discussing how we can improve maternal health.

My name is Elizabeth Howell. I am an obstetrician gynecologist and a health services researcher. I serve as Professor in the Departments of Population Health Science & Policy and Obstetrics, Gynecology, and Reproductive Science and direct the Blavatnik Family Women's Health Research Institute at the Icahn School of Medicine at Mount Sinai.

As I recently shared in my TEDMED talk, the first time I witnessed a maternal death was during my residency training and I will never forget it. I was coming back on duty to cover the labor and delivery unit and it was chaos when I got off the elevator. All I could see was a swarm of doctors and nurses hovering over a patient in the labor room. They were all desperately trying to save a woman's life.

The patient was in shock. She had delivered a healthy baby boy about an hour before I came to the hospital. Suddenly she collapsed, became unresponsive, and had profuse uterine bleeding. By the time I got to the room, multiple doctors and nurses were there and the mother was lifeless.

The resuscitation team tried to bring her back, but despite everyone's best efforts she died. What I remember most about that day was the father's piercing cry. His cry went through my heart, and the heart of everyone on that floor. This was supposed to be one of the happiest days of his life. Instead it turned out to be the worst day.

This tragedy happens to hundreds of families every year in the United States. Approximately 700 women die from a pregnancy-related cause each year. Our maternal mortality rate is higher than other high-income countries, and the numbers are far worse for women of color. Our rate of maternal deaths has increased over the last decade while other countries have reduced their rates. Yet we spend more on healthcare than any other country in the world.

The leading causes of maternal deaths in the United States include cardiovascular conditions such as cardiomyopathy and stroke, hypertension, hemorrhage, embolism and infection. In addition, data indicate that maternal deaths from substance use disorders and mental health are climbing. Maternal mortality involving opiates doubled over the last decade.

A maternal death is just the tip of the iceberg. For every death, over 100 women experience a severe complication related to pregnancy and childbirth resulting in thousands of women every year experiencing one of these events according to the CDC. These complications, called severe maternal morbidity, include life threatening events such as stroke, blood clots, end organ damage (e.g., kidney failure), receiving a blood transfusion, having a hysterectomy, or experiencing another tragic complication. The CDC reports that severe maternal morbidity is increasing and has doubled over the last two decades.

The uncomfortable part of this story is the fact that the majority of maternal deaths and a significant proportion of severe maternal morbidity are preventable. In fact, a recent CDC report that summarized findings from nine state maternal mortality review committees found that over 60% of the deaths were preventable making quality of care a critical lever to address the rising rates of maternal mortality. By quality of care I'm not just referring to the care provided by physicians, nurses, midwives, and other providers, but also the systems in place that make it possible –

or more difficult – for women to receive evidence-based care. This holistic view also encompasses coverage, hospital system policies and practices, health care resources, and more. If we raised quality of care for pregnant women before, during, and after pregnancy, and implemented standardized care procedures across hospitals in the United States we could significantly lower rates of these tragic events.

The good news is that there are efforts at the national and state level to address quality of care, standardize care, and improve outcomes for pregnant women. At the state level perinatal quality collaboratives are working to improve quality of care for mothers and babies. Members identify health care processes that need to be improved and use the best available methods to make change. There are success stories in specific states but more resources are required to achieve better outcomes. At the national level the Alliance for Innovation on Maternal Health (AIM) is a national partnership that aims to reduce maternal deaths and severe maternal morbidity by engaging hospitals, health systems, state-based public health systems, consumer groups, community organizations, and others to implement evidence-based maternal safety bundles (standardized care practices). This data driven quality improvement initiative targets some of the most preventable causes of maternal death (high blood pressure, hemorrhage, and venous thrombotic disease). The AIM program is currently in 27 states and has the potential to reach the majority of US births. But the use of these bundles in many places around the country is missing or spotty and reflects the fact that quality of care differs across our nation.

Quality of care differs greatly for women of color. Black women are three to four times, and American Indian women are three times more likely to experience a pregnancy-related death than are white women. Although many want to think that income differences drive these disparities it goes beyond class. A black or African American woman with a college education is nearly twice as likely to die as a white woman with less than a high school education and she is two to three times more likely to experience severe maternal morbidity.

These disparities are even more pronounced in some cities. For example, in New York City black women are 8 to 12 times more likely to die from a pregnancy-related death than are white women. I am sure some of you have heard the heartbreaking story in ProPublica about the CDC epidemiologist, Dr. Shalon Irving, who died three weeks after giving birth to her first child. Dr. Irving was a brilliant epidemiologist who was committed to studying racial disparities in health. This was her first baby; she was 36; and she was African American. She had a complicated pregnancy but left the hospital with a healthy baby girl. Three weeks later she died from complications of hypertension. She was seen four or five times after her delivery by healthcare professionals. However, she was not listened to and the severity of her condition was not recognized.

Shalon's story is just one of many examples of racial and ethnic disparities in healthcare. There is growing recognition that social determinants of health – like racism, poverty, education, and segregated housing contribute to these disparities. But Shalon's story highlights an additional underlying cause – quality of care, lack of standards in postpartum care. She was seen multiple times by clinicians after the birth of her daughter and before her death but she still died. Quality of care in the setting of childbirth is an underlying cause of racial and ethnic disparities in maternal mortality and severe morbidity and something we can address now.

Research by our team and others has shown that for a variety of reasons, black women tend to deliver in a specific set of hospitals and those hospitals have worse outcomes for both black and white moms regardless of patient risk factors. This is true in the United States overall where three quarters of all black women deliver in a specific set of hospitals while less than one-fifth of white women deliver in those same hospitals. Both black and white women have worse outcomes in those hospitals. In New York City, a woman's risk of having a life-threatening complication in one hospital can be six or seven times higher than in another hospital. Black and Latina mothers are more likely to deliver in hospitals with worse outcomes. In fact, differences in delivery hospital explain nearly one half of the black-white disparity and one-third of the Latina-white disparity in severe maternal morbidity.

Our poor performance on maternal mortality and the glaring racial disparities that exist require immediate action. I am pleased today to provide testimony in strong support of legislation aimed at reducing maternal mortality and morbidity and that specifically addresses the longstanding racial and ethnic disparities in maternal mortality and morbidity in our country. There are a number of important elements discussed in these bills that are essential to achieving our goals: 1) development and testing of patient-centered maternal health quality measures that address health disparities before, during, and after pregnancy, 2) authorization of the AIM program to ensure best practices across hospitals and health systems for the care of pregnant women, 3) extension of Medicaid for 12 months postpartum to ensure access to needed care, 4) development and expansion of state and regional perinatal care quality collaboratives, 5) care management and coordination to address the social determinants that contribute to disparities, 6) infrastructure to support better data collection and measurement, and 7) support for implicit bias training for healthcare professionals. I suggest expanding the last element to include support for training students, trainees, and healthcare professionals on patient-centered communication strategies, shared decision-making skills, and actions to address both implicit and explicit bias.

I would like to end my testimony today by emphasizing the fact that quality of care in the US health care system is an underlying driver of our high maternal mortality and morbidity rates and the racial and ethnic disparities that exist. If we raised the quality of care universally to what is supposed to be the standard, we could bring the rates of deaths and severe maternal morbidity down dramatically. The question is: are we as a society ready to value pregnant women from every community? We must do better.

I thank you for the opportunity to provide testimony. I look forward to your questions.

References

Howell EA, Egorova NN, Balbierz A, Zeitlin J, Hebert PL. Site of delivery contribution to black-white severe maternal morbidity disparity. *Am J Obstet Gynecol.* 2016 Aug;215(2):143-52.

Howell EA, Egorova N, Balbierz A, Zeitlin J, Hebert PL. Black-white differences in severe maternal morbidity and site of care. *Am J Obstet Gynecol.* 2016 Jan;214(1):122.e1-7.

Building U.S. Capacity to Review and Prevent Maternal Deaths. (2018). *Report from nine maternal mortality review committees.* Retrieved from http://reviewtoaction.org/Report_from_Nine_MMRCs.

CDC Pregnancy Mortality Surveillance System. https://www.cdc.gov/reproductivehealth/maternalinfanthealth/pregnancy-mortality-surveillance-system.htm.

CDC Severe Maternal Morbidity in the United States https://www.cdc.gov/reproductivehealth/maternalinfanthealth/severematernalmorbidity.html.

Mangla K, Hoffman MC, Trumpff C, O;Grady S, Monk C. Maternal self-harm deaths: an unrecognized and preventable outcome. *Am J Obstet Gynecol.* 2019 Mar 5. [Epub ahead of print].

Howell EA. Reducing Disparities in Severe Maternal Morbidity and Mortality. *Clin Obstet Gynecol.* 2018 Jun;61(2):387-399.

AIM Program – Alliance for Innovation on Maternal Health https://safehealthcareforeverywoman.org/aim-program/.

Ms. ESHOO. Thank you, Dr. Howell.

Members may notice that I am allowing witnesses to go past their 5 minutes, but I think every word that they have to be instructive to us is really essential.

Dr. David Nelson, it is your turn to testify. You have 5 minutes, and thank you again for being here.

STATEMENT OF DAVID NELSON, MD

Dr. NELSON. Chairwoman Eshoo, Chairman Pallone, Ranking Member Walden, Ranking Member Burgess, and members of the Energy and Commerce Subcommittee on Health, thank you for inviting me today. I am an obstetrician and gynecologist with fellowship training in maternal-fetal medicine. I am the chief of obstetrics at Parkland Hospital in Dallas, Texas. Parkland is one of the largest single public maternity services in the country. Last year, we delivered 12,671 women. This is more deliveries than 10 States in our country.

As the medical director of this service, I would like to share my appreciation of this committee for their efforts and celebrate the Preventing Maternal Deaths Act that encourages State programs to establish Maternal Mortality Review Committees. However, as you know, our work is not done. A single preventable pregnancy-related death is one too many. Mr. Johnson's testimony last year to this committee and Shalon's mother's testimony today emphasized this issue.

So what are the next meaningful steps? To answer this question, I offer two themes: 1, access to prenatal care, and 2, use of relevant quality data. The significance of access to care depends on how the issue of maternal mortality is framed. The findings of the Texas Maternal Mortality Review Committee from last year were that the majority of the pregnancy-related deaths could be prevented. Similar to other reports, there was a significant racial disparity. Women of color were significantly more likely to die when compared to non-Hispanic White woman, and the majority of these deaths under review were Medicaid-funded at delivery.

So how can we address pregnancy-related deaths that are potentially preventable among women of color and receiving Medicaid funding? I offer our experiences from Parkland Hospital as one strategy. Parkland is unique. It represents a public hospital serving almost exclusively medically indigent women. Of the more than 12,000 women delivered last year, 90 percent were Medicaid funded. At Parkland, there has been a concerted effort to improve access to prenatal care. And today there are 10 clinics located throughout Dallas County. These clinics are in the neighborhoods where our patients live and are often colocated with pediatric services to enhance patient use.

Of the more than 12,000 women delivered in 2018, 97 percent accessed prenatal care. These clinics also serve as the medical home for our patients with important followup for services like blood pressure surveillance and depression screening after delivery. The system has administrative and medical oversight that is seamless. The same protocols are used by nurse practitioners at all 10 sites, and this guarantees consistent care that is standardized for referrals of high-risk women to a centrally located clinic.

Not all complications, though, can be identified before delivery. At the hospital a multidisciplinary team of nurses and providers work together according to standardized protocols. Individualized care is stratified based upon medical acuity and risk for complications. For example, we have standardized management strategies for response to obstetric emergencies like hypertension and hemorrhage. This emphasizes a culture of safety with continuous quality improvement. Recently, we have implemented an urgent request to the bedside function with our nursing partners to electronically track and monitor a timeliness to a patient's bedside for immediate care.

These efforts dovetail Parkland's participation in the newly formed regionalization program known as Maternal Levels of Care, as well as the Alliance for Innovation in Maternal Health. These initiatives share similar principles with California Maternal Quality Care Collaborative. Putting this together, access to prenatal care is considered one component of a comprehensive public healthcare system. It is community-based and extends to the inpatient care setting for a standardized approach.

An example of how access to prenatal care translates to improved outcomes, the maternal mortality rate during pregnancy and that delivery for the 3 percent of women that did not access prenatal care is more than 25-fold higher than those that had prenatal care access at our hospital.

Moving to the second theme, how do we measure quality? An obvious method is to track rates of maternal mortality. This unfortunately is easier said than done, and our hope is the recent passing of the 2018 legislation is a key step forward in this effort.

Another method of assessing quality is measuring rates of severe maternal morbidity, or SMM rates. These are unexpected outcomes that result in significant consequences to a woman's health like hysterectomy or transfusion. These rates are almost universally derived from hospital billing codes simply because no other data sources are available. We must consider the potential unintended consequences of tracking such metrics, especially transfusion, because this can become a perverse surrogate of quality. If a provider hesitates or, worse, withholds a transfusion of blood, then a patient may have a risk of mortality. It is critical we use relevant data to guide our policies.

Thank you again for this opportunity to share our experiences from Parkland and our efforts to establish access to care. Also thank you for your understanding of the importance of the relevant quality data. Ultimately these efforts can lead to safer deliveries of mothers and their infants for the future generations of our country.

Thank you.

[The prepared statement of Dr. Nelson follows:]

UTSouthwestern Medical Center, David Nelson, MD, Assistant Professor, Department of Obstetrics and Gynecology, Division of Maternal Fetal Medicine, September 6, 2019

Chairwoman Eshoo, Chairman Pallone, Ranking Member Walden, Ranking Member Burgess, and distinguished members of the Energy and Commerce Subcommittee on Health, thank you for inviting me to speak with you today on behalf of Parkland Hospital and the University of Texas Southwestern Medical Center on the hearing entitled, "Maternal Health: Legislation to Advance Prevention Efforts and Access to Care."

For introduction, I am trained as an Obstetrician-Gynecologist as well as having sub-specialty fellowship training in Maternal-Fetal Medicine. Currently, I am an Assistant Professor at the University of Texas Southwestern Medical Center and serve as the Chief of Obstetrics at Parkland Hospital in Dallas, Texas. Parkland Hospital is one of the largest single, public maternity services in the country with 12,671 women delivered at our facility last year. This delivery volume at Parkland Hospital represents approximately 1 out of every 300 new Americans born each year, and in total, represents more births than occurred in ten separate states in the country last year.

I would like to share my appreciation of this committee for their efforts and celebrate the federal legislation, Preventing Maternal Deaths Act, signed into law on December 21, 2018, that encourages state programs to establish Maternal Mortality Review Committees (MMRC). By supporting multidisciplinary local expert review, and aligning with community advocates, this is a meaningful step forward in addressing the national crisis of maternal mortality in the United States; however, as you know our work is not done. A single preventable, pregnancy-related death is one too many, and as Mr. Charles Johnson stated last year to this committee that, "No statistic that [sic] can quantify what [it] is like to tell an 18 month old that his mother is never coming home." So, what are the next meaningful steps in advancing maternal health and prevention of mortality? As a provider of maternal care services, I offer two themes which in my view are two important pieces to help solve this puzzle and prevent this tragedy: (1) access to prenatal care, and (2) use of relevant quality data to ensure well-informed decisions.

First, the significance of "access to care" depends upon how the issue of maternal mortality is framed. In 2013, the 83rd Texas Legislature established the Maternal Mortality and Morbidity Task Force for my home state of Texas. The most recent findings of this MMRC were reported in September 2018. This effort, chaired by Dr. Lisa Hollier—immediate past-president of the American College of Obstetricians and Gynecologists (ACOG)—identified that the majority of pregnancy-related deaths could be prevented. And, similar to other reports, there was a significant racial disparity with women of color significantly more likely to die when compared with non-Hispanic white women. Notably, the majority (68%) of maternal deaths in Texas under review were Medicaid-funded at delivery. So, how can we address pregnancy-related maternal deaths that are potentially preventable, among women of color, and receiving Medicaid-funding? I offer our experiences from Parkland Hospital as one strategy.

Parkland Hospital is unique as it represents a public hospital serving almost exclusively medically-indigent women. Of the 12,671 women delivered last year, 90% were Medicaid-funded. At Parkland, there has been a concerted effort to improve access to and use of prenatal care for decades. The goal has been to establish a program of seamless care beginning with enrollment during the prenatal period and extending through delivery at Parkland into the postpartum period. Today, 10 prenatal clinics are strategically located throughout the 909 square-miles of Dallas County to provide convenient access for entry into prenatal care. These 10 clinics are located in the neighborhoods where our patients live and are often co-located with comprehensive medical and pediatric services to enhance patient use. Indeed, of the 12,671 women delivered in 2018 at Parkland Hospital, 97% accessed prenatal care prior to delivery. Importantly, we were then able to identify conditions placing mothers and their infants at high-risk for complications including hemorrhage, infection, hypertension, diabetes, and HIV long before the mother presented for delivery. Moreover, these 10 clinics serve as the "healthcare home" for our patients.

Also, these same clinics serve as the follow-up location after delivery for important postpartum services to include postpartum depression screening, mental health care, and family planning services.

Because the entire clinic system as well as the hospital is operated by Parkland, administrative and medical oversight is seamless. The same prenatal protocols are used by nurse practitioners at all 10 clinic sites to guarantee consistent, protocol-based care that includes standardized referrals of high-risk women to a centrally-located prenatal clinic specifically designed for women with high-risk pregnancy complications. This high-risk pregnancy clinic includes specific programs for women with conditions such as diabetes, infectious disease, placental abnormalities, and hypertensive disorders to just name a few. Each clinic is staffed by maternal–fetal medicine faculty with special interests in such complications. Importantly, Parkland has a closed medical staff, and all attending physicians are employed by the University of Texas Southwestern Medical Center Department of Obstetrics and Gynecology, whose members adhere to agreed-on practice guidelines using an evidenced-based outcomes approach. Many of these strategies can be found in the textbook *Williams Obstetrics*—now in its 25th edition—which is the most popular obstetric textbook worldwide. This reference text has been based at our institution for the last 40 years, and 17 of the faculty help co-author the current edition. We are fortunate to have such talented, local expertise to provide care for our patients as well as train future healthcare providers to include advanced practice providers, nursing students, medical students, resident physicians, and fellows.

Not all high-risk complications can be identified within the prenatal period. Within the hospital setting, a multidisciplinary team of nurses, advance practice providers, resident physicians, Maternal-Fetal Medicine fellows, and faculty work together according to standardized protocols alongside obstetric anesthesiologists, certified registered nurse anesthetists, and pediatric teams. Individualized care is stratified within labor and delivery based upon medical acuity and risk for complications. For example, we have standardized management strategies for response to obstetric emergencies—such as hypertension and obstetric hemorrhage—that have been in place for decades. This culture of safety emphasizes careful attention for hypovolemia due to blood loss. Dr. Jack Pritchard, recognized last year by Ranking Member Burgess, proudly established the "30/30 rule" for observation of blood counts and urine output using simple testing with reliable results. This grounded, and effective, approach has been honed over generations with continuous quality improvement and focus on patient-centered outcomes for safety. Recently, we have implemented an "urgent request to the bedside" with our nursing partners to electronically track and monitor timeliness to a patient's bedside for immediate care. These efforts dovetail Parkland Hospital's participation in the newly formed regionalization program known as "Maternal Levels of Care" as well as the Alliance for Innovation on Maternal Health (AIM) Plus program in Texas. Both are now national initiatives to standardize readiness, recognition, response, and reporting of high-risk conditions placing mothers at risk for death and share similar principles with the California Maternal Quality Care Collaborative organization.

Putting this all together, this geographically-based public health prenatal care program specifically targets all populations of pregnant women to identify the high-risk conditions *before* a woman presents for delivery. Although this reduces her individual risk, it does not eliminate the potential for unanticipated obstetric emergencies. When such unexpected, life-threatening events arise, prompt identification and mobilization of resources is exercised. These same principles are part of the foundation of the AIM collaborative endorsed by our national professional organizations, such as ACOG. And more recently, we are encouraged by the August 21, 2019, release of The Joint Commission 13 new elements of performance (EPs) applicable to Joint Commission-accredited hospitals due to take effect July 1, 2020. These new requirements are within the Provision of Care, Treatment, and Services (PC) chapter at PC.06.01.01 and PC.06.01.03 for management of hemorrhage as well as hypertension and mirror much of our existing practices as described. Taken altogether, "access" to prenatal care is considered one component of a comprehensive and orchestrated public health care system that is community-based and extends to the inpatient care setting using evidenced-based, standardized practices that are monitored for quality assurance.

Turning now to the second theme, how do we then measure such quality? An obvious method is to track rates of maternal mortality. This unfortunately is easier said than done and putting our collective arms around maternal mortality data is only the beginning. At present, much of the data tracking for maternal mortality is limited to use of coded death data from maternal death certificates. The use of such coded data is fraught with potential error due to miscoding. As noted last year in this committee, half (50.3%) of obstetric-coded deaths in Texas during 2012 actually showed no evidence of pregnancy within 42 days. To be clear, this is not an indictment of the current processes involved in compiling such data, or of those that have dedicated their life to this important effort, but rather a point to emphasize that it is extremely difficult to confirm cases from afar. Moreover, this underscores the need for significant resources to accurately collect such critical information. Compare this effort to the existing infrastructure already used for other recognized significant public health issues. One example is tuberculosis (TB). For Dallas County alone, there are more than 50 dedicated staff within the Dallas County Health Department tracking, reporting, and actively managing cases of TB. These heroes within the DCHD provide follow-up, chart abstraction, reporting, and daily direct observed therapy located at a patient's home, place of employment, or even under a bridge. The same level of infrastructure has not yet been put forward for maternal death. We need sustained support to actively identify these complex cases, and ultimately, provide good quality data to make well-informed decisions. Our hope is that the recent passing of the 2018 Preventing Maternal Deaths Act is a key step forward in this effort.

A second method of assessing "quality" of maternal care is measuring rates of severe maternal morbidity (SMM), or *near-misses*. These are unexpected outcomes that result in significant short- or long-term consequences to a woman's health, such as hysterectomy and transfusion. These SMM rates are also almost universally derived from hospital billing codes–simply because no other data sources are available. Moreover, we must consider the potential unintended consequences of tracking such "SMM" metrics, especially transfusion of blood. Blood transfusion is the single greatest contributor to the SMM rate both at Parkland Hospital and nationally. In 2014, blood transfusion accounted for more than 80% of the SMM rate in the United States. We caution, however, that this can become a perverse surrogate of quality. If a provider hesitates, or worse, withholds a transfusion of blood to a patient to avoid the "label" of SMM, then there is an unintended risk of mortality. Indeed, the reason obstetric hemorrhage is deadly is because of failure to promptly restore a woman's circulating blood volume. This can have far-reaching consequences in quality measurement across hospitals. For example, a hospital with a high rate of transfusion could be considered inferior to a hospital with a low rate of transfusion. Is it possible that this evaluation is upside down? The hospital with the higher transfusion rate may actually be higher in quality than the hospital with a low rate of transfusion as measured by mortality. We must be careful to not inadvertently worsen mortality while trying to avoid a surrogate of morbidity by careful selection of quality metrics.

In closing, thank you again for this opportunity to share our experiences from Parkland Hospital and our efforts to establish prenatal care access. Also, thank you for your understanding of the importance of relevant quality data and reporting. To advance the national effort in improving both maternal mortality and morbidity, it is critical that accurate, relevant clinical data are reported and are used to guide decisions for healthcare policy. Ultimately, these efforts can lead to safer deliveries of mothers and their infants for the future generations of our country.

Thank you,

David B. Nelson, MD, FACOG
Chief of Obstetrics, Parkland Hospital
Dedman Family Scholar in Clinical Care
Assistant Professor, Maternal-Fetal Medicine
Department of Obstetrics & Gynecology
University of Texas Southwestern Medical Center
Dallas, Texas

Ms. ESHOO. I thank you, Doctor.

Usha Ranji, you are recognized for your 5 minutes of testimony.

You can proceed, and thank you.

STATEMENT OF USHA RANJI

Ms. RANJI. Good morning, Chairwoman Eshoo, Ranking Member Burgess, and members of the committee. I am Usha Ranji, Associate Director of Women's Health

Policy at the Kaiser Family Foundation, a nonprofit, nonpartisan organization that provides health policy analysis.

Thank you for inviting me to testify about the role of Medicaid coverage for pregnant and post partum women. I will highlight three main areas: research on the importance of health coverage for babies and mothers; the role of State policy decisions on access to care during and after pregnancy; and some of the current efforts to close gaps in post partum coverage.

Medicaid is the primary source of health coverage for low-income women and the major financier of maternity care. In the mid-1980s in response to rising rates of infant mortality, Congress and States saw an opportunity to use Medicaid to improve birth outcomes by expanding the program to more low-income pregnant women and children. Today, the program finances more than 4 in 10 births nationally and more than half in many States.

Research shows that women with Medicaid coverage consistently fare better than uninsured women on several measures of access, including greater use of timely prenatal care. More recent research suggests that Medicaid expansion is associated with a narrowing in racial and ethnic disparities in infant outcomes. Our work at KFF finds that low-income women with Medicaid use care at rates that are comparable to their privately insured counterparts, and there is broad agreement that access to care before and after a pregnancy is essential for prevention, early detection, and treatment of some of the conditions that raise a woman's risk for pregnancy complications.

Medicaid plays a critical role in promoting access to that care. Maternity care is one of the benefits that all States must cover under Medicaid. Eligibility for Medicaid is based on decisions that States make within Federal guidelines. Federal law requires that all States cover pregnant women with incomes up to 138 percent of the Federal poverty level, which is just under $30,000 a year for a family of three, but most States cover pregnant women with higher incomes, recognizing the importance of coverage during the perinatal period.

Yet after a woman gives birth, there is no requirement to continue Medicaid coverage beyond 60 days post partum. Historically many women would become uninsured in the months following pregnancy as a result. But policymakers have opportunities to improve coverage for post partum women and their families. States across the country have made different decisions about whether to expand Medicaid under the ACA.

In the 14 States that have not changed their Medicaid program eligibility levels, post partum women cannot stay on the program unless they requalify as parents. However, in these States eligibility for parents is much stricter than for pregnant women. For example, in some States, a new mother would lose Medicaid coverage 2 months after giving birth if she and her partner have income above $4,000 a year.

Federal subsidies are available to help——

Ms. ESHOO. Can you say that one more time?

Ms. RANJI. Sure. When we look at the eligibility criteria for parents, it is much lower than it is for pregnancy under Medicaid, and it is State-determined, and in all

States, it is actually lower for pregnancy, and in some States, it is as low as $4,000 a year for a family of three.

Ms. ESHOO. Wow.

Ms. RANJI. Federal subsidies are available to help some lower-income mothers purchase private marketplace insurance. But when a mother's income falls between her State's Medicaid level for parents and the poverty line, she does not qualify for either Medicaid or private insurance subsidies.

Today, a handful of States are exploring options to improve Medicaid coverage for women after pregnancy. All States can set and raise the income eligibility levels for parents, and that is without adopting the Medicaid expansion.

Earlier this year, Illinois approved extension of post partum coverage under Medicaid to 1 year. Policymakers in Missouri and California have also proposed extending coverage for mothers in need of substance abuse treatment and mental healthcare, respectively. These are a few examples of efforts to enhance care and coverage for low-income moms.

Madam Chair, members of the committee, the research is clear. Having health coverage before, during, and after pregnancy promotes access to care. And lack of coverage is associated with poor health outcomes. Furthermore, our understanding of the health needs of women shows that the post partum period has evolved beyond one visit, yet in more than a dozen States, Medicaid coverage ends 2 months after childbirth, even though for a mom, her need for care does not end then.

In short, there is strong empirical evidence to support what families across the country already know and experience on a daily basis, that a mother's ability to care for her own health and wellbeing is integral to her ability to do the same for her children.

Thank you.

[The prepared statement of Ms. Ranji follows:]

MEDICAID AND HEALTH COVERAGE FOR LOW-INCOME WOMEN IN PREGNANCY AND AFTER CHILDBIRTH, USHA RANJI, MS, ASSOCIATE DIRECTOR, WOMEN'S HEALTH POLICY THE KAISER FAMILY FOUNDATION, PREPARED FOR THE COMMITTEE ON ENERGY AND COMMERCE, SUBCOMMITTEE ON HEALTH, U.S. HOUSE OF REPRESENTATIVES

Introduction

Good morning, Chairwoman Eshoo, Ranking Member Burgess, and Members of the Committee. I am Usha Ranji, Associate Director of Women's Health Policy at the Kaiser Family Foundation. Thank you for inviting me to testify about the role of Medicaid coverage for pregnant and postpartum women. The Kaiser Family

Foundation, KFF, is a non-profit organization that provides non-partisan health policy analysis, polling, and journalism (Kaiser Health News) to inform policymakers, the media, the health policy community and the public. We are not associated with Kaiser Permanente or Kaiser Industries. In my testimony today, I will summarize KFF's research on Medicaid and postpartum coverage (Appendix 1) and address the following key points:

- Research shows that coverage before, during, and after pregnancy facilitates access to care that supports healthy pregnancies as well as positive maternal and infant outcomes after childbirth.
- Medicaid is the primary source of health coverage for low-income women, and a major financer of maternity care, covering more than four in ten births in the U.S. Research finds that for low-income women, Medicaid is comparable to private insurance in terms of many measures of access to care.
- States set eligibility criteria for Medicaid within federal guidelines. The federal minimum income level for pregnancy-related eligibility is effectively 138% of the federal poverty level, but many states set higher thresholds, recognizing the importance of coverage during the perinatal period. Pregnancy-related coverage ends after 60 days postpartum. Infants born to women with Medicaid coverage for pregnancy are eligible for Medicaid for the first year of life.
- Even without expanding Medicaid under the Affordable Care Act (ACA), states can expand access to Medicaid by broadening parental coverage. Prior to having the option to expand Medicaid eligibility under the ACA, 17 states and DC set income thresholds for parents that were at the poverty level or higher.
- Today, eligibility for women after childbirth varies because policymakers have made different decisions about whether to expand Medicaid as well as whether to increase income thresholds for parents - even in states that have not adopted the Medicaid expansion.
- These state choices affect women's ability to stay on Medicaid after pregnancy ends. In expansion states, many postpartum women can remain on the program and those who do not qualify for Medicaid typically qualify for subsidies to assist with the costs of obtaining private insurance in state Marketplaces.
- To retain Medicaid coverage after pregnancy in the 14 non-expansion states, postpartum women need to requalify under their state's parent eligibility criteria, which are much lower than the income thresholds for pregnancy (from 17% to 100% of the federal poverty level).
- Women with incomes at or above 100% of poverty can qualify for ACA marketplace subsidies in all states, but in states with lower parental coverage thresholds, women with incomes between the state Medicaid eligibility level

for parents and 100% of poverty may have no pathway to affordable coverage. This has implications for their ability to access needed health care services during this important life stage.

- Some states are undertaking efforts that rely on Medicaid to strengthen postpartum care and coverage for women. There are multiple initiatives under way to target services to different groups who have had a Medicaid funded birth and who may be more vulnerable, including those affected by substance use and mental health challenges.

Research shows that coverage before, during, and after pregnancy is important to facilitate access to care that supports healthy pregnancies, as well as positive maternal and infant outcomes after childbirth. Research finds that for low-income women, Medicaid is comparable to private insurance in terms of many measures of access to care.

Efforts to improve coverage for pregnant women began in the mid-1980s in response to rising rates and stark disparities in infant mortality and low-birthweight. Led by the Southern Regional Taskforce on Infant Mortality, governors saw an opportunity to use Medicaid to play a role in improving birth outcomes by providing coverage to uninsured, low-income pregnant women as well as expanding eligibility for children. The federal government then raised the eligibility floor for Medicaid coverage and provided states with incentives to extend coverage for pregnancy even above the minimum requirement. This led to a substantial increase in Medicaid's coverage of low-income pregnant women, infants, and children up to age six and declines in the uninsured.[16]

Research has shown that people with Medicaid coverage fare much better than their uninsured counterparts on several measures of access to care. One synthesis[17] of peer-reviewed literature concluded that the expansions for pregnancy eligibility contributed to "improvements in prenatal care use," while more recent analyses of federal data from the Pregnancy Risk Assessment Monitoring System (PRAMS) found significantly higher rates of timely and adequate prenatal care among pregnant women covered by Medicaid compared to uninsured women.[18,19] Mothers covered by Medicaid are much more likely than those who are low-income and uninsured to have a usual source of care, recent doctor and dental visits, and other preventive services, such as screenings for breast and cervical cancers.[20] Our own work at KFF finds that low-income women with private insurance use care at rates that are comparable to their privately-insured counterparts and significantly higher than those

---

[16] Rowland, et al. The Key to the Door: Medicaid's Role in Improving Health Care for Women and Children." *Annual Reviews of Public Health*, 1999.

[17] Howell E, "The Impact of the Medicaid Expansions for Pregnant Women: A Synthesis of the Evidence." *Medical Care Research and Review*, March 2001.

[18] MACPAC, "Access in Brief: Pregnant Women and Medicaid," November 2018.

[19] Wherry, L.R. "State Medicaid Expansions for Parents Led to Increased Coverage and Prenatal Care Utilization among Pregnant Mothers." *Health Services Research*, December 2017.

[20] Long S et al., "How Well Does Medicaid Work in Improving Access to Care?" *Health Services Research*, February 2005.

who are uninsured.[21] Low-income women in Medicaid were also significantly less likely than those who are privately-insured to report that cost was a barrier to care.[22]

Today, there is continued need to improve maternal and infant health and a growing urgency to develop policy and programmatic responses to the rise in maternal mortality and morbidity and the wide racial and ethnic disparities in maternal outcomes.[23] Medicaid plays a major role in health coverage for all low-income women, but particularly for women of color because they are more likely to be low-income (Figure 1). There is greater recognition that access to health care *throughout* a woman's reproductive years, including before and after a pregnancy, is essential for prevention, early detection, and treatment of some of the conditions that place women at higher risk for pregnancy-related complications, including cardiovascular disease, diabetes, and chronic hypertension. And, there is strong empirical evidence to support what families across the country know and experience on a daily basis - that a mother's ability to care for her own health and well-being is integral to her ability to do the same for her children.[24]

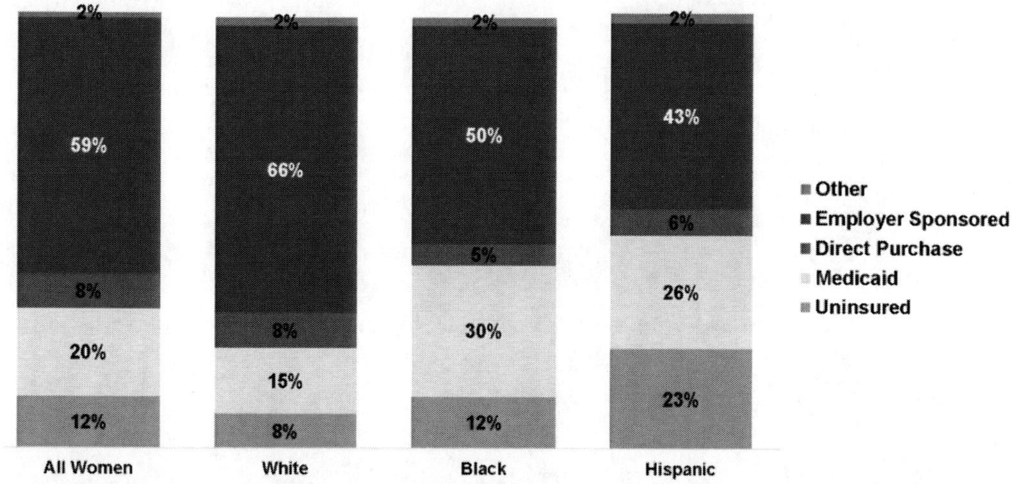

Notes: Data reflect coverage in 2017 among women 15-49. "Other" includes those covered under the military or Veterans Administration as well as nonelderly Medicare enrollees.
Source: Kaiser Family Foundation analysis of Census Bureau's American Community Survey.

Figure 1. Health Insurance Coverage Among Women of Reproductive Age, by Race/Ethnicity.

Medicaid is the primary source of health coverage for low-income women, and a major financer of maternity care, covering more than four in ten births in the U.S.

Medicaid has historically prioritized coverage for children and pregnant women. Children make up 43% of the Medicaid population overall, and among adult women

[21] Kaiser Family Foundation, Medicaid's Role for Women, March 2019.
[22] Kaiser Family Foundation, Medicaid's Role for Women, March 2019.
[23] Centers for Disease Control and Prevention, "Racial/Ethnic Disparities in Pregnancy-Related Deaths — United States, 2007–2016." *MMWR,* September 6, 2019.
[24] Georgetown University Health Policy Institute Center for Children and Families, Health Coverage for Parents and Caregivers Helps Children, March 2017.

on the program, two-thirds (67%) are in their reproductive years (19 to 49). The program now finances more than four in ten (43%) births nationally[25] and more than half in some states (Figure 2).[26]

While maternity care is a mandatory benefit that states must cover, states have discretion to determine the specific scope of maternity care benefits under Medicaid. All states cover prenatal care and delivery services. States that have expanded Medicaid eligibility under the ACA must cover all preventive services recommended by the United States Preventive Services Task Force (USPSTF) and Women's Preventive Services Initiative (WPSI) for beneficiaries that qualify as a result of the expansion. These include many pregnancy-related services, such as prenatal visits, screening tests, and folic acid supplements. It also includes coverage for breastfeeding supports that extend to the postpartum period, with coverage for lactation consultation and breast pumps. Many states cover substance use treatment and home visiting services, and just a few now cover doula services.[27]

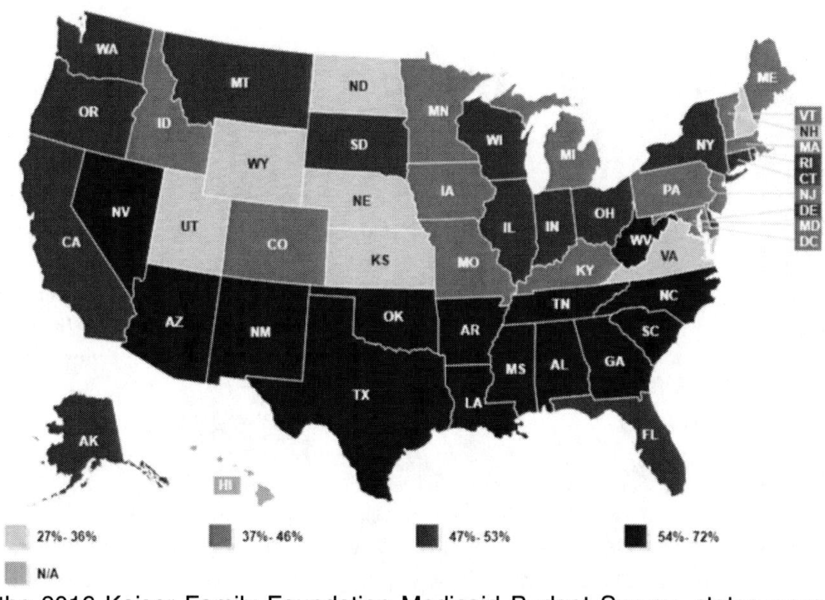

Note: In the 2016 Kaiser Family Foundation Medicaid Budget Survey, states were asked to report the share of all births in the state that were financed by Medicaid in the most recent 12 month period for which data were available. States reported data from 2010-2016, which varied by calendar year, state fiscal year, and federal fiscal year.

Source: Kaiser Family Foundation. Implementing Coverage and Payment Initiatives: Results from a 50-State Medicaid Budget Survey for State Fiscal Years 2016 and 2017.

Figure 2. Medicaid is the Leading Financer of Maternity Care in Many States.

---

25 Centers for Disease Control and Prevention. "Births: Final Data for 2017." *National Vital Statistics Report*, November 7, 2018.

26 Kaiser Family Foundation, State Health Facts: Medicaid Enrollees by Enrollment Group, 2014.

27 Kaiser Family Foundation, Medicaid Coverage of Pregnancy and Perinatal Benefits, April 2017.

Under federal law, women who receive pregnancy-related services under Medicaid cannot be charged for any share of the cost of care, but after the postpartum period, that can change. A large body of evidence shows that even nominal cost sharing impedes access to care for low-income women and families. For low-income mothers, the lower cost sharing and absence of deductibles under Medicaid can be a major advantage over private insurance.

States set income eligibility criteria for Medicaid within federal guidelines, and most extend coverage to pregnant women above the federally-required minimum of 138% of poverty, recognizing the importance of coverage during the perinatal period. Pregnancy-related coverage ends after 60 days postpartum. Infants born to women with Medicaid coverage for pregnancy are automatically enrolled in Medicaid for the first year of life.

Federal law requires that all states extend eligibility to pregnant women with incomes up to 138% of the federal poverty level (FPL), which equals $29,435 for a family of three; however, most states go beyond this minimum threshold, ranging from 138% to 380% FPL (see Table 1 in the Appendix).

Pregnancy-related coverage for the mother must last through 60 days postpartum[28] and the infant is eligible for Medicaid for the first year after birth. Following the 60 days postpartum period, the decision about coverage for women is up to the states and depends in part of whether the state has opted to expand Medicaid as allowed by the ACA or where they set parental income eligibility levels. Wisconsin, for example, has not expanded Medicaid under the ACA, but extends parental coverage to 100% FPL, which is higher than most other non-expansion states.

Infants born to women who had Medicaid during pregnancy are automatically enrolled in Medicaid for their first year. This allows access to numerous preventive services for many low-income families, including newborn screenings, immunizations, and well child visits. Notably, research finds that when mothers have Medicaid, there is greater retention of coverage for children as well.[29]

Historically, many postpartum women would become uninsured in the months following pregnancy because they had no pathway to coverage. Even today, the availability of Medicaid coverage for women in the postpartum period varies considerably by state.

Prior to implementation of the ACA, many women with Medicaid during pregnancy would become uninsured after the 60 days postpartum period ended.

---

[28] Pregnancy coverage under Medicaid ends for the woman on the last day of the month that is 60 days after the pregnancy ends.

[29] Sommers BD. "Insuring children or insuring families: do parental and sibling coverage lead to improved retention of children in Medicaid and CHIP?" *J Health Econ,* November 2006.

After this time, women would need to requalify for Medicaid as a parent, and all states set much lower income eligibility thresholds for parents, compared to pregnant women. Women with incomes above their state's parental eligibility level would likely be disenrolled from Medicaid after the postpartum coverage ended.

There is significant instability in health coverage among low-income women, a phenomenon known as "churning," due in part to the volatility of employment and income levels for this population. A national study of women's insurance coverage during the perinatal period in the pre-ACA era found that more than half of women covered by Medicaid or CHIP at the time of delivery were uninsured at least one of the six months following delivery. This was far higher than the rate for women who had private insurance at the time of delivery (55% Medicaid compared to 35% private).[30]

Even without expanding Medicaid under the ACA, states can expand access to Medicaid by broadening parental coverage. Prior to having the option to expand Medicaid eligibility under the ACA, 17 states and DC set income thresholds for parents that were at the poverty level or higher.

In states that have implemented Medicaid expansion, there is alignment between the minimum income eligibility level for pregnancy and the expansion threshold at 138% of poverty. As a result, qualifying postpartum women in these states with incomes up to 138% of poverty can retain Medicaid coverage after pregnancy-related coverage ends. Continuous Medicaid coverage can promote greater continuity of care by allowing postpartum women to remain within the same provider network and care system that she saw during pregnancy. Those with higher incomes can qualify for federal subsidies in the Marketplaces up to 400% of poverty. There is a pathway to coverage and assistance for most postpartum women in expansion states.

Women with incomes above 100% of poverty can qualify for ACA marketplace subsidies in all states, but in states with very low parental coverage thresholds such those in many non-expansion states, women with incomes between the state Medicaid eligibility level for parents and 100% of poverty may have no pathway to affordable coverage. This has implications for their ability to access needed health care services during this important life stage.

In the 14 states that have not changed their Medicaid program eligibility levels, postpartum women need to requalify for Medicaid under the parental eligibility category to stay on the program after pregnancy coverage ends. However, Medicaid income eligibility levels for parents are much lower than for pregnant women, ranging from 17% to 100% of poverty in those states (Figure 3).

---

[30] Daw, et al. "Women in the United States Experience High Rates of Coverage Churn in Months Before and After Childbirth." *Health Affairs*, April 2017.

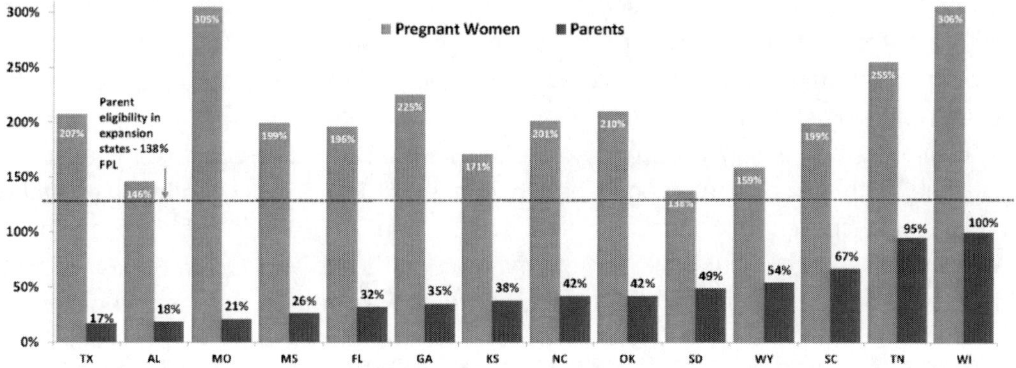

Note: For pregnant women, reflects highest eligibility limit for pregnant women under Medicaid, CHIP, or the unborn child option. For "Parents," eligibility limits calculated as a percent of the Federal Poverty Level (FPL) & are calculated based on a family of three for parents. In 2019, the FPL was $21,330 for a family of three. Thresholds include the standard five percentage point of the FPL disregard.

Source: Based on national survey conducted by Kaiser Family Foundation (KFF) with the Georgetown University Center for Children and Families, 2019.

Figure 3. Medicaid Eligibility Thresholds for Pregnant Women Compared to Parents in Non-Expansion States, 2019.

Marketplace premium subsidies are only available for those with incomes between 100% and 400% of poverty. Therefore, if a postpartum woman's income is above the state's Medicaid eligibility level for parents but below the federal poverty line ($21,330 annually for a family of three), she would not qualify for either Medicaid or private insurance subsidies. As a result, many women in non-expansion states become uninsured after pregnancy-related coverage ends (60 days postpartum) because they do not have access to Medicaid or federal subsidies. We refer to this group as falling into the "coverage gap."

Some states are now undertaking efforts that rely on Medicaid to strengthen postpartum care and coverage for women. There are multiple initiatives under way to target services to different groups of women who have had a Medicaid funded birth and who may be more vulnerable, including those affected by substance use and mental health challenges.

Some states are seeking to extend Medicaid coverage to postpartum women with related health challenges. For example, policymakers in Missouri have submitted a waiver application to the federal government to help finance a Medicaid extension for postpartum women in need of substance use treatment. The CDC found a four-fold increase in the number of women with opioid use disorder at labor and delivery between 1999 and 2014.[31]

The American College of Obstetricians and Gynecologists (ACOG) recommends that postpartum women with substance use disorders should have access to and continue use of treatment services, including pharmacotherapy. The postpartum period can be a particularly susceptible time for relapse, with loss of insurance and access to care considered a potential trigger for relapse. CMS currently has a funding opportunity for up to 12 states to develop programs to care for pregnant and postpartum women with opioid use disorder.

California has approved a policy to extend Medicaid coverage for a year to any individual with a maternal mental health condition. For a new mother who needs medications, for example, to manage postpartum depression, this extension of Medicaid coverage could fill an otherwise unaffordable gap, particularly since Medicaid would not impose cost sharing charges. Postpartum depression can occur anytime in the first year after delivery, making the frequency of well child visits during that year a chance for identifying and screening for maternal depression. Recognizing this opportunity, in 2016 CMS approved coverage of postpartum depression screening for women during well child visits. Under the CMS initiative, if the woman is enrolled in Medicaid, treatment services can be covered under Medicaid. If a woman is uninsured, for example in a non-expansion state, in order for Medicaid to cover the treatment under the child, the treatment must involve the child, such as family therapy.

Earlier this year, Illinois enacted an extension of Medicaid postpartum coverage to one year for women with incomes up to 200% of poverty. The state is in the process of applying for an 1115 waiver to procure federal financing assistance.

These are just a few examples of the ways that states can leverage Medicaid to enhance care and coverage for low-income pregnant women and after childbirth when they have become mothers.

For women, the need for health care services does not end two months after childbirth, even though their health coverage might. The year after a delivering baby is a not only a medically vulnerable time for many women, but even for those who appear to be healthy, postpartum care in the year after having a child is critical. The evidence on this is clear — having health coverage promotes access to care, especially for low-income people, and the lack of coverage is associated with poorer health outcomes. The availability of coverage to postpartum women, particularly for those who are low-income can improve their use of critical services and lead to better outcomes for women and their families.

Appendix

See attached Appendix: Kaiser Family Foundation, "Expanding Postpartum Medicaid Coverage."

---

[31] Centers for Disease Control and Prevention, "Opioid Use Disorder Documented at Delivery Hospitalization." *MMWR,* August 10, 2018.

Ms. ESHOO. Thank you, Ms. Ranji.

Those are some startling numbers, that it sounds like you have a child and then the system becomes punitive.

The witnesses have now concluded their opening statements. We are going to move to Member questions. Members each have 5 minutes to ask questions of our witnesses, and I will start by recognizing myself for 5 minutes.

There are many layers to this, but I want to go back to where we began with Ms. Irwin and many of the things that she said in her testimony to us. She said that we need to hold healthcare professionals accountable for improving the quality of care and ensuring equity.

Her daughter has had, I think, more education as one person than most Members sitting on this dais. So she was not low income. She was not uneducated. And it seems to me that racial bias is alive and well in this area of giving birth and what happens post partum.

Let me ask Dr. Harris: What is the AMA doing about this? I mean, it seems to me that you can track the hospitals where women of color frequent those hospitals than others. I think the statistics are really very clear. This is not a foggy picture. We heard Dr. Nelson talk about their very purposeful training.

So what is the AMA doing before you came to the witness table? Have you targeted the hospitals? Is it red light and siren to do something that addresses this? Maybe you can just briefly explain to us what the AMA is doing, and if you are not, what you plan to do, to be fair.

Dr. HARRIS. Thank you, Chairwoman.

From the AMA's standpoint, we would see our audience as impacting the physician community. Certainly, I heard from Dr. Howell, though, that there is value in hospitals developing standards. And it would be the recommendation that those standards include some metrics for evaluation.

Ms. ESHOO. That hasn't before begun yet, in terms of AMA partnering with hospitals and doctors?

Dr. HARRIS. No, we have not worked with hospitals to develop any specific metrics. But we are starting internally, as I mentioned earlier. We have just hired Dr. Aletha Maybank. She is our first——

Ms. ESHOO. That is a first step. It's a first step.

Dr. HARRIS [continuing]. Chief health equity officer.

And that is building on the work that we already have been working on from our Commission to End Disparities.

Ms. ESHOO. Thank you.

Obviously, the causes of pregnancy-related deaths differ. The doctors on the panel, what I want you to instruct us about, because we know heart disease and stroke cause most of the deaths overall. Obstetrics emergencies, severe bleeding, amniotic fluid, embolism cause the most deaths at delivery, but severe bleeding, high blood pressure, and infections are the leading causes in the week after delivery, and weakened heart muscle is the leading cause of deaths 1 week to 1 year post partum.

This is in our memorandum from the committee staff.

How best do you recommend to us to pursue each one of these categories? And for the life of me, I don't understand why the doctors that are trained in this—I mean, this is a specialty, as our ranking member is—that these deaths are a result of these areas, and, as you said, Dr. Howell, they are preventable. Where have we gone wrong? Have they forgotten what they learned? Is their training not up to snuff?

Can you be instructive to us on that, Dr. Howell?

Dr. HOWELL. Sure. Sure. So you bring up a really important point, which is what we are pushing for through ACOG and the Alliance for Innovation on Maternal Health. We need standardized care practices based on evidence-based medicine——

Ms. ESHOO. And that is not the case now?

Dr. HOWELL. Well, we do. So AIM has started a few years ago. And it is growing in numbers. It now reaches 27 States, and these are partnerships with hospitals and health systems, departments of health, caregivers to try to work together to improve quality and safety. And we don't just target the most preventable causes like hypertension, you know, blood clots, et cetera. We also target additional things.

We have come up with an AIM bundle on how we might address reducing disparities in hospitals and health systems with some key steps that we recommend. We also have, as part of this effort—it is very much a data-driven effort—so we have quality—we have measures and metrics that we are trying to use to utilize and examine how hospitals are doing, which we think is a very important part. So we can't only implement, but we have to evaluate to make sure what we are doing is the most meaningful way.

So that is one big effort that has been going on for about, I believe AIM started in about 2015, and it is very much a partnership.

Ms. ESHOO. Well, thank you very much.

My time is up, but I also think the American Hospital Association has to lean in on this as well because the statistics can be traced right back to where women of color, what hospitals they go to, and the number of deaths there or the tremendous complications that follow. But my time is up.

So the Chair will now recognize the distinguished Dr. Burgess, the ranking member of our subcommittee, for his 5 minutes of questions.

Mr. BURGESS. Thank you.

Dr. Nelson, you look like you wanted to say something. Can I give you a moment to respond to previous discussion?

Dr. NELSON. I agree with Dr. Howell that part of the issue is our view. We have not had the full view that we need to see. There are the issues surrounding pregnancy, delivery, and the now subsequently post partum. One of the issues we need to recognize is the process measures that need to be in place, meaning our response that is consistent to emergencies like hypertension and hemorrhage, things like a massive transfusion protocol where we directly get blood to the patient's bedside that needs help, processes like simulation to train our team members in a safe environment. And then we need performance measures that are meaningful to track data and identify quality and sincere efforts to improve that space. That, I think, is a major step forward for us collectively that we are trying to see.

Mr. BURGESS. And since you are talking about it—and, once again, I want to thank you. You were very kind to show me around the new unit at Parkland Hospital. They have just moved in to new facilities, and so it is different from what it was back in the 1970s when I was there, but I was impressed that there are some of the things that I learned in the 1970s that are still appropriate today, but you have also made things different in a number of ways. And one of the ways that really impressed me was the availability of, I guess, an emergency bleeding cart that would be just footsteps away—and you had several of them strategically positioned throughout the labor and delivery units so that the response time could be significantly reduced. Dr. Howell in her written testimony talks about coming into a scene where somebody is exsanguinating an hour after delivery. We had a hearing last year—Mr. Johnson, whose wife had a bleeding complication after cesarean section—can you speak to that and how the urgency with which the situation is responded to has helped you in managing this crisis?

Dr. NELSON. Yes, sir. And Dr. Howell is absolutely right. Time is of the essence in these emergencies. Our labor and delivery suite is over the size of a football field. There are 44 labor and delivery rooms, and in partnership with the Maternal Levels of Care Program for Texas and in alignment with the AIM program, we have four hemorrhage carts on our unit. These are carts that contain specific resources, specific instrumentation, and needs that a nursing team or physician team might need to immediately respond to a hemorrhage event. We debrief after every time we utilize a massive transfusion protocol, meaning every time we activate a massive resource allocation to a patient, we debrief with the team to understand if there are opportunities to learn from the nurses or physicians. We use multidisciplinary simulation where we train in an environment with nursing—nurse midwives, anesthesiologists, and team members. We formalized a checklist that is consistent with the AIM platform. We have the hemorrhage cart that we mentioned. We also perform daily huddles for every scheduled surgery that we have performed, and because our service deals with a fair number of women with what is called placenta accreta spectrum disorder, or morbidity—placentas, we actually have a dedicated team of maternal-fetal medicine faculty and public surgeons for those cases.

Mr. BURGESS. For people who don't know, that can be one of the scariest situations you can encounter. So let me ask you this, and one of your predecessors, Dr. Norman Gant, who was the chairman of OB/GYN when I was a resident back in the 1970s, I forget what he was haranguing us about one day, but he was famous for doing that, and he was giving us the business about how he was worried that his residents were giving care without caring, and he wanted us to be sure to delve into the interpersonal part of the relationship with the patient and being certain we listened to the patient and heard the patient. Some of that strikes me as—when Mr. Johnson was here last year and gave his testimony about the problems his wife had after a cesarean section and when we listened to Ms. Irving talk about her daughter's problems, I mean, there were some significant things that happened, and I don't want to say there were care lapses, but I am sorry, a diastolic blood pressure of 118 millimeters of mercury, that is not an appointment to clinic tomorrow. I mean, that is something that needs—something needs to be acted upon. So are we empowering people to make the decisions that need to be made when they encountered these points?

And either Dr. Howell or Dr. Nelson, since you are the clinical specialists.

Dr. NELSON. I absolutely agree accountability is critical, and tracking that accountability is one issue. The urgent requested bedside function we actually have in place to track time from the blood pressure to when a response was seen. To add on to the comments from Dr. Howell and some of our other panelists, there is absolutely an issue of racial disparity in our services. At Parkland alone, we have a diversity inclusion officer. We have an instructorled course once a month on this issue, and every new hire has to go through that because of our environment served. That is a commitment that we have at our organization.

Mr. BURGESS. And I would just stress that, because of the environment served, you are basically what would be described as an inner-city hospital, and you deal primarily with the indigent population of Dallas County, Texas?

Dr. NELSON. Yes, sir.

Mr. BURGESS. Thank you for being here today. Thanks all of you for your testimony. It has all been very enlightening.

I will yield back.

Ms. ESHOO. The gentleman yields back.

I now would—let's see. Where is—a pleasure to recognize the gentlewoman from California, Ms. Matsui, for her 5 minutes of questioning of the witnesses.

Ms. MATSUI. Thank you very much, Chairwoman Eshoo and Ranking Member Burgess, for holding this very important hearing. Like our witnesses here today, I am deeply concerned about the rates of maternal death and severe maternal morbidity in this country that is supposed to be one of the most developed countries in the world. And a special thank you to Ms. Irving for sharing your family's loss. I am so sorry.

Keeping our mothers and babies safe and healthy is vital. As a cosponsor of last year's Preventing Maternal Deaths Act, I am pleased that we are building on this effort to address outstanding racial and ethnic disparities that exacerbate poor maternal health. Extending Medicaid coverage for maternal health services across continuum of care is a critical next step, and strengthening the quality measures and training programs will help protect our mothers and babies when care is delivered. I thank the committee for prioritizing the hearing on this issue. Several of you pointed out in your testimony the uncomfortable truth that a significant portion of severe maternal disease and death is preventable. It is clear how critical Medicaid coverage is to ensure access to care and avoid preventable maternal health complications.

Dr. Howell, you touched upon how quality of care pertains to both clinician practice and system policies. In your holistic view, what is the link between coverage and quality of care?

Dr. HOWELL. So coverage is essential, and I think we heard from Ms. Ranji about how important coverage is, you know, preconception, antenatal, during delivery, and post partum, and the growing awareness that a third of these deaths are happening in the post partum way-out period. We are talking about cardiomyopathies. We are talking about suicides. We are talking about women dying from things that we could do something about, but we have not been giving adequate access to care. So it is instrumental, and it is a key link.

Ms. MATSUI. OK. In Sacramento, we have been looking at, through a Black Child Legacy Campaign since 2015, on this whole area of maternal death, prenatal, post partum activity, and we have come across quite a lot of activities that have really increased our chances here in Sacramento County, and we are really pleased to see that most of the country is sort of looking at how we are doing it too.

In Sacramento, we also have cultural brokers at one of our FQACs, the WellSpace Health, that helped to engage and support pregnant women by integrating medical care, parental education, and community resources for housing and transportation into a prenatal program for families. It has to be all-inclusive, as you know. This comprehensive model has led to rates of premature and low birth rate that are significantly below the national average.

Dr. Harris, it sounds like the AMA is doing some interesting work around social determinants. Can you elaborate on how you envision health plans integrating social and environmental health data—environmental data to better address a mother's unique needs, and how will this lead to healthier babies?

Dr. HARRIS. Absolutely, and thank you. And the structural and social determinants of health are critical as we understand how to address this issue and actually other healthcare crises. We have to look at transportation. Is there access to get to prenatal visits? We have to look at other social supports to make sure that our pregnant moms get to their prenatal visits. For moms who are pregnant and diagnosed with depression, we have to make sure that they have access to psychiatric care and care for therapy, and so addressing housing and education and employment are all critical as we address actually this issue, but really all health issues.

Ms. MATSUI. Sure. Both you and Ms. Ranji made it clear that mental healthcare throughout the pregnancy is paramount to improving the health of mothers and their babies. Would you both expand on the transmaternal mortality with regards to mental health? What is the link between depression and pregnancy and maternal outcomes? You want to take this one, Ms. Ranji?

Ms. RANJI. Thank you. I will let Dr. Harris and my colleagues comment on the clinical aspects, but I will say what we have heard from all the other witnesses is that maternal mental health is a very serious issue. It is a contributor to the maternal mortality and morbidity rates that we have been seeing, and that that is—what we know is that is an issue that does not resolve in perhaps 2 months' time, that that is an ongoing chronic condition that could require various levels of care depending on a woman's individual situation. And so access to care and services is likely needed for an extended period of time.

Ms. MATSUI. OK. I wanted to follow up. Dr. Nelson, what mental healthcare services are offered to women through your clinic's healthcare home model, and why is mental healthcare both before and after birth so vital?

Dr. NELSON. I appreciate you asking that. Mental health is critically important. In Texas, in our maternal mortality reviews from 2012 to 2015, there were 33 suicides, and 85 percent were post partum. In 2013, I published a paper screening 17,000 women with post partum depression. We identified rates consistent with other populations served. Only 22 percent made it to a psychiatrist that were identified to screen positive. From that our service identified an opportunity. We now have mental health counselors placed strategically in all 10 clinics similar to the home you described. Recently, we have actually exercised telehealth and telemedicine with virtual visits. Last year, 1,100 phone calls were made by those mental health counselors to the patients at their home and at their work for those that can't access the clinic directly.

Ms. MATSUI. Oh, that is wonderful. Thank you very much, and I know I have run out of time.

I yield back.

Ms. ESHOO. The gentlewoman yields back.

Pleasure to recognize the ranking member of the full committee, Mr. Walden, for his 5 minutes of questions.

Mr. WALDEN. Thank you, Madam Chairwoman.

And, again, thanks to all our witnesses for your testimony.

Dr. Howell, as I mentioned in my testimony, we have more to do on maternal mortality and morbidity, but we took a good first step, I think, in the last Congress with H.R. 1318, the Preventing Maternal Deaths Act, which, as you know, became law. That bill reauthorized key CDC programs to improve data collection reporting around maternal mortality. That will help support State review committees like the ones set up in my home State of Oregon to study these issues.

Dr. Howell, you are set up in New York, as I understand it, but your organization does national research. How has the work of the State review committees informed Alliance for Innovation on Maternal Health maternal safety and quality improvement initiatives?

Dr. HOWELL. So the maternal mortality reviews around the country are key and essential to the program for AIM because they teach us about each death and where are the preventable moments, what are the things we really need to work on to prevent a death. And then that information is brought to the perinatal collaboratives using some of the tools that AIM has brought together, and that is the way we can implement. We learn from the deaths. We take data and information. And then we act on it. And I think that is why these partnerships with the CDC/AIM are so important, but we need all States to have Maternal Mortality Review Committees. We need them all to review their deaths. We need them to submit them to the CDC so that they can have a central system for monitoring. And so we still need to continue to improve our data acquisition and management.

Mr. WALDEN. But it is fair to say where it does exist, it is working? You are seeing the information flow which allows then a positive response?

Dr. HOWELL. So I think it is mixed in the sense that, yes, there are places that it is really working and you are seeing a lot of movement and you see a lot of positive energy around this. Sometimes the resources are not fully there yet, and so some places are not able to actually do as well as others.

Mr. WALDEN. OK. Good. Dr. Harris, it is important to look at every factor related to maternal mortality and morbidity, but one piece I am worried about is the mental health, as has been discussed here already. And in your testimony, you mentioned that depression in pregnancy is associated with poor maternal outcomes, including maternal death. We have tried to take the lead in this committee on reforming America's mental health laws, but we all know there is more work to be done, especially for mothers with post partum depression. And I must say as a footnote, I was deeply disappointed in my own State. The Governor and the legislature actually cut mental health support funding in my State, and why I cannot imagine, but I, in town halls and other meetings I had this August, I learned the legislature just did that, and it is stunning. You say it occurs in nearly 15 percent of births. That is staggering, especially considering some of the dire outcomes we now know about. Are the State Maternal Mortality Review Committees capturing these outcomes, and are there ways that we can do better?

Dr. HARRIS. Actually, I will have to defer to my colleagues who are obstetricians to maybe talk more about whether or not that data is captured, but I will say, if it is not captured, that is certainly an opportunity gap. We have, as you notice, I think, from the last 30 years or so had a mental health system, no infrastructure, severely underfunded, and we certainly need to catch up, if we can, overall but particularly in this issue. You heard Dr. Howell talk about suicide. I think for many years there was a misperception that depression was normal after the birth of the baby, that it was the baby blues. And so it is critical that we end—there are some emotional swings that do occur, but those are not what we are all talking about with the diagnosis of a major depression, and we have to make sure that the major depression is treated if it is identified within the first visit.

Depression is a chronic disease, and it will need treatment as sometimes for a lifetime, but certainly it is not just a take a pill and your depression will be cured. So this is a huge issue, and we certainly have a long way to go. Funding for mental health overall, and certainly as regards to post partum moms.

I will say one more thing, and there is some great research—I don't have time, but I think we provided this to the committee staff from the Center on the Developing Child at Harvard University. It talks about the importance—of course, we all know the importance of brain development in the first 2 to 3 years, but moms who are depressed are perhaps not interacting with their children in a way, and it may impact even the architecture of their brain development. And, of course, later there are all sorts of negative impacts from that. So many nuances to the importance of mental healthcare for pregnant moms.

Mr. WALDEN. That is a really important point that could easily be overlooked, is that in relationship. Thank you.

Thank you all for your testimony, and we will keep you in our hearts. Thank you.

Ms. ESHOO. The gentleman yields back. Thank you.

I now have the pleasure of recognizing the gentleman from Massachusetts, Mr. Kennedy, for his 5 minutes of questions.

Mr. KENNEDY. Thank you, Madam Chair. Thank you for calling this important hearing. Thank you to all of the witnesses for being here for the work you do every day and for lifting up the voices that need to be heard. It is easy to study the stats to hear some of these stories, to learn about the inequities and implicit bias, to look into the eyes of a spouse, a parent, child, and to talk to a survivor and become, candidly, a bit dejected, to begin to question why we can't in this Nation protect mothers like the rest of the world can, to ask why nearly a thousand American women die from pregnancy and childbirth every year, and why do another 65,000 nearly die or bear those scars for a lifetime?

The tragic truth is that we already know the answer to these questions: a long and pernicious history of racism calcified in ourinstitutions, including our healthcare sector; economic inequality that leaves entire communities relying on unfunded, unprepared hospitals already stretched too thin; and the politically motivated decision by many States to reject Medicaid expansion that leaves thousands of women uninsured less than 2 months after giving birth.

So, to begin with, Ms. Irving, words will never suffice, and there is nothing we can say or do that will make up for the preventable loss of your daughter. Please know that we will carry her story with all of us. In your testimony, you told us about implicit bias training and that it isn't enough, and you are absolutely right. What systematic reforms would you like to see in our healthcare system beyond that mandatory training?

Ms. IRVING. I would really like to see some type of a program/policy standardized—what would you call them—I guess, standardized policies that are tied to either accreditation or funding. That is, I think, the only way you are going to get people to move off the dime. The implicit bias training is great, but you need to have some kind of evaluation on whether or not that is making a difference in the lives of patients, mothers who are coming there. And if it is not, if it is going—if it is causing harm, then they need to be held responsible, whether it is funding cuts, whether it is accreditation that is withheld, or however you want to put it, but there has to be an incentive for folks to do the right thing.

Mr. KENNEDY. Thank you.

Ms. Ranji, nearly half American counties do not have a single practicing OB/GYN, and there are stark divides across access to care within cities like Washington or Boston. Would adding doula services as a covered benefit under Medicaid—as, by the way, a bill introduced by my colleague Ayanna Pressley, the Healthy MOMMIES Act, would do, with increased access to care and reduced rates of preventable maternal deaths or complications?

Ms. RANJI. Thank you for the question. Currently, you raise the issue of doula services. Currently, doula services is covered under in, as far as I know, two States, Oregon as well as Minnesota, under Medicaid. It is a benefit that is not available to many women covered by Medicaid across the country. It is an area that has been of interest in many States. New York is also piloting a program, and several other States have considered recently adding doula services. Doula services are an important—could be an important source of support for pregnant and post partum women. Doula services expanded beyond just labor and delivery. I am not familiar with the research necessarily tying it to rates of maternal mortality or morbidity or the effect of that, but there is a lot of research, particularly the Listening to Mothers Survey, that has looked at women's perceptions around doula care and have found it very useful. And perhaps some of my clinician colleagues here could speak to working with doulas.

Mr. KENNEDY. Thank you, and just very briefly here, question for each witness, if I can. Can any of you tell me how many post partum women die annually from suicides or accidental overdoses?

Dr. NELSON. I can speak to the Texas maternal mortality review. From 2012 to 2015, overdose was the number one cause, and from 2012 to 2015 in Texas, there were 33 suicides.

Mr. KENNEDY. No national figures, though?

Dr. NELSON. I do not have that, no.

Mr. KENNEDY. Nobody? And to be clear, we do not have any idea how many women die in this country after giving birth from suicides or accidental overdoses because it has never been studied, and it is not reported. So we can't address something we don't know to be a crisis if we don't even know how big a crisis that it is, yet I think we can all acknowledge that it certainly is one, Doctor, given the statistics that you indicate. But we also can't wait for years for these studies to take place before we act, and that is why we need to have perinatal mental health providers in these conversations and why we need to have guaranteed Medicaid coverage for a full year after birth.

Grateful to all of you for being here today. Thank you for your attention to a critical health crisis in our country.

I yield back.

Ms. ESHOO. The gentleman yields back, and thank him for his questions.

I gave birth to two children, in 1969 and 1971, which means they are both older than I am now, but when I complained to my doctor post partum after each birth how depressed I felt, I was told that is just the way it is. So I just place that on the table for everyone to think about, and now I would like to recognize the gentleman from Michigan, Mr. Upton, who served as the chairman of our full committee and with special leadership qualities.

Mr. UPTON. Thank you, Madam Chair. I know that we all appreciate today's hearing. I want to do what we can, particularly on a bipartisan basis, to resolve this.

Every one of our districts is different. All of our States are different. My district has a central city of Kalamazoo, hundred-some thousand people and some rural counties as well. In the past, we have had some counties without hospital to help so people literally had to go out of their county that they reside in if they were going to deliver at a hospital, and, obviously, that happens. Michigan has got pretty rural areas, particularly in the UP, and we had pretty high death rate, maternal, in Kalamazoo back in the 1990s. And we worked very closely with HHS and got some special money to grant to really target Kalamazoo to see what we could do to alleviate some of those terrible statistics that are there, which go right along with what you have been saying. Women of color, Hispanics, Medicaid births at our hospitals generally are over 50 percent and have been for some time, whether it be either in an urban setting or maybe a rural hospital as well. And I am—Dr. Nelson, I have heard of Parkland Hospital. I don't know how many hospitals are in Dallas, and it seems like you have done a remarkable job trying to really reach out with the satellites and others.

I guess the question is a little bit of a followup to Chairwoman Eshoo to Dr. Harris. So, when you see these statistics that are out of sorts, bad, things that none of us would accept, what efforts— what collaborative efforts—and I guess, Dr. Howell, I ask you to be part of this since you are with Mount Sinai, so thinking about the hospital situation—what efforts are you taking on yourself to say, "What can we work with?" How do we work with the AMA and others to try and duplicate a success that we have seen—I would call it a success—of what we have seen at Parkland? Maybe if the three of you could chat a little bit about that.

I have got one last question for Ms. Ranji at the end as well, but if you could just expand on that a little bit. Because we see these statistics, what are you going to do? What is happening? Where is the leadership to try and get it done?

Dr. HOWELL. So, in New York, we have had a lot of work around this for the last 4 to 5 years when we recognized that we were doing so poorly as a State and the significant racial and ethnic disparities that existed. So, at the State level, we have had a collaborative across all the States trying to implement some of the AIM bundles, three of those bundles in hospitals across the State. And in New York City, the Department of Health had a lot of efforts trying to work on quality improvement, implicit bias training to do so.

At my own institution, we have done a lot of similar things that Dr. Nelson has mentioned in terms of trying to standardize care, building a culture of safety and equity. We have had implicit bias trainings and required it of our obstetricians, gynecologists. We have had all sorts of different things.

But one other point I would just like to quickly raise is, a lot of the research that I have done has really been looking at New York City hospitals, and part of the story here is some hospitals don't have the resources, have the know-how to be able to implement these bundles and do these things. It takes resources. You need protected time because you need a partnership between physicians and nurses, a physician and nurse leader to champion these efforts. And so, while it is in part healthcare professionals in the way that they treat patients, another big part of this story is the place matters, and where you deliver matters. And the resources, the staffing, some of the basic bread and butter of high-quality, efficient hospitals is just not there, and that is something else we need to be thinking about.

Mr. UPTON. So, just to comment. So all of us here support community health centers, all of us, everyone on this committee. It has been a great bipartisan effort for many, many years. And I know I have been to all of my community health centers. I am going to be meeting with some of my folks from Michigan this afternoon. I am going to follow up with questions based on this hearing. I know that they are very active, and I applaud what they are doing, and we are going to push them hard. And I would just—my remaining time, Dr. Harris, if you can help, particularly in your leadership role now, I think that would be terrific.

My last question, Dr. Ranji, so one of the things that has come up, some States have that 1115 waiver to extend the time beyond 60 days that a woman might be able to be able to get some care under Medicaid. Some States have it, some States don't. A couple of the bills that we are talking about today, in fact, have that coverage, which I think is good. I think it is very good.

What is the impact on the States, because, again, Medicaid is run by the States, so they have to make the application. So what is the reaction of the States going to be if, in fact, we do this thing that I think most of us could support?

Ms. RANJI. Well, Federal legislation would allow uniformity for——

Mr. UPTON. So they wouldn't have to apply for the waiver? They would automatically—if they want do it, they do it.

Ms. RANJI. Right. Allow availability of coverage across the country.

Mr. UPTON. So my time is expired, but let me just say, so how many States you think right away would—how many States have it now, and how many States would say, "Sign us up"?

Ms. RANJI. I can't tell you how many States would say, "Sign us up." I should say Illinois earlier this year did approve that policy and is, in fact, seeking a Federal waiver to secure Federal financing, but again, if it was written into Federal legislation that would allow—that would be uniform across the country.

Mr. UPTON. Thank you, and all my time is expired. I yield back.

Ms. ESHOO. I thank the gentleman, and he yields back. It is now a pleasure to recognize the author of the MOMMA's Act, Congresswoman Robin Kelly, for her 5 minutes of questioning.

Ms. KELLY. Thank you, Madam Chair. Again, good morning, and thank you all for being here to share your expertise, your insights, your experiences surrounding this critical issue of maternal health.

Ms. Irving, thank you so very much. It can't be easy, but I just want to thank you over and over again.

And Dr. Harris, thanks for all of your support. We could not have written the bill without the expertise and support of the AMA, ACOG. We really appreciate everybody.

In recent years, as you have heard today, the number of American moms dying from pregnancy and childbirth has climbed drastically while globally the rate has declined. New American moms are twice as likely to die today than in 1985, and it is very scary to me. My husband and I have four children between us, three girls, only one has had a baby yet, and it is interesting or scary to think that it was safer for me to have a baby than my next two daughters, who I think are going to give me grandchildren.

After almost 35 years—never know—the situation should be getting better, not worse. As with nearly all health disparities, women of color, especially Black and Native American moms, as we have heard, bear the burden of this crisis and continue to die at much higher rates. In some places that disparity grows even larger, such as my State of Illinois. One of these mothers was Kira Johnson, the daughter-in-law of TV's Judge Glenda Hatchett. Kira raced cars, flew planes, spoke five languages. She died soon after giving birth to her second son, Langston.

While each death is tragic, the reality of the situation foretells more tragedy. According to ACOG's research, more than half of all maternal deaths are preventable. In Illinois, it said 75 percent of them are. It is clear that we can and must do more to protect mothers' lives. Conditions like hemorrhaging and preeclampsia can and should be prevented. We must understand the need to listen to women and their health concerns. Just last month, I held a field inquiry in Chicago on maternal mortality. Over and over again I heard the same problem: Women are not being listened to, especially women of color.

The hard truth is that no law can legislate away racism. No laws can change the hearts and minds of people who operate on, deliver care to, or just look at people of color from the lens of unconscious bias. But our laws can change how care is delivered within our hospitals by equipping our providers with standardized emergency obstetrical protocols. Our laws can support providers across their training continuum with tools that help them become more reflexive about how their own biases play out in the care they provide to women of color. Our laws can extend care to mothers who are Medicaid beneficiaries throughout the entire post partum period. Our laws can support full collection of consistent data about who dies on the way to motherhood and why.

Knowing this, I introduce the MOMMA Act, which builds on recent successes and data standardization and protocol development to prevent deaths and also establishes a National Maternity Mortality Review Committee, expands Medicaid coverage for new moms to a full year, and seeks to address the racial disparities in maternal mortality.

As chairwoman of the Congressional Black Caucus Health Braintrust and cochair of the Congressional Caucus on Black Women and Girls, a prime importance to me is equitable healthcare access and delivery and the healthcare system's impact on those who, before the ACA, historically experienced barriers to care, whether due to cost, geographic isolation, insurance coverage, and especially due to forms of exclusion, such as race and the residuals of racism.

The time has come for action. We have already lost too many mothers to this crisis, and there are too many kids growing up without mothers because of preventable maternal deaths, and I think that is something this committee needs to look at: How long do we postpone? How long do we keep talking about this as mothers continue to die? It is incumbent upon us to honor their lives with action, action that will prevent another mother from need- lessly dying or another family from being torn apart. We see the inequity. We are calling it out, and we are here to eliminate it.

I would also like to enter into the record a statement from Stacey Stewart, president and CEO of March of Dimes, and from Advocate Aurora Health. Thank you, again.

And I yield back.

Ms. ESHOO. The gentlewoman yields back.

It is a pleasure to recognize the gentleman from Illinois, Mr. Shimkus. I didn't like the news that went out with your name attached to it, but we have, let's see, 16 months left to work with you, so take it away. You are recognized for 5 minutes.

Mr. SHIMKUS. Thank you, Madam Chairman. I appreciate that. I like the news. My wife likes the news. So I have been on the ballot since 1988 for every 2 years. So it is time to not be on the ballot. So thank you for those kind words, and we will get the chance to work together more.

Ms. Irving, we grieve with your loss. Thank you for being here.

I am encouraged that this committee is continuing its efforts to understand and address underlying causes of our Nation's maternal mortality challenges. As we have mentioned a couple times today, the President signed H.R. 1318, which is Preventing Maternal Deaths by our colleagues Herrera Beutler and Diana DeGette from the full committee. This legislation enhanced Federal efforts to support State Maternal Mortality Review Committees to improve data collection. I am going to talk about why that is important. I am glad my colleague, Congresswoman Kelly, is here from Illinois because these are most recent stats based upon having started to gather more and better information.

In fact, in October last year, October 2018, Illinois Department of Public Health released its first maternal morbidity and mortality report, which found that, during 2014 and 2016, there were 231 pregnancy-associated deaths, with the pregnancy-associated mortality ratio being highest for women living in rural counties and in the city of Chicago, 60 to 56, respectively. You know, obviously, we mourn every death, and one is too high, but that is just the stats that now we can now dig into and figure out what is going on.

Understanding that this issue affects a broad and diverse population, it is important to make sure any Federal legislation considers the unique needs of States and the localities as opposed to a one-size-fits-all solution. For example, Illinois has a waiver to cover mothers up to 200 percent of the Federal poverty limit. And the ACA exchange coverage begins at 100 percent of the Federal poverty limit, and this is due—Ms. Ranji, are you concerned that additional Federal legislation affecting patients at these income levels could complicate State efforts, or worse, end up punishing States for having made such investments by simply bolstering States and dedicating their resources elsewhere?

Ms. RANJI. Thank you. You know, the Federal legislation or a Federal—as I said before, would add a uniformity to the policy and make it——

Mr. SHIMKUS. Yes, that is exactly why I am asking the question, because if the State of Illinois is better than the Federal legislation, then you are penalizing Illinois for what it is trying to do internally to address these concerns.

Ms. RANJI. Well, States would still retain the option and flexibility that they have now——

Mr. SHIMKUS. We have to make sure that that is available in the legislation. We can't assume that that is going to be the way the legislation comes out. We have to—that is part of the package.

Ms. RANJI. Certainly that would have to be part of the terms if that was——

Mr. SHIMKUS. Right, and that is our concern.

Ms. RANJI. I would just add that, you know, I think what we have talked about today is that coverage is one part of this whole conversation, and that is one area that States have been making efforts in, as has been discussed. You know, States as well as providers and you alluded to differences in provider availability in different regions. Provider States all have a role in this.

Mr. SHIMKUS. And States follow the money, just like anybody else, and so the FMAP does drive decisions by States, and I think we have to understand that and make sure that these kind of contradictory, sometimes competing messages are direct into the way in which we want them to perform.

Let me go to Dr. Howell real quick. In your testimony, you mentioned specific elements of legislation to combat maternal mortality, specifically those elements pertaining to data collection and support for implicit bias training for health professionals.

As a member of the Communications and Technology Subcommittee, we discuss the potential benefits of using Big Data and machine learning, algorithms and such, but also note that the data we often rely upon to inform decisions is inherently biased. You know, that old garbage-in/garbage-out debate that we have all the time. I am curious if you or others on the panel could expand on or offer examples of effective ways to limit the negative impact this bias has on patient care.

Dr. HOWELL. I think you bring up a really good point about data quality, and I want to echo that if you just use vital statistics alone to figure out the maternal deaths, you are going to miss a lot of the mental health and the—you know, the late deaths because it was not a reliable system. The pregnancy check box, which was introduced in 2003, was introduced differently across all the different States, and so, again, you are not dealing with apples-to-apples comparisons.

That is why Maternal Mortality Review Committees are so essential, because we are really collecting data from multiple sources on each death. So we really understand what is the underlying cause, what were the contributing factors. And then now we have the CDC trying to have the MMWR program, which is surveillance, 33 States are part of it, to actually collect this information from the MMRCs so that there is now a national understanding of what is going on. We need to get that all the way up to 50 States, but that is the way to have better quality data around maternal deaths.

Mr. SHIMKUS. Thank you, Chairman.

Ms. ESHOO. I thank the gentleman. Excellent questions and highly instructive answers.

I now would like to recognize Dr. Ruiz from California for his 5 minutes of questioning.

Mr. RUIZ. Thank you. While it is stating the obvious, I would be remiss not to say that is abhorrent that the United States of America is one of only three countries where maternal mortality is on the rise, along with Afghanistan and Sudan, and it is unacceptable that 60 percent of pregnancy-related deaths are actually preventable. Even worse is the fact that the CDC found that Black women were three to four times more likely to die from a pregnancy-related cause than White women. This is one of the reasons that I have been working on legislation to address health disparities in women's health equity. The Women's Health Equity Act will create a centralized, independent interagency council in the executive branch to facilitate coordination between Federal agencies on women's health issues.

The problem is that you have different agencies working in silos, and they are not communicating being efficient in what they are doing, and they are not opening up the resources as well as they could be with efficiency between all the different governmental agencies addressing this issue. This will enhance coordination and communication between the agencies when addressing women's health issues and health disparities.

The interagency council would focus on collecting and analyzing programs currently in place and give recommendations on how to better coordinate their efforts. The council would also be responsible for monitoring, evaluating, and providing recommendations to address women's health equity and health disparities. It would also streamline programs and activities within Federal agencies that are working towards the same goals.

Dr. Harris, do you agree that the lack of coordination on the Federal level is hampering efforts to truly address health disparities?

Dr. HARRIS. Well, what I would say is you bring up a great point about the importance of getting out of our silos, and interagency coordinating councils are a proven method to do that in other disease and public health crises. And so I would say that any opportunity where folks get out of their silos and work together and agencies coordinate their efforts better is a step in the right direction. I would say, from the AMA's standpoint, we would hope that there would be physician input into any of that agency coordination.

Mr. RUIZ. Well, just to let you know, AMA has been very active in contributing their input into this legislation. Dr. Howell, what are your thoughts on that?

Dr. HOWELL. I agree with what Dr. Harris said, that, you know, us working together, collaborating, and sort of figuring out the next steps, having the voices of many parties, including physicians, in this discussion is really important.

Mr. RUIZ. Excellent. So, you know, I grew up in a farmworker community where residents were largely poor, with English as a second language. And as a kid growing up and later as a doctor who practiced medicine there, I saw firsthand how critical cultural competence is to delivering effective, high-quality care, and it is not just understanding terms from a different culture; it is a cultural sensitivity where you can understand the practice of truly trying to understand a person's background in order to provide the best therapy and increase compliance and increase success of those recommendations. The Giving Voice to Mothers study released this summer surveyed women in the United States in an effort to learn more about mistreatment during birth and found that 17.3 percent of women experience one or more types of mistreatment, including but not limited to privacy violations, being shouted at or scolded by healthcare providers, or having treatment withheld.

Women of color were more likely to report an experience of mistreatment, with 33 percent of indigenous women, 25 percent of Hispanic women, 22 percent of Black women reporting an experience of, at least, one form of mistreatment. We have heard on our panel today about at least one terrible example of what can happen when a patient doesn't receive the care she is saying that she needs. These experiences further perpetuate mistrust in healthcare systems and influence women's desires to access care.

Dr. Harris, in your experience, how can we imbed improving the experience of care in efforts to improve the quality of care?

Dr. HARRIS. Another important topic, and thanks to the committee members for raising this. There is this whole universe of how we understand and work with others, so you mentioned two terms: cultural competency, cultural sensitivity. I even use the term cultural humility. So we have to appreciate all of these issues in the context. Several of the committee members have mentioned implicit bias, unconscious bias, another part of that universe.

What we know is all of us have unconscious and implicit biases and how should we—but unfortunately there is no gold standard at this point, and one of the things that AMA wants to do is look at not necessarily developing a gold standard, but what might be the components of a great program to get it all.

Mr. RUIZ. I would love to work with you on that. Just in closing, Chairwoman, we can't look at maternal mortality disparities if we don't look at the overall health disparities in our system, because a pregnant woman doesn't exist only when she is pregnant, right? So you have to look at her health and her experience with her health, because that is one of the leading factors of health outcome, is her health prior to being pregnant. And just recently, for example, as an example of how we have these inherent biases, September 6th, JAMA Open Network published an article that showed that, out of over 800,000 women and men under Medicare, they found that Black and Hispanic women were diverted from EMS, from the emergency department designated for them, took a longer trip to send them to the safety net hospital elsewhere——

Ms. ESHOO. Thank you, Doctor, your time has expired.

Mr. RUIZ [continuing]. Which, you know, has dire consequences.

Ms. ESHOO. The gentleman yields back.

I would like to recognize Mr. Guthrie of Kentucky for his 5 minutes of questioning.

Mr. GUTHRIE. Thank you, Madam Chair. I appreciate it very much.

And thanks, Ms. Irving, for telling your story. We had a hearing on this for some bills that we did pass and signed into law. There was a husband in your seat, and he was talking about his wife, and he made the same arguments that you made. He said his wife— I think it was either a business consultant or private equity. His wife I think was a Ph.D., athlete, UCLA, if I remember—delivered at UCLA Hospital—and then had complications and went back. I don't know how many days it was. It was several days, and she was just dismissed with "you are exaggerating" or whatever.

And so what we are saying here—I know we are implicit bias, cultural bias, and we are using those terms, and they are absolutely accurate. But what we are saying is—you said it wasn't lack of education, it wasn't lack of insurance, it wasn't lack of access. I think Dr. Howell said that, if you control for education, insured, African-American women or women of color are treated different than less educated and within coverage for Whites, so what we are saying is, African-American women or women of color are showing up in front of healthcare professionals, and healthcare professionals are treating them differently. We need to do—if it is commission, if it is the agencies, if it is cross-referencing that we can do in Washington, we need to do that to make sure that this is taken care of.

Dr. Harris, you are the only one here representing healthcare profession. What is going on? Is the AMA trying to address this internally? I know we are here in Washington trying to address it, but we know there is a problem. We know it is lack of—there is bias, and what do you think it is, and what is AMA trying to do to address that?

Dr. HARRIS. I think we are trying to find the answers to those questions, and as I mentioned earlier with our new work and, by the way, this is building upon work for many years that the AMA, our commission to end health disparities—again, I just talked to Dr. Aletha Maybank this morning, and we talked about the possibilities. Now we are just getting our center up and running, but this is one of the areas where we want to focus on, we want to understand why, and then what are the solutions that physicians can implement.

Of course, as you know, I am a psychiatrist by training, so I am trained to listen maybe in a different way, but, as I said in my testimony, for whatever reason, many of them are racism, discrimination, implicit/unconscious biases, women are not being heard, particularly African-American women are not being heard. So the fact that we are talking about that is the first step, and I know at the AMA that we are going to move forward and try to find solutions and spread that to the medical community. Of course, our partners at ACOG are here, and we will work closely with them.

Mr. GUTHRIE. I want to correct the record. I think she was a UCLA athlete. She was—Cedars-Sinai was the hospital. So I want to make sure I have that corrected, the previous witness, it was her—so Parkland, though, you have 90 percent Medicaid, and you have this extensive program, and so I think what Dr. Howell said, in New York City, you have hospitals—and I understand that. It is absolutely a fact: You have hospitals that have better outcomes, and hospitals, others. And you are saying it is more women of color go to their—they are kind of divided up in where they go to get their service. But what I don't understand—getting back to the healthcare professionals, why aren't they just showing up—are they showing up at your hospital, Dr. Nelson, saying, "What are you doing? How can we replicate it and move forward?"

It looks like we are here doing a mandate from Congress, and if Congress needs to mandate it, we need to mandate it. But it seems like within the healthcare profession, they would be flooding to what you are doing, or in New York, some of the hospitals go into the hospitals having better outcomes, and just, what are you doing different? Because when we did the bill last year, we found that, in high-risk pregnancy, some hospitals didn't even have high-risk kits available when they were doing high-risk deliveries, just the basic stuff. And it is hard for us to fix—when they are not even doing the basic stuff—from Washington.

So, Dr. Nelson or Dr. Howell, whoever wants to talk about that, it is disturbing that the healthcare profession is not addressing this better than they are? Not saying you are not.

Dr. NELSON. Well, I think, to speak first, you are absolutely correct and that the first issue that Dr. Harris mentioned is we have to recognize we have a problem, and collectively we have to agree that we have a problem and this includes issues within high-resource settings and low-resource settings. And one of the steps forward that I am proud of is the regionalization of care that we have provided in Texas, and that is not to say we are closing hospitals in rural communities. We support that. It is really to identify women with prenatal care that have a high-risk condition, identify their needs, and get them to a facility that has resources——

Mr. GUTHRIE. I understand what you are doing, but are other hospitals flocking to you from other cities and trying to understand what you are doing and replicate it?

Dr. NELSON. That model is one of the opportunities, and it dovetails AIM, and it dovetails the California initiative. These are standardized practices that we can all collectively agree to in the medical community to say——

Mr. GUTHRIE. Because you being 90 percent Medicaid, you are not at the top of the chain in terms of financing?

Dr. NELSON. But the principles——

Mr. GUTHRIE. It can be replicated.

Dr. NELSON. The principles of care are the same, and that is emergent response to emergent conditions, and time is key.

Mr. GUTHRIE. Right. Thank you.

My time has expired, and I yield back.

Ms. ESHOO. I thank the gentleman, and he yields back.

Pleasure to recognize the gentleman from North Carolina, Mr. Butterfield, for his 5 minutes of questioning.

Mr. BUTTERFIELD. Thank you very much, Madam Chair.

Thank you to all of the witnesses for your testimony today.

Let me begin with you, Ms. Ranji. Thank you for coming today, and thank you for your words.

As you pointed out in your testimony, research shows that health coverage before, during, and after pregnancy is important to support healthy pregnancies and positive outcomes. Medicaid, that favorite word that we all talk about, Medicaid, I wish it was available in every State in the Union with respect to its expansion, but Medicaid is a vital program for many families in my district and all of our districts. I am glad the committee is looking at bills that would extend Medicaid eligibility for pregnant women to 1 year post partum. A maternal-fetal medicine specialist at Duke University in my district shared with my staff recently that extending Medicaid coverage to 1 year post partum would be life-altering and potentially lifesaving for her patients, many of whom have not had regular care until finding out that they were pregnant. Extending Medicaid coverage for new moms is a vital step to ensure these women can continue to be cornerstones of our families.

Ms. Ranji, simply put, healthy moms lead to healthy babies. Is that an overstatement?

Ms. RANJI. There are certainly a lot of research that connects the health of moms with the health of their children and as well as coverage that access to coverage for moms also connects to access to coverage for children.

Mr. BUTTERFIELD. Could you describe for me the long-term positive benefits that 1-year post partum Medicaid coverage would have on moms and their children?

Ms. RANJI. Well, like I said, in several States now, women do lose coverage after 2 months, and so extending to 1 year would provide access—seamless access so that women could continue to see the same providers and follow up on many of the issues that—clinical issues that my colleagues have talked about today. Cardiac-related health, maternal mental health, and again, coverage provides access to a provider and being able to continue and follow up on all of those issues that, again, that we know don't resolve within 2 months usually.

Mr. BUTTERFIELD. Thank you. Many of the witnesses, Madam Chair, today have commented on the disgraceful and disturbing fact that African-American women are three to four times more likely to die from a pregnancy-related cause than their counterparts. Black women are also more likely to have complicating conditions, like uterine fibroids and hypertension, among others, which can cause severe maternal morbidity and have potentially life-threatening and lifelong consequences.

There have been countless stories of women dying or becoming ill because their symptoms were ignored or treatments were not offered. What should we do—and let's try you, Dr. Howell, on this if we can. I just looked at your bio. It looks like you are well suited to handle this. What should we do to educate providers about conitions like these that disproportionately impact women of color and how to identify and treat them?

Dr. HOWELL. So, again, a very important point about risk status for women when they enter our healthcare system, antenatally as well as on labor and delivery. So risk stratification is an important part, and it is something that we use also in our AIM bundles to understand who is most at risk and to make sure those people are getting what they need and when they need it. So I think in addition to just pure clinical care and thinking about the best way to optimize care for individual patients, we also need to think about some of these other issues around communication strategies, decsionmaking, shared decisionmaking, listening to patients to better understand their story, and recognizing and teaching healthcare providers that there is a bias not to listen to women in general, which we have heard in our own focus groups across race and ethnicity, but it is more pronounced for women of color. So I think those are some of the steps that we need to take.

Mr. BUTTERFIELD. Thank you. Thank you very much.

Madam Chair, since Dr. Ruiz went over 1 minute, I will go under 1 minute, and maybe we can cancel each other out. Thank you.

I yield back.

Ms. ESHOO. I always knew you were a good man, always. Mr. BUTTERFIELD. Yes. He is my friend.

Ms. ESHOO. Yes. Well, you are both my friends.

The gentleman yields back, and now it is a pleasure to recognize the gentleman from Virginia, Mr. Griffith, for his 5 minutes of questioning.

Mr. GRIFFITH. Thank you very much, Madam Chair.

And clearly somebody said it earlier, we have to identify that we have a problem, and clearly that has been identified, and we heard the testimony last year of Mr. Johnson. We heard your testimony today, Ms. Irving, and those losses where the mothers were just—they just weren't paid attention to. And that clearly is a concern.

But I was struck, Dr. Howell, by one paragraph in your testimony, and I am going to repeat that paragraph because I think it is helpful, and then I am going to ask you a question.

Quoting your testimony: "Research by our team and others has shown that, for a variety of reasons, Black women tend to deliver in a specific set of hospitals, and those hospitals have worse outcomes for both Black and White moms regardless of patient risk factors. This is true in the United States overall where three quarters of all Black women deliver in a specific set of hospitals while less than one-fifth of White women deliver in those same hospitals. Both Black and White women have worse outcomes in those hospitals. In New York City, a woman's risk of having a life-threatening complication in one hospital can be six or seven times higher than in another hospital. Black and Latino mothers are more likely to deliver in hospitals with worse outcomes. In fact, differences in delivery hospital explain nearly one-half of the Black/White disparity and one-third of the Latina/White disparity in severe maternal morbidity."

So here is my question, with their choosing a specific set of hospitals, how do we fix those hospitals, and should we have some way of getting the information out if we can't fix those hospitals that these hospitals are far more dangerous? Doesn't solve all the problems, but your testimony indicates that one-half of the disparity is because of specific hospitals. Nothing else that we are doing here at the Federal level or the State level, but the specific hospitals they are choosing? How do we fix them?

Dr. HOWELL. So I think what is interesting about the work we have done in New York City is that it is not the traditional hospital characteristics, so it is not percent Medicaid. The median percent Medicaid in New York City hospitals is like 80 percent, so we are talking about a highly—60 percent of our deliveries are covered by Medicaid. So it is not volume. It is much more—we don't really understand why there is such a variation, other than having to go in and talk to hospitals, and that is what our research team is doing. So we are going into hospitals who have low rates and hospitals that have high rates to try to understand what the differences are. And what we are finding is that it is things like staffing. It is things like culture—the culture of the institution and the way that they treat adverse events. It is things like communication and the emphasis. It is quality and safety on labor and deliveries and the use of evidence-based practices, but it is also whether there is any focus on equity and diversity and how they think about it.

So more work needs to be done to understand these variations, especially in large urban centers where you have high volume, but that is one key, important piece because, in certain hospitals, regardless of what you look like, your risk is higher to have one of these severe complications, and that is an important part of the story we are talking about today.

Mr. GRIFFITH. And so, while we look at these bills—and I think this was the same point that Mr. Guthrie was making just a minute or two ago, and he and I hadn't talked about what we were going to discuss, but he started hitting some of that same testimony.

While we are working on this legislation, that is an area we need to focus on. And right now, while there is some studies in these bills, I don't think the bills are really focused on that area, and maybe we need to give some more money to the NIH to focus in on that so that we can figure out what the problem is. Maybe they need to be doing what Dr. Nelson is doing in Texas, but maybe that doesn't work in New York City because what works in Texas might not work in New York City, but we still need to figure out, if that is half of the problem, then it ought to be addressed in some of our bills as more than just a casual line in a study.

Would you not agree, Dr. Howell?

Dr. HOWELL. I think that it is one important part of something that needs to be addressed. So, yes, I do agree that it is one more element that we need to look at and a very important one in New York City.

Mr. GRIFFITH. And, Dr. Nelson, you would be more than happy to talk with anybody who wants to figure what you are doing right.

Is that correct?

Dr. NELSON. Yes, sir.

Mr. GRIFFITH. And you would be willing to work with these hospitals that in the testimony are just listed as—and I am not asking for names today—a specific set.

Dr. Howell, real quick. I just have a few seconds left. Should we identify for the public those specific set of hospitals where your risk is higher?

Dr. HOWELL. So I think that, Dr. Nelson, I think we both agree that measurement is a key. Quality measures that are important and that women can use to help choose hospitals I think is an important measure, but we have to be very careful about the development of appropriate risk-adjusted quality measures so we do not penalize the hospitals that take care of the sickest and the hardest cases, and I think that is a really important part of doing really well-done, quality measure development in maternal health that focuses on both the patients—patient-centered, thinking about experience—as well as on disparities.

Mr. GRIFFITH. Thank you.

I am out of time. If the chairlady would like to give you time, Dr. Nelson, she can. But I am out.

I have to yield back.

Ms. ESHOO. Well, the gentleman yields back, but I think that his question to you is really very, very important. All of the collection of the data is essential so that you have something that is foundational, but we already know where women of color deliver and die. So there has to be—I think there needs to be a red-light- and-siren team that gets into these hospitals, and I also think that we should consider the accreditation of that hospital based on the morbidity rates.

So I don't know if that is what the—where the gentleman was going, but it certainly is my sentiment.

Mr. BURGESS. Would Dr. Nelson respond to that?

Ms. ESHOO. Certainly.

Dr. NELSON. So one of the comments of sharing, in all seriousness, sharing our experiences and what we do as practices is actually part of the outreach and one of the things that we actually stress as part of the regionalization of care. We actually have an outreach team going to lower-level facilities to talk about emergent response to hypertension and labor management. So that actually is one of the existing programs we currently are using right now.

Ms. ESHOO. I mean, I don't know if El Camino Hospital in Mountain View, California, knows what you are doing. And I am not saying that they have a problem. It is marvelous what you are doing, but this needs to be under a national umbrella, and I don't think anyone is arguing with that.

It is a pleasure to recognize the gentlewoman from California, Ms. Barraga´ n, for her 5 minutes of questioning.

Ms. BARRAGÁN. Thank you, Madam Chairwoman.

And thank you all for being here today, for sharing your stories. The statistics are quite tragic, completely unacceptable in a country like ours.

I first learned about the issue of racial health disparities when I was in the White House. I was an intern, and the New England Journal of Medicine came out with a study. It showed that they had sent an African-American woman, a White woman, a Latina woman to similar doctors, same doctors, complaining of the same symptoms, and they were all treated differently, and that is when I first learned of it.

And I think one of the points made by my colleague Dr. Ruiz is critically important. It is certainly overall health and making sure we are all getting access to equal care, but that we are being listened to.

And, Ms. Irving, I want to thank you for coming and sharing your story of your daughter, and the testimony that you provided is something that we all needed to hear. And that is why I am glad we are having this hearing today to kind of look at these bills and see what can be done.

It sounds to me there is not one fix. It sounds like there is going to be a series of things that need to be done to be fixed, to fix this issue and to make this wrong right.

And so I thank you all for coming.

Dr. Howell, two of the bills that we are being presented with and are looking at are H.R. 1898, the MOMMA's bill that my colleague Ms. Kelly has, and H.R. 2902, which is a bill that my colleague Alma Adams has. Have you had a chance to look at those bills? I would like to know if you believe those bills might help eliminate some of the implicit bias among the medical professionals.

Dr. HOWELL. So I did get a chance to look at those bills. I don't have my notes. Could you just repeat the names of the two you wanted me to talk about real quickly?

Ms. BARRAGÁN. Sure. The MOMMA's Act.

Dr. HOWELL. Yes.

Ms. BARRAGÁN. And the other one is the Maternal Care Access and Reducing Emergencies Act.

Dr. HOWELL. Got it. So, yes, I did have chance to look at all of the bills, which, again, I think there are elements that are key for this issue.

The MOMMA'S Act, authorizing the AIM program, which I told you is the key to having standardized care practices implemented in hospitals and health systems across the United States currently reaching 27 States, so potential to reach more than 50 percent of all U.S. births, very important. We need to authorize that.

Second, Perinatal Quality Collaboratives, Maternal and Infant Health Quality Collaboratives are so important as a tool to improve quality of care. And these are partnerships with hospitals and health systems and Department of Health.

As you have heard from my colleague, very important to extend Medicaid for 12 months post partum. You know, there are so many cases of women who have gestational diabetes. They go on to have a risk. They are seven times more likely to have type 2 diabetes, but if we don't capture them in that post partum period, they could go on and be much sicker the next time they get pregnant, as well as cardiovascular complications that are so important.

Then, finally, the Regional Centers of Excellence to address implicit bias and culturally competent care, which we have had a discussion about, which I think is a really important piece, again, I would expand it to think about patient-centered communication, shared communication. It is not just bias. That is the problem. But we are not doing a good enough listening to our patients, communicating with our patients, and understanding their perspectives. So having centers of excellence that really focus more broadly with a focus on explicit and implicit bias, I think, are important.

And I think that the Maternal CARE Act has very similar themes to it. The Maternal CARE Act, though, does talk a fair amount about care coordination and its importance to target social determinants of health, which I think is an important piece. It calls for a medical home demonstration project, which I think is of interest.

My one thought I would just share is that CMMI Innovation project looked at group prenatal care versus birth centers, which is predominantly midwifery care, versus maternity home care for prenatal services to see if we could lower adverse birth outcomes, lower costs, and improve satisfaction. And the other two models performed better than the maternity home model.

So that is evidence that I think we have to include in these discussions. There is no question that care coordination in general seems to really do a good job targeting disparities, and it may need to be a piece, but we need more evidence to make sure, because this early evidence is not telling us it may be the best step forward.

Ms. BARRAGA´ N. Thank you, Dr. Howell.

I also want to mention I think another component is making sure that we get more people of color into the medical profession that are there to listen, that are there to understand. I am proud to have Charles Drew University Medical School in my district, which is a historically Black graduate institute that is a district that is 88 percent Latino/African American, that is bringing more and more people into the fold, into these professions and certainly, if I had more time, would ask about your opinion, but I wanted to certainly say that I think this is another angle we can certainly improve in as well.

Thank you very much, and I yield back.

Ms. ESHOO. The gentlewoman yields back.

It is a pleasure to recognize the gentleman from Florida, Mr. Bilirakis, for his 5 minutes of questions.

Mr. BILIRAKIS. Thank you, Madam Chair. I appreciate it so much.

And thank you to the witnesses here who are testifying. Very informative.

Dr. Howell, we can't solve what we don't understand. That is why, last Congress, this committee passed bipartisan legislation, the Preventing Maternal Deaths Act, which provides funding through the CDC for States and other entities to develop Maternal Mortality Review Committees so we can start collectively understanding and reducing our rate of maternal mortality.

CDC recently announced it is funding the first round. It is funding the first round of grants to support 25 States, their efforts to combat maternal mortality through the creation of Maternal Mortality Review Committees. As States prepare their implementation efforts, what should this committee be paying the most attention to?

Dr. HOWELL. Well, I think it is wonderful that the CDC is now sponsoring 25 perinatal quality collaboratives. I think the data is at a key point.

I also want to say one thing, though. You are absolutely right. What we don't understand, we can't really address, but there are models of success. We have heard a lot about Parkland today. If we look at California Collaborative and what they have done, by using Maternal Mortality Review Committees, gathering the information around deaths, then using that information to drive quality improvement. And they have done a number of the bundles, the same bundles we are talking about for AIM. They started—hemorrhage, hypertension, venous thromboembolic disease—and they have actually lowered deaths in hospitals that adopted these bundles by, like, 21 percent for the hemorrhage-related deaths and their mortality rate, while the rest of the United States has been going up, theirs has been going down. So we have evidence that, when we tie data to quality and improvement, we can really make a difference.

The important lesson about California, though, is—an additionally important lesson—is that their disparities, however, did not decrease. So they lowered mortality for White women and they lowered it for Black women, but that gap is still there. And now they are trying to target a lot of the things that the rest of us are trying to target around health equity, combining quality improvement, what the data tells us with cultural humility, and sort of trying to understand communities, getting them involved to help tackle this problem, which is something that the AIM bundle also tries to do. The ACOG partners with community organizations to get their input about how best we implement these bundles not only in hospitals and health systems, but we get communities on board as well.

Mr. BILIRAKIS. Thank you.

Are there concerns within the research community regarding the integrity of the data being collected in States, and if so, what are those concerns, and how might they be addressed? Are there any concerns with regard to the integrity of the data?

Dr. HOWELL. Well, there are certainly concerns with the use of what I had mentioned about if you only base maternal mortality rates on vital statistics data only that you are only getting a slice of the picture, and it is not a great way of monitoring our trends across the Nation. The CDC now uses vital stats. It combines it with State discharge abstract data, which gives a better estimate, but still the best estimates are the data from the Maternal Mortality Review Committees that actually get multiple sources of data to figure out how this death occurred, what were the contributing causes, and then feeding that back up to the CDC through their MMWR program is probably the best way for us to get data on this that we can use for improvement.

Mr. BILIRAKIS. Very good.

Thank you. Last week, the CDC released a report titled "Racial and Ethnic Disparity in Pregnancy-Related Deaths." In the report, CDC suggested that steps still need to be taken in order to better integrate care delivery between hospital and pre- and postcare services for mothers and their newborns, as well as better management of high-risk patients.

How might this committee consider addressing these specific challenges highlighted by the report? And can you highlight any States or entities that can be looked at as models—again, best practices in these areas?

Dr. NELSON. So I think that I would echo. Much of what Dr. Howell just mentioned, I think, is reflective in that effort. California has been a model for a lot of the programs, but the same principles are true within the AIM domain. Parkland Hospital publishes *Williams Obstetrics* as a textbook. It is the most popular textbook worldwide. We have 17 authors on our faculty, including myself, and these principles are the same. The important part of this is disseminating that level of scholarship and information to the community centers, to the communities at large, and the providers in those communities.

Mr. BILIRAKIS. Well, thank you very much.

And I yield back, Madam Chair. Thank you.

Ms. ESHOO. The gentleman yields back.

It is a pleasure to recognize the gentlewoman from Florida, Congresswoman Castor, for her 5 minutes of questioning.

Ms. CASTOR. Well, thank you.

And, Chairwoman Eshoo, I want to thank you very much for organizing this hearing here today on the maternal health crisis in America.

It is good to see so much engagement by the committee this morning, right, our first committee meeting back after the district work period.

First off, I want to say I am really proud to be a cosponsor of Representative Kelly's MOMMA's Act. And I am so glad that she joined the committee this year. She is a champion on this issue, and her voice is vital to this discussion, and it is needed. It is just horrendous what is happening with disparities when it comes to maternal health in the United States of America.

And I want to thank the witnesses for being here and for providing your expertise. Already I have seen Members making long lists of how we can improve the bills that are before us today.

Ms. Irving, I thank you very much for sharing the story of your daughter. You are very brave to do so, and I know she would be very proud to know that you are carrying on her work.

I am also grateful to the advocates across America who engage every single day, whether it is the March of Dimes or it is the American College of Obstetricians and Gynecologists or Every Mother Counts, the folks in the trenches, making sure that—whether they might be Healthy Start—making sure that women and families have every opportunity to have healthy children.

In the Tampa Bay area, I am very fortunate. We have a terrific Healthy Start REACHUP initiative led by Lo Berry. They are one of the national leaders. But what they tell me is, while they have years of experience and they are making progress, they are not able to reach everyone. We are still not able, after so many years, to ensure that women of childbearing age get the services, get the support that they need. I mean, in America, it is so disjointed, Medicaid and maybe private health insurance and maybe you are uninsured and you are trying to find a community health center, but that community health center doesn't provide care. It is still not enough.

And I was really taken by the comments of Dr. Ruiz and Representative Butterfield, who highlighted this really is a continuum of care that is in crisis, and add on top of it the disparities, the racism that continues, the social stigma probably in many different groups. We have got to do so much more. So I will look forward to as we get into the markups on these bills how we can really tackle this continuum of care.

I am also fortunate, back in Tampa, we are home to the University of South Florida. Dr. Judette Louis is the chair of the College of Medicine's Obstetrics and Gynecology Department. She shared, again, the sobering statistics. In Florida, Black women are nearly three times more likely to die from pregnancy-related causes than White women. She said that, yes, the Maternal Mortality Review Committees and the perinatal quality collaboratives are helping, but so much needs to be done.

I want to start my questions with Ms. Irving. You have listened. These folks are very smart. Members of Congress have had some insightful questions. What would your daughter want to highlight after listening to everyone here today? What would your daughter say, "Boy, that is absolutely right"? What would she have wanted to highlight to this?

Ms. IRVING. I wish I knew. My daughter was a brilliant person. I think the most, what she might say or start off saying is, this is not a new phenomenon. This has been going on for decades. Why can't we get it right? There are things that can be done but are not being done. I think she would probably say that behind every one of these statistics, there is a woman who is loved, who is missed. And look at the domino effect. Look at the families. Look at the children that are suffering because we can't get it right.

She would want us to look at making sure that there are the standard care policies and procedures in place, and there is some accountability behind it so that we can make sure that folks are being listened to.

I listened to all of your talk and things about people come in, and it is the hospitals, and there are certain hospitals where you can't go or where you won't get the same amount of care. That wasn't the case for Shalon. The case was that she wasn't heard. She came in. She presented with the symptoms. It wasn't that she was making it up. She came in with swollen legs. She wasn't voiding. She was gaining weight. She gained 7 pounds in one week, and she was there three times that week. Her blood pressure was off the chart. She was not only not listened to, she wasn't—her symptoms were not addressed. She was there. She was in a very, very good hospital. She had great doctors in that hospital. She had gold-plated insurance. She was not an ignorant woman. She knew what was wrong, and she kept saying it: "I don't feel well. This is not—this is not me. There is something going on here."

But she was dismissed with the "Oh, it is fine. You just had a baby. Give it time. Don't worry about it."

I think my daughter was just so tired at that point. She didn't stand up and say, "Look, I am going to the emergency room, or I am going to call another doctor, or I am going to another hospital or whatever until somebody listens to me."

With a newborn baby with colic, with respiratory distress, she just was tired. And she needed someone to advocate for her. She needed someone to realize that they had to take care of her at that time, and so I think she would just be off the chart right now because that is not happening.

Ms. CASTOR. Well, let that be a lesson for all of us as we move these bills. Thank you.

Ms. ESHOO. The gentlewoman yields back.

I now would like to recognize the gentleman from Missouri, Mr. Long, for his 5 minutes of questioning.

Mr. LONG. Thank you, Madam Chairwoman.

In this final round of *Jeopardy!* today, we only have one category left, and that is "Who said it?" So in the category of "Who said it?" for $1,000:

"After delivering another perfect baby, I was sitting next to Kira by her bedside in the recovery room. That is when I first noticed blood in her catheter. I notified staff immediately. A series of tests were ordered, along with a CT scan to be performed stat. I understood 'stat' to mean the CT scan would be performed immediately.

"Hours passed, and Kira's systems escalated throughout the rest of the afternoon into the evening. We were told by the medical staff at Cedars-Sinai Kira was not a priority, and we waited for the CT scan to be done. We waited for the hospital to act so she could have her recovery. Kira kept telling me, 'Charles, I am so cold. Charles, I don't feel right.' She repeated these same words to me for several hours. After more than 10 hours of waiting and watching my wife's condition deteriorate, after 10 hours of watching Kira suffer in excruciating pain needlessly and begging and pleading them to help her, the medical staff at Cedars-Sinai finally took action.

"As they prepared Kira for surgery, I was holding her hand as we walked down the hall to the operating room. Kira looked at me and said, 'Baby, I am scared.' I told her without doubt everything would be fine. The doctor told me I would see her in 15 minutes. Kira was wheeled into surgery, and it was discovered that she had massive internal bleeding caused by a horrible medical negligence that occurred during her routine c-section. She had approximately three liters of blood in her abdomen. Kira died at 12:22 a.m., April 17th, 2016. Langston was 11 years old.

"As someone who experienced firsthand what it was like to have your spouse die in front of you, I do not have the words to describe the loss my family has suffered. My boys no longer have their mother. Kira was the most amazing role model and mother any boy could ever wish to have. I no longer have the love of my life, my best friend."

Of course, those were the words of Charles Johnson IV, who I believe was of means. Kira was of means. It wasn't someone that didn't have good prenatal care. It wasn't someone that had—didn't have a—it was a preplanned c-section.

We are talking here today, and I hear a lot of people talking about access to prenatal care, which of course is vitally important, but cases like this, cases like Ms. Irving's, all I want to do is come down there and hug your neck. I can tell you that.

But I am the only Missouri Member that is on Energy and Commerce. So, consequently, I am the only Missouri Member that is on the healthcare subcommittee. So I feel an obligation to travel the State for healthcare issues. I visited just during this break a week ago—it may have been a week ago today, I am not sure of the timing—but Kansas City Children's Mercy hospital. Went through the neonatal. Went—you know, and I do that quite often. I go to St. Louis Children's up there.

Our oldest daughter is a pediatrician, and I know when she does her rounds at the hospital that, you know, all that she wants to do and you think all any doctor would want to do is love these babies and make sure they get a good start and love the mothers, and so whatever we can do on this committee.

I mentioned earlier in my little outburst when we had the outburst in the hall—which I apologize to you all that that went on for any length of time during your testimony—I am a member of the Black Maternal Health Caucus. And I deeply care about this issue. The timing didn't work out to bring up H.R. 4215 today, the Excellence in Maternal Health Act. Nobody's fault, just the timing didn't work out.

But I am an original cosponsor of that, and I just want to thank you all for being here today and your heartfelt testimony. I have said a lot of words today, but there is no words to say, to express what an unbelievable issue this is and the things that happen, but if your testimony here today, Charles' testimony back in September of 2018, I believe it was, we have had a lot of important, lot of big hearings, a lot of memorable hearings in Energy and Commerce. Mark Zuckerberg from Facebook is an example of—Dorsey, Jack Dorsey of Twitter, you know, the rooms were packed, a lot, you know, but no hearing ever moved me like Charles Johnson's testimony that day, and your testimony here today is right along there with it.

So God bless you and thank you for being here, and thank all of you for being here, and if there is anything that me, my staff, the committee can do, please keep us apprised, any suggestions, ideas. We will be honored and glad to work with you.

I yield back.

Ms. ESHOO. The gentleman yields back.

It is now a pleasure to recognize the gentlewoman from Delaware, Ms. Blunt Rochester, for her 5 minutes of questions.

Ms. BLUNT ROCHESTER. Thank you, Madam Chairwoman.

And thank you so much to the witnesses for your testimony. I especially want to acknowledge Representative Kelly for her leadership in this important issue.

I held a townhall meeting in the past month over the recess, and a midwife stood up and shared her perspective on the role that she plays. And one of the things that she focused on was the social determinants of health, particularly in maternal mortality. And she said that she was caring for a soon-to-be mother, many of which are told go out and get some exercise, but they don't feel safe walking around their neighborhoods, or who are being told to eat nutritious diets but don't live within blocks of a grocery store selling fresh fruits and vegetables.

And as we transition our health system, you know, I think it is critical that we think about the social determinants of health and all those things that surround it.

And so my first question is to Dr. Harris. Can you talk about the social determinants of health and how we can address this challenge of maternal mortality by dealing with the social determinants of health?

Dr. HARRIS. Thank you.

And I can. I can say that the AMA is very committed to addressing these issues because, if you look at that circle of care and you look at the fact that maybe health outcomes are impacted, and we know they are impacted some by physicians and hospitals, but we see a huge impact related to the social determinants of health: transportation, housing, whether or not you have a job. You mentioned whether or not you live in a food desert, and I know now and my colleagues can talk about whether or not you live in a maternity care desert.

So those are all pieces that we plan to focus on as we build out the work of our Center for Health Equity, but I will say we have current policies that raise the importance of social determinants of health. So, wherever we go, I mention that and, in my own work, that it is not enough for us to say to exercise. Physicians should say that, but we have to make sure there are equitable opportunities for exercise, to access healthy, nutritious foods. So that work will be included in the work of our Center for Health Equity.

Ms. BLUNT ROCHESTER. Thank you.

This questions is for the panel, and it is one that has plagued me for a long time.

And, Ms. Irving, first of all, thank you so much for sharing your testimony and for sharing your daughter's story. And it is at the heart of my question. I don't understand why. I can talk about the social determinants of health and understand that there is a disconnect sometimes between access to healthcare or the kind of healthcare, but your daughter, you know, smart, understood health.

I watched a Jon Stewart piece last night about maternal mortality, which is interesting, and he said that—they showed a clip of a father, an African-American man, who said his wife died because he was afraid to be perceived as the angry Black man if he spoke up for her.

So I am curious. Can you explain to me for those African-American women that are experiencing this and it is not an issue of access to healthcare, education, a doctor, can the panel, can someone help me understand? What is it? What is going on?

Ms. IRVING. I will start off and then turn it over, but I had the same issue, and I suffer now from regret that I wasn't that angry Black woman, and I think my daughter kept me from doing that because she would say, "Mom, just calm down. Just let them handle it. It is going to be OK."

But it wasn't OK, and I wish now that I had stood up and said, "Look, you are going to do something right now."

But I think it might have had the negative effect, because then I would have pushed them away, and it might—well, it would have—I can't see how it would have turned out any worse than it did, but that is what a lot of Black women or Black men face when you are coming in because you are looked at as a threat. Then, if you start getting loud, the next thing you know, you could be put out of the hospital because you are not communicating in a way that is acceptable.

Ms. BLUNT ROCHESTER. Doctor.

Dr. HARRIS. So that is an important part. I would say that is the other end of folks examining their own implicit biases. I have not had a child, but I have often been the only African-American woman in a room, and I think people of color, particularly African-American women, because there are issues around discrimination based on gender and race, end up self-editing sometimes and being extra careful so that we are not the angry Black woman or the angry Black man.

And I think as we have this conversation, we have to talk about that more. It only comes, I think, with some practice and some experience and, frankly, some privilege that you feel more comfortable raising issues. And that should not be the case.

Ms. BLUNT ROCHESTER. You are right.

Dr. HARRIS. And so I will say that was part of our discussion, will be part of our discussion at the AMA. But it really needs to be part of this society's discussion to look at, I think, the biases and the racism and discrimination in all contexts.

Ms. BLUNT ROCHESTER. I know I am out of time, and it is just something that has plagued me. I know people like Serena Williams, Beyoncé have gone through this, and it is not even—it is beyond privilege.

Thank so you much for having this hearing, and I will send questions in writing. Thank you.

Ms. ESHOO. The gentlewoman yields back, and you ask a very heavy question, but a necessary one.

It is a pleasure to recognize the gentlewoman from Indiana, Ms. Brooks, for her 5 minutes of questioning.

Mrs. BROOKS. Thank you so much, Madam Chairwoman.

And I also want to thank the ranking member because this is something that we have been focused on for a couple of Congresses, and we must do more. We rarely in this body, I think, have an opportunity like we have now to educate those medical providers of the future.

And one thing that you mentioned, Ms. Irving—and I want to thank you so much for sharing your horrible, very, very sad story, but the power of your testimony, the power of your written testimony, which I read this morning and was quite moved this morning, even before you spoke—you mentioned something that I don't think that we have talked about enough, although Dr. Burgess mentioned it. In his medical training, he had a doctor who talked about care, about caring, and you mentioned med schools.

And I think the hearing we had last Congress and the hearing we are having this Congress from all of the incredible professionals here that are studying it, that are working on it, that are trying to improve—Indiana has the third-highest rate of maternal mortality. Now, yes, we just instituted that review committee. Luckily our new, or fairly new, head of State Department of Health is an OB/GYN, and this is a top priority, Dr. Kristina Box, top priority now for our State, but we have got to start earlier. The review committees are after the fact. We have got to study the data. We have to collect the data to understand the problem.

But what would you all like to see our med schools do, our nursing programs do, our—we haven't really talked. That is one aspect we haven't really talked about.

Maybe starting with you, Ms. Irving.

Ms. IRVING. I think the training that we have talked about before as far as the implicit bias training, et cetera, is good to start early. They must recognize that every patient should be treated as an individual. Even though we have standards of care, you look at the patient as a whole. And I haven't been to medical school. So I don't know what the training is, but you have to have that "it could be my mother, it could be my wife, it could be my daughter" and look at each patient through those lenses and work on it from that point.

Mrs. BROOKS. Thank you.

Dr. Harris, how do we take what Ms. Irving is hoping and praying that folks like you all implement?

Dr. HARRIS. I think that is critical, and the AMA 5 years ago looked at the issue of training the next generation of physicians, and we awarded 11 $1 million grants and have since then developed a consortium of other medical schools that can share best practices, and I will say a couple of those medical schools are specifically focused from our grant, although they were already working in these areas, on two issues that have been raised.

One is the social determinants of health. So we have medical students now getting trained and understanding and appreciating the importance of social determinants of health. And we have a couple of other medical schools that are talking about health disparities, making sure that the future workforce is a diverse workforce so that the faces of our physicians match the faces of our patients, and then, of course, from those learnings we are spreading that out to the consortium of medical schools, and then hopefully that will be spread out to the entire medical school community.

So we are committed and do agree that we need to raise these issues early in training of physicians.

Mrs. BROOKS. Dr. Nelson, I want to commend Parkland.

And thank you, Dr. Harris.

Has the med school community reached out, and are they studying your model in Parkland, and how do we do a better job getting—because it is not just doctors. It is nurses. I am sure there were many nurses that didn't listen to your daughter's needs, not just doctors—doctors, nurses, others. How about the medical training? I don't just mean med schools.

Dr. NELSON. Correct. That is what I was going to build upon. So I am a faculty at the University of Texas Southwestern Medical Center. And we are one of the largest obstetrics and gynecology programs in the country. We have 72 residents in our current existing program. And part of our responsibility is to talk about and begin the training that you heard here. It also extends to the training that we have within our nurse midwives, our advanced practice providers with nurse practitioners, and nursing students who are responsible for training the next generation.

And this is the part that becomes really difficult, is translating the importance and advocacy that we are hearing that we need to share in fighting for our patients and hearing their voice, is something that is our responsibility to carry forward.

Mrs. BROOKS. Thank you all. My time is up, but I certainly hope that our med schools take the opportunity to actually listen to your testimony, to read it and to listen to it. I think it would be incredibly instructive.

With that, I yield back.

Ms. ESHOO. The gentlewoman yields back.

I now would like to recognize the gentleman from Maryland, Mr. Sarbanes, for his 5 minutes of questioning.

Mr. SARBANES. Thank you, Madam Chair.

I want to thank our witnesses for your testimony today. Extremely compelling and in certain instances certainly heart-wrenching. So thank you for being here.

Ms. Ranji, I wanted to talk a little bit more about the situation that women can find themselves in when they have to make a switch to different coverage because of the expiration of Medicaid coverage, and we have heard from many of you and it is well documented that the Medicaid, current Medicaid pregnancy coverage only covers women for 60 days after they give birth, and then, at that point, what happens can range from losing coverage completely, potentially being able to enroll through a marketplace plan on one of the exchanges, et cetera.

Obviously, getting some coverage after that 60 days is better than having no coverage. But I think it is important to recognize that forcing women to change plans during what is a very, very critical time can also generate negative consequences. So I would just like to ask you a few questions about that phenomenon, which is referred to in shorthand as churning.

If a woman gains Medicaid coverage as a result of her pregnancy, what are the coverage options after that coverage ends 60 days post partum? What is the range of things that could happen there?

Ms. RANJI. Right. Well, it really depends where you live. And this is what, when it comes to post partum coverage, there is a lot more variation across the States for low-income women. So, like you said, some women are able to continue on Medicaid. Some may be able to get subsidies to purchase private insurance. Some may be uninsured. But the phenomenon that you refer to, churning, certainly has an impact.

We know that disruptions in conversation are relatively frequent for low-income women around the time of delivery, and we know that churning can negatively affect access to care. It can really result in delays in care, having to switch providers, identifying a new provider network. And down the road that can lead to delays in things like preventive services like cancer screenings, et cetera.

So churning is relatively common among this population when you have to switch plans.

Mr. SARBANES. I mean, in fact, that is exactly the moment in time when someone's condition might change in a way where, if there was a continuous perspective because the coverage was lasting for a longer duration, that change would be captured in terms of the care plan for that particular individual. But because there is a transition happening to a different coverage, potentially involving different providers, involving a different set of benefits as to what is covered and what is not covered, the system will miss the opportunity to identify the kind of care that should be delivered. Then you can end up having drastic consequences from that. Is that correct?

Ms. RANJI. Well, and being able to stay with the same coverage plan can allow you to stay with the same provider and provide that continuity of care from a relationship that a woman may have formed with—during the prenatal period—with the provider, being able to continue with that provider or with that group of providers could streamline her access to follow up on conditions and obtain preventive services.

Mr. SARBANES. I would also imagine that it's going to be easier to deploy strategies for more sensitivity to the patient population, and we have heard testimony about the importance of that today. If the coverage situation is not one that is in flux, it is just better if you have got a longer period of time in which to deploy these strategies to get out in front of some of the biases, discriminatory practices, and other things that we have heard testimony about today.

So, clearly, there are strong arguments in favor of extending the Medicaid coverage period substantially. And that is at the heart of a number of the proposals that we are hearing about today.

Thank you all for your testimony. I appreciate it, and I yield back.

Ms. ESHOO. The gentleman yields back.

It is a pleasure to recognize the gentleman from Montana, Mr. Gianforte.

Mr. GIANFORTE. Thank you, Madam Chair.

Ms. Irving, I just want to say I am sorry for the loss of your daughter. And I want to thank you for being here to tell your story. Unfortunately, Montana has a higher maternal death rate than the national average, and our State faces unique challenges in this space.

Dr. Howell, in your testimony you state that maternal deaths from substance use disorders and mental health are climbing. Unfortunately, methamphetamine use is an epidemic in Montana. How does drug addiction impact maternal deaths, and what changes can we make to help mothers who are facing a drug addiction?

Dr. HOWELL. So, just as substance-use disorders are growing across our country and we are having an opiate crisis, that also affects maternal deaths, as well as from other areas. And, although this is not my area of expertise, I will just share that I think that the risk factors and some of the issues are lack of treatment centers for opiate abuse and also lack of access to opiate replacement therapies.

Mr. GIANFORTE. So our specific problem is methamphetamine.

Dr. HOWELL. So that is not my area of expertise, but I think some of the general things that we know about substance-use disorder can be applied in the maternal healthcare setting and that we don't recognize that there are other options, and there are treatment alternatives and that there is not enough being done. I would defer also to my colleague, if he has more to add.

Mr. GIANFORTE. Dr. Nelson.

Dr. NELSON. So we have a robust perinatal intervention programs that covers opioids as well as methamphetamine use. This requires intense multidisciplinary care. It involves case management, addiction medicine, obstetricians, and pediatricians. And it has implications related to the care of the mother during the pregnancy. It can also have implications to the baby at delivery as well.

Mr. GIANFORTE. OK. Thank you.

Today is World Suicide Prevention Day, and unfortunately Montana leads the Nation in suicide, number one. We understand the impact that a lack of access to mental health services has on our communities. To ensure that people have access to these services they need in the face of this crisis, I recently introduced a bipartisan bill to designate 988 as the National Suicide Prevention Hotline. This is an essential resource for anyone facing mental health crisis. I look forward to working with my colleagues to get this bill through committee, and I hope it will be available to help mothers that we are discussing today.

Dr. Howell, again, if we could, can you describe what is being done especially in rural areas to address the increase in maternal deaths for mental health complications such as post partum depression?

Dr. HOWELL. So I am not an expert on rural healthcare, coming from New York City. But I can comment that I think a lot of the things that you were hearing about—depression is a major issue for pregnant women and post partum women. You have heard rates of around 15 percent, and so it is a major issue, not only for breastfeeding, maternal-infant bonding, but everything you can think about for both the mother, the child, and the family, and so we have to do a better job around mental health.

Now, in rural areas, just like there are major access issues in cities around mental health, as you have heard, but there is also additional barriers, and so the use of telemedicine, the use of new techniques around cognitive behavioral therapy on, you know, internet platforms, sort of thinking outside of the box is the way that we have to move forward to sort of broaden our ability to reach patients from everywhere around the country.

Mr. GIANFORTE. And that is really essential, particularly in our rural communities. We are not going to have a specialist in every discipline, in every community. Telehealth is one way to do it. So I appreciate your comments there.

Dr. Harris, Montana has seven federally recognized American Indian Tribal Governments. You mention in your testimony that CDC recently released a report that American Indian women are two to three times more likely to die from pregnancy-related causes than White women.

Can you talk a little bit about the key drivers of this disparity in our Native American population?

Dr. HARRIS. So I would imagine that it is about access, it is about bias, all the issues that we have discussed today. We want to make sure that we appreciate all of the issues faced by those who are not of the same community. Again, that is why we stress the importance of a more diverse physician workforce, making sure that those in rural areas have access to healthcare. You mentioned telemedicine. Making sure that everyone, again, has affordable, meaningful coverage.

So I think all of those drivers are the same or similar. They won't be absolutely the same for Native American women as African-American women, and I appreciate your point on methamphetamine being an issue in your State, and I think that is why certainly we need to do all that we can to address opioids, but I think there is an opportunity here to make sure we have an infrastructure for substance abuse disorders in general and not just regarding opioids.

Mr. GIANFORTE. Yes, thank you, Doctor.

And just in closing, Madam Chair, if I could, I want to echo the comments of Ranking Member Walden in his call for additional hearings, and I would just suggest that, if we do that additional hearing, that we might include the Native American voice at the table because the Tribal communities are not represented here today and possibly IHS, Indian Health Services, as well as we continue to look at these issues.

With that, I yield back.

Ms. ESHOO. I think that is an excellent suggestion from the gentleman. And we have two Members of Congress, women Members of Congress, for first time in the history of the Congress, that are Native Americans. So, thank you.

Now I would like to recognize the gentleman from California, Mr. Cárdenas, for his 5 minutes of questioning.

Mr. CÁRDENAS. Thank you so much, Madam Chairwoman.

And also I would like to thank Ranking Member Burgess for having this important hearing on this very important and heart-breaking issue.

I want to also thank all of the panelists for providing your expertise, especially Ms. Irving. You are someone who should have never had to learn so much about this issue and to endure what you have had to endure. So thank you for coming in and enlightening us.

Ms. Irving, I would like to thank you for sharing with us today what you have been going through, and I know it is not about you. It is about making sure that we do better for the families and the women of today and tomorrow. So thank you for enlightening us. As a parent and a grandparent, I can only imagine the pain that you have gone through, and I certainly agree with those who have been calling you very brave, but I would also like to point out that I truly do believe that you are an embodiment of what it is to have faith. And by being here today, you are putting that faith into action.

And I believe that it is incumbent upon us on this side of the room to act responsibly and to do whatever we can to make sure that we pay heed to your advice and the wisdom of all of you so that we can actually take action swiftly and accurately so that less pain is endured by families going forward.

I do have a question for you. Could you please describe for us what high-quality, fair, and respectful post partum care for your daughter could or should have been, should she still be with us?

Ms. IRVING. I think for the first time what should have happened is she should have been able to see her doctor within a week after giving birth. Just like the baby went in 2 or 3 days after birth, there should be a mandatory 1 week, let's come in, let's check you out, let's see how you are doing. She should have been able to call up a doctor or go in and see the doctor right there.

Instead, what she had was she saw a nurse practitioner a couple of times, and that nurse practitioner left and said she came back to see the doctor, but the doctor never showed up at all. So I would think the doctors would follow their patients and make sure that they see the patient and make sure that their symptoms or concerns are addressed right then and there.

Mr. CÁRDENAS. Thank you. What you just described is proper standards of care in the moment, case-by-case, not just theoretically. So thank you so much.

Dr. Howell, we have heard about some of the systematic barriers to care that Black women face. And we know that Hispanic women face many of the same obstacles, as do Native Americans, et cetera. Yet reporting on the rates of maternal mortality for Hispanic women has been inconsistent, and it is difficult to find clarity on what it is telling us.

Can you speak to this issue and what the potential consequences to this lack of data might be?

Dr. HOWELL. Yes. So a perfect example is the national statistics do not suggest that Latina women have an elevated rate. Our pregnancy mortality review done in New York City revealed, when I said that they were 8 to 12 times higher for Black women, for Latina women it was 3 times higher. And it shows you that, when you get more granular data and when you invest in maternal mortality reviews that actually collect data from multiple sources, you can get better data on race and ethnicity. You can get the causes. That allows to us actually see a true story.

Without the data, you don't know. And that is what happens, when you have a vital statistics system that doesn't collect the stuff in a good way. That is why I think it was underreported.

Mr. CÁRDENAS. Thank you.

One of the things I would like to personally comment on that I want to thank all the women who are here in this committee room and also the men, but the women vastly outnumber the men who are guests and experts apprising this important committee on this very, very critical issue.

And I personally want to add to that, that I believe that when this side of the room looks more like that side of the room, I think that, especially when it comes to issues facing women and families, we are going see much quicker, much more accurate results out of what happens in the decisionmaking of this elected body.

I am not casting aspersions on us men or what have you, but what I am saying is, when there are women in the room, you enlighten us in a way that I—and you think of things and approach in a way that I just can't, and I just want to thank you for doing that at every opportunity and certainly today.

Thank you very much. I yield back.

Ms. ESHOO. I thank the gentleman for most especially for those comments, as well as the others.

It is a pleasure to recognize the gentleman from Georgia, Mr. Carter, for his 5 minutes of questions.

Mr. CARTER. Thank you, Madam Chair.

And I want to thank each and every one of you for being here today. This is an extremely important subject.

And especially I want to thank you, Ms. Irving, for being here. Yours is quite a compelling story, and we just cannot say enough about your courage and your work, and we thank you very much for that.

Ladies and gentlemen, I am from the State of Georgia. This is obviously—maternal mortality is a national problem. There is no question about that, but in the State of Georgia, it is a serious problem. In fact, we have the unenviable, unenviable position of being the number one State in the Nation in maternal mortality, and for what reason we can't figure out. But that is what really is driving us to try to do something about this, and I have been doing it. I have been doing it in my district. I have held many roundtable discussions with different groups about why is this and how can we address this situation and how can we make things better, because we all want to make it better. Regardless of which side of the aisle you are on, you want to make it better.

This is not a Republican, this is not a Democrat issue. It does not discriminate against anyone, and we have to work toward a solution, and I have to tell you that I am really proud the last session that Representative Jamie Herrera Beutler, her bill, Preventing Maternal Deaths Act, passed. And that is good. It was signed into law. We need more bills like that, and I am really proud of that.

I will have to tell you I am a little bit disappointed that we don't have some Republican bills that we are talking about here. In fact, we don't have even much Republican input in these bills. And I hope that that is going to change for a couple of reasons.

First of all, we have been out in our district for the past 5 weeks, and I have been proudly proclaiming that not only do I serve on the oldest and the most diverse as far as subject matter is concerned committee in Congress but also the most bipartisan committee, and I consider it to be the most bipartisan committee. So I am a little disappointed—I have to express that to the chair-person—we don't have more Republican bills.

Having said that, I do have to tell you I do have a bill I am working on with Representative Katherine Clark of Massachusetts that has to do with Medicaid. It is a Medicaid demonstration project that tests how we might be able to enhance access to care by better utilizing birth centers. All throughout our testimony today, what we have heard about is access to healthcare. That is extremely important in the solution to this problem. We all understand that. And birth centers, I think, are not being utilized to the point that they could be, and I hope that it is something, and I thank Ms. Clark for working with me on this, and it is something that I want to work with her on.

Ms. Ranji, I will ask you first. Again, one of the things that we have heard during this testimony has been access to healthcare. And I would just ask you, is there a better place or a place for a better use of birth centers, that we could possibly use them in a potential solution or a partial solution to this national health problem?

Ms. RANJI. Well, thank you for the question.

Just as Medicaid policies vary between States, it is a similar situation with birth centers, and so while birth centers themselves are not my area of expertise, I know the availability and the certification and the licensing procedures and practices vary between the States. I could certainly see that there would be room for growth of presence in birth centers and coverage under Medicaid, but, again, the availability and access, those vary a lot between localities, and the financing policies would then have to be worked out with it on the State level.

Mr. CARTER. One thing I will inform you about is that I represent South Georgia. You know, there are two Georgias. There is Atlanta and everywhere else, and I am in everywhere else. So birthing centers are extremely important for us and particularly in the rural areas. So that is why I look at that, and I am excited this bipartisan bill that Representative Clark and I are working on.

Dr. Nelson, I want to ask you. Currently I am the only pharmacist serving in Congress. So I have a very—an interest in opioid epidemic and a very strong interest in how it is impacting maternal health.

And I just wanted to ask you, could you very quickly help us to understand, when you have a mother who is going through an opioid addiction, how they are handled and treated during the pregnancy?

Dr. NELSON. So the problem of opioids is also a major crisis for this country. In 2017 alone in Parkland, we delivered 69 women with opioid disorder. In 2018, I personally toured Dr. Giroir and Dr. Adams, the Assistant Secretary of Health and the U.S. Surgeon General, through Parkland Hospital to see our program. Our program is comprehensive, and the challenges are both related to the maternal care, the risks to mom, but also the neonatal opioid withdrawal syndrome risk to the baby. And that is a chronic, life-changing opportunity for us to have resources provided for a pregnant mother and her unborn child.

Mr. CARTER. Real quickly, just how do you get over the stigma— or not stigma, but the obstacle of a mother who is addicted that doesn't want that to be known, so she doesn't reach out for care? I know that has got be a problem and something we have got to address as well.

Dr. NELSON. I agree that stigma is important. Our service as physicians is to be a healthcare home for those patients and to provide them access, and that is a complex issue related to interfacing the legality of some of those circumstances. But our first and foremost effort should be providing access to care to those women and getting them resources to potentially even get better.

Mr. CARTER. Great. Thank you all for being here. This is a most important subject, especially for the State of Georgia and for our country.

Thank you, and I yield back.

Ms. ESHOO. The gentleman yields back.

It is a pleasure to recognize Mr. Engel from New York, who is the author of the Quality Care for Moms and Babies Act.

Thank you for your solid work, Mr. Engel. And you are recognized for 5 minutes of questioning.

Mr. ENGEL. Thank you. Thank you, Madam Chair.

And thank you for holding this very, very important hearing.

And thank you to all the panelists. Thank you so much. We appreciate everything that you have done.

Ms. Irving, I want to single you out because what you are doing today takes an enormous amount of courage, and so God bless you and know that we support you, and what you are doing today will save the lives of countless other people tomorrow. So thank you for having the courage.

I want to thank the chairwoman and the—Chairman Pallone for holding today's subcommittee hearing on the Nation's maternal mortality crisis and which includes my bipartisan, as the chairman said, bicameral legislation, the Quality Care for Moms and Babies Act. The bill would bring together diverse stakeholders to develop care quality benchmarks for women and children, as well as to also find existing and new quality collaboratives.

Quality collaboratives are on the front lines of the efforts to end this crisis. The New York State Quality Collaborative has developed resources to address the leading causes of maternal deaths in New York, which include hypertension and hemorrhaging. These resources were distributed to over 126 birthing hospitals in New York.

So I urge Members on both sides of the aisle to support this commonsense, bipartisan legislation. I would also like to ask for unanimous consent to submit a letter of support from many organizations, including March of Dimes, the American College of Obstetricians and Gynecologists, in support of Quality Care for Moms and Babies Act.

Dr. Howell, it is always good to see more New Yorkers in Washington. I get lonely over here. So please come back, and thank you for the great work that you do and that Mount Sinai does as well. Mount Sinai, of course, is very well known in New York and very well respected.

So I want to personally thank you, Dr. Howell, for your service on the New York State Task Force of Maternal Mortality, and it is my understanding that the task force issued a report this past March in which it recommended expanding the New York State Perinatal Quality Collaborative and as you know, as you mentioned, which I appreciate you mentioning it, I am sponsoring the Quality Care for Moms and Babies Act with my friend, Congressman Steve Stivers. It is a bipartisan bill. Our legislation authorizes funding for existing and new perinatal quality collaboratives.

Let me ask, you Dr. Howell. Can you again share—I think it is worth repeating—why developing and sustaining perinatal quality collaboratives is an important tool for addressing racial and ethnic disparities in maternal health outcomes?

Dr. HOWELL. It is a very important tool for us to use across the United States, as well as in New York, because it allows us to build—have partnerships with physicians and nurses, with departments of health, hospitals, and health systems to target specific processes based on the evidence that we can target together to improve, and we have done it in a number of different situations, not only in terms of the bundles that you have heard about but in terms of trying to lower our cesarean section rates, in terms of our elected delivery rates. We have done it on the NICU side.

So it is these groups that can take the shared learning and utilize that to help make improvements in hospitals, and your bill supports that, and I think it is a really wonderful and important part of this story that we need to advocate for.

Mr. ENGEL. Well, thank you, and I have high hopes that we will pass the bill and pass it on the floor and hopefully get it passed in the other body and have the President sign it into law. So thank you for everything you are doing.

Dr. Harris, let me ask you. In your written testimony, you note that the quality of maternal care can vary greatly by provider and facility. Given that public health programs cover most births in the U.S., with Medicaid alone covering 43 percent of them, I believe obviously these programs are uniquely situated to improve maternal health.

To that end, the Quality Care for Moms and Babies Act would direct the development of a core set of maternal and infant health performance measures for Medicaid and CHIP that promote best practices.

So let me ask you, Dr. Harris, how would the creation of this measure core set affect the quality of care and reduce maternal morbidity and mortality, especially for women of color?

Dr. HARRIS. Mr. Engel, Congressman Engel, if you don't mind, I would like to let Dr. Howell talk about the specifics of that, of the core metrics, and how they would help. But from sort of the 30,000-foot view, it is very important to have the data. Data then informs. And that is, again, why the AMA is very supportive of these review committees. You have heard a lot today, but there is no sort of one-size-fits-all solution, and patients are unique.

And as Dr. Howell mentioned earlier, California has done a great job of reducing mortality but not African-American women. So we still need to look at the data and why overall mortality decreased but not African-American women.

So I think the opportunity there is to get that data, get the data specifically for African-American women. And then, once we get that data, it is important to have funding to implement what we find in the data. So I would say that from a 100,000-foot view and let Dr. Howell talk about specific measures that should be included to improve those disparities.

Mr. ENGEL. Well, thank you.

If the chairwoman will indulge, we will have Dr. Howell.

Dr. HOWELL. So, I think it is incredibly important that we develop quality measures in maternal healthcare that are both patient-centered and address disparities. We have done work showing that hospital performance on primary, low-risk cesarean or hospital performance on elective delivery is not correlated with hospital performance on severe maternal morbidity.

So the current group of quality measures don't really provide information to mothers about the different facilities in terms of safety, and they weren't correlated either with neonatal morbidity at term. We need better quality measures that can serve and we can give to the public so that they can better understand what is going on.

So your bill that advocates for quality measure development I think is really instrumental and a very important piece. And having quality measures also target disparities and address disparities is another piece, because previous data shows that the quality measures in obstetrics are not really doing that either.

Mr. ENGEL. Thank you.

Thank you, Madam Chair, for your indulgence. And thank you for all the great work you are doing.

Ms. ESHOO. Thank you for your work, Mr. Engel, and this sounds like a resounding—we recognize endorsements, don't we, when they occur? I think I just heard one.

I now would like to recognize the gentleman from Illinois, Mr. Rush, who is—I am really pleased to be joining him in his congressional district in a handful of weeks where he is conducting a field hearing on this very issue.

And you are now recognized for 5 minutes for your questions.

Mr. RUSH. I want to thank you, Madam Chair, and I certainly want to applaud you for holding this critically important hearing.

Ms. Irving, I feel you. I understand some of what you are going through. I am reminded just this very day that, some 10 years ago, this very same committee, subcommittee, had a hearing on post partum depression. I had introduced a bill entitled the Melanie Blocker-Stokes Postpartum Depression Act of 2007, and her mother, Melanie Blocker-Stokes' mother, Ms. Carol Blocker, sat at this very same table that you are sitting at some 10 years ago.

Melanie was one of my constituents who had been seeing a series of doctors post partum, and none of them diagnosed the depression that she was going through. And she ultimately, on a bright Saturday morning, spring Saturday morning, went up to a hotel in Chicago, on near the north side of Chicago, and leaped to her death from the 10th floor, and the cause of it was post partum depression.

So here you are, another mother in a line of mothers who are coming to this Congress asking and pleading and bringing your pain to this—to our presence, to this table, asking us to help, and I want you to know that some of us are determined to provide the help that you are seeking and other mothers are seeking.

My bill was—the language of my bill was included in the ACA Act, in the Obamacare, and I was very pleased with that, but we have such a long, long way to go in order to deal with it. So I applaud you, and I commiserate with you, and I just—you know, your pain is a pain that generations will remember and will bear until we are able to solve this problem of maternal mortality.

I want to move to questioning, if I have got a few moments here. And I want to ask Dr. Ranji. Dr. Ranji, I am curious about doulas and the effect on the healthcare system of doulas, and can you explain to us why you think that doulas can improve health outcomes, and also can you address what are some of the cultural and economic variants to presenting a nationwide system that would include doulas?

Ms. RANJI. Well, the research shows that women and moms have expressed, in many surveys, have expressed interest in having doulas care, more support during the prenatal, labor, and delivery, and post partum periods. There is, you know, some sense—we talked earlier, the panel was talking about the ability to be able to, sometimes for patients being able to challenge providers or ask for what they need, and there is some research showing that women have said that maybe if they had more support, for example, with assistance of a doula, that that might be part of expanding her ability to be able to recognize and sort of understand what her options are.

Currently, under Medicaid, only two States, as far as I know, Oregon and Minnesota, include coverage for doulas, but there are some other States that have certainly been considering it, and New York is one that has a pilot program going in certain parts of the State where they are also considering, at least are doing for some women, expansion of coverage for doulas.

Mr. RUSH. So do you know of any—what are some of the barriers that you see that we may face in terms of implementing or creating a doula care system?

Ms. RANJI. Right. Well, some of the barriers include sort of administrative and procedural barriers. Right now, you know, Medicaid reimburses licensed medical practitioners, and the sort of doula training standards and doula certification and licensing is still an area that is in work. It is not an area that I have focused on, but there is a lot of published research out there that I certainly will also be able to share with you, if that is of interest.

Mr. RUSH. I want to thank you, Madam Chair.

I yield back.

Ms. ESHOO. I thank the gentleman for his work on this issue, and I look forward to the hearing in your district.

Now I would like to recognize Ms. Schakowsky of Illinois, who is a member of our full committee and is waiving onto the Health Subcommittee today where she served for many years.

So you are recognized for your 5 minutes of questions.

Ms. SCHAKOWSKY. Thank you so much, Madam Chair, for allowing me to waive onto today's hearing. And it is such an important one.

I want to thank all the witnesses. And I want to give a special thank you to my friend and colleague from Illinois, Robin Kelly, who has been such a champion of this issue for our State.

Illinois has been one of the most extreme pregnancy-related death disparities in the Nation. According to data from our Department of Public Health, Black women are six times more likely to die of pregnancy-related conditions as White women. It is just totally unacceptable.

And I want to say a really special thank you to Ms. Irving, and I am so grateful that you have shared your daughter, Shalon's, story with us today, and I just want to add when I read the article that was given to us that this is the third child and the last child that you have also buried. So I am so sorry for that.

I fully believe the words of your testimony, that this disparity, quote, "has to do with the appallingly way Black women are or aren't attended to or listened to," unquote. I am complete—I am fully supportive of extending Medicaid coverage for the post partum care up to—from 60 days to 1 year, as the bill that we are considering today proposes, and though that will make a transformative change, that is certainly not enough.

Ms. Irving, I wanted to ask you a question. Here you have such an educated daughter in the healthcare field. She is a doctor herself. What did the physicians tell her as she continued to suffer after the birth of her daughter that somehow indicated that they must not have been hearing her?

Ms. IRVING. Every time she went to the doctor's office—and there were probably at least five times, three times I know of, in 1 week—each time it was a dismissive "You just had a baby, give it time, you will feel better."

Ms. SCHAKOWSKY. Did they do any of the tests that would have indicated what the problems were?

Ms. IRVING. On the last day that she went, which was the 24th, 5 hours before she collapsed, she went in, and they gave her a test for preeclampsia, but since she didn't have any blurriness of vision, they said, "Well, we can rule that out."

And they gave her a test for blood clotting. She said, "I have had blood clots. I know what they feel like. This is not a blood clot." And, of course, it wasn't a blood clot. But her blood pressure was still off the roof. I think if I am correct it was 174 over 119, and she was sent home, and 5 hours later she collapsed.

Ms. SCHAKOWSKY. You also said in your testimony that essentially that no one is really immune, regardless of education, et cetera.

Ms. IRVING. No.

Ms. SCHAKOWSKY. And that the issue of racial disparities is certainly a huge problem.

I wanted to ask Dr. Howell a question. I am interested in the idea of holding hospitals accountable for maternal care, maternity care through a value-based care model. Do you believe that bundled payments for an entire episode of maternal care could give health systems more incentives and greater control to improve the pregnancy-related outcomes from beginning to end, with regard to racial disparities in particular?

Dr. HOWELL. I think we need more work on alternative payment models to think about maternity care and incentivize clinicians and hospitals correctly. I do worry about unintended consequences, specifically that certain hospitals will be penalized if we don't do this right in terms of the fact that they have the highest-risk patients and we are not recognizing that. So I think there is a lot of work to be done in this space. I don't have the perfect solution yet because I want to make sure that we think about those unintended consequences as we move forward.

Ms. SCHAKOWSKY. So do you think bundled payments may be one thing that at least should be explored so that, from prenatal care through the full year, maybe issues like post partum depression be considered in a bundle of payments?

Dr. HOWELL. I think they should be explored. I think that the measures that they would be accountable for would need to be partnered with new quality measures that are really well developed and so that we have the right things. Some of those measures would also be targeting disparities. So, if you measure the success based on those quality metrics that look at patient-centeredness and disparities, it might be a promising avenue, but, again, always remembering that we can't penalize those hospitals that take care of the sickest patients. So we have to make sure that we are accounting for that in our models.

Ms. SCHAKOWSKY. We also want to make sure that diversity in the workforce is there so that everyone is represented at every level of care. Thank you so much.

And, again, Ms. Irving, thank you so much very much.

I yield back.

Ms. ESHOO. The gentlewoman yields back.

I want to, on behalf every member of the subcommittee, I want to thank each witness.

Ms. Irving, there really aren't words. You are a source of inspiration to us to move ahead in your daughter's name, in your name, in your granddaughter's name, and I think that if—I think as she is watching and listening from heaven, she is—you can hear the "Bravos" from there. Thank you. Thank you.

You really have, you have touched all of us, and we are not going to rest until we have solid legislation that addresses this and that this statistic in the United States of America piercing the conscience of our country, and I think it is a combination of things, women being undervalued, women not being listened to. In the history of humankind, no man has given birth to a child, and so I remember the doctor saying to me, "Well, they are the blues, but they will go away." So we have a lot of work to do. Thank you.

Thank you to you, Dr. Harris, Dr. Howell, Dr. Nelson, Ms. Ranji. This has been an outstanding hearing.

Mr. RUSH. Madam Chair, if I just could for 10 seconds.

Ms. ESHOO. Sure.

Mr. RUSH. Ms. Irving, I was just looking at some notes. Melanie was also in the healthcare area. She was a pharmaceutical sales manager. So she was very aware of health issues with doctors. Her husband was a physician, and she had a daughter, only child, and her name was Summer. So your granddaughter's name is Soleil. So there are so many similarities here.

I wanted to note that for the record.

Thank you, Madam Chair.

Ms. ESHOO. OK. I would like to remind Members that, pursuant to committee rules, they have 10 business days to submit additional questions for the record to be answered by the witnesses.

And I know that you will all cooperate, give straightforward, succinct answers. OK?

And I ask each witness to do so promptly to any questions that you may receive.

I now want to ask unanimous consent to enter into the record the following: a statement from the March of Dimes; a statement from the American College of Obstetricians and Gynecologists; a statement from the American Hospital Association; a statement from America's Health Insurance Plans; a report from the Center for American Progress on racial disparities and maternal mortality; a coalition letter from the American College of Nurse-Midwives, et al.; a statement from the Premier Healthcare Alliance; a statement from Gauss Surgical; a report from Premier Incorporated on maternal health trends; a report from ProPublica and NPR on maternal mortality.

So I ask for unanimous consent. Mr. GUTHRIE. No objection.

Ms. ESHOO. So ordered.

[The information is available at the conclusion of the hearing.][32]

Ms. ESHOO. And this will conclude our hearing today. The subcommittee is adjourned.

[Whereupon, at 1:25 p.m., the subcommittee was adjourned.]

[Material submitted for inclusion in the record follows:]

STATEMENT FOR THE RECORD SUBMITTED BY STACEY D. STEWART, PRESIDENT AND CEO, MARCH OF DIMES, HEARING OF THE HOUSE ENERGY & COMMERCE COMMITTEE'S SUBCOMMITTEE ON HEALTH, "IMPROVING MATERNAL HEALTH: LEGISLATION TO ADVANCE PREVENTION EFFORTS AND ACCESS TO CARE," TUESDAY, SEPTEMBER 10, 2019

March of Dimes, a unique collaboration of scientists, clinicians, parents, members of the business community, and other volunteers representing every state, the District of Columbia and Puerto Rico, appreciates this opportunity to submit testimony for the record for the hearing, "Improving Maternal Health: Legislation to Advance Prevention Efforts and Access to Care." March of Dimes applauds you for holding this hearing to consider policy proposals to address our nation's maternal health crisis.

Each day, in thousands of delivery rooms across the country, mothers cradle newborns wrapped in the iconic pink and blue stripped receiving blanket. They will bundle their new baby girl or boy in the same blanket as they go home for the first time, and swaddle their infant in the soft flannel during the early sleepless nights. Tragically, more than 700 infants will keep their hospital receiving blanket, but will not have their mothers to lovingly wrap them in it. In the United States, 700 mothers die from pregnancy-related causes each year, and more than 50,000 others experience dangerous complications that could have killed them - making the United States the most dangerous place in the developed world to give birth.[33] For women of color, the dangers of giving birth are even more acute. Black mothers of all ages are more than three times as likely to die from pregnancy-related complications as their white

[32] The Center for American Progress report has been retained in committee files and also is available at https://docs.house.gov/meetings/IF/IF14/20190910/109919/HHRG-116-IF14-20190910-SD006.pdf.

[33] March of Dimes. *Nowhere to Go: Maternity Care Deserts Across the U.S.* October 2018. Available at https://www.marchofdimes.org/materials/Nowhere_to_Go_Final.pdf.

peers.[34] The rates of pregnancy-related death for black and native women over the age of thirty are four to five times higher than their white peers.[35]

Our nation is in the midst of a crisis in maternal and child health. Virtually every measure of the health of pregnant women, new mothers, and infants is going in the wrong direction. Preterm birth rates are rising. In many communities, infant mortality rates exceed those in developing nations. Nations such as Slovenia and French Polynesia have a better infant mortality rate than the United States.[36]

Striking disparities exist among the health of mothers and babies of different racial and ethnic backgrounds. Black children face the highest child mortality rate among racial/ethnic groups – more than two times higher than the rate for Asian children and 1.5 times higher than the rate for white children.[37] There are dramatic variations in key measures like well-visits for women and infants among different racial and ethnic groups, as well as geographic areas.

Maternal Mortality and Severe Maternal Morbidity Are a Public Health Crisis

Women across the United States are tragically dying or suffering serious consequences from pregnancy-related causes. Despite the fact that many countries around the world have successfully reduced their maternal mortality rates since the 1990s, the U.S. rate is still higher than most other high-income countries,[38] and the U.S. maternal mortality rate has doubled in the past 25 years.[39] A significant racial and ethnic disparity in maternal mortality exists in the United States, with black women being three times more likely to die from pregnancy-related causes compared to white women.[40,41] These disparities cannot be explained by differences in age or education. According to the latest data from the Centers for Disease Control and Prevention (CDC), maternal mortality rates among black women with a

---

[34] Petersen EE, Davis NL, Goodman D, et al. Vital Signs: Pregnancy-Related Deaths, United States, 2011–2015, and Strategies for Prevention, 13 States, 2013–2017. MMWR Morb Mortal Wkly Rep 2019;68:423–429. Available at: http://dx.doi.org/10.15585/mmwr.mm6818e1.

[35] Petersen EE, Davis NL, Goodman D, et al. Racial/Ethnic Disparities in Pregnancy-Related Deaths — United States, 2007–2016. MMWR Morb Mortal Wkly Rep 2019;68:762–765. Available at: http://dx.doi.org/10.15585/mmwr.mm6835a3external.

[36] Central Intelliegence Agency. World Factbook: Infant Mortality Rate. Access May 2019. Available at https://www.cia.gov/library/publications/the-world-factbook/rankorder/2091rank.html.

[37] America's Health Rankings Health of Women and Children Report. March 2018. United Health Foundation. Available at https://assets.americashealthrankings.org/app/uploads/ahr_hwc_2018_report_summary_022818a.pdf.

[38] WHO. Trends in Maternal Mortality 1990-2015. Available at: http://www.who.int/reproductivehealth/publications/monitoring/maternal-mortality-2015/en/.

[39] CDC. Pregnancy Mortality Surveillance System. Available at: https://www.cdc.gov/reproductivehealth/maternalinfanthealth/pmss.html.

[40] Creanga AA, Berg CJ, Syverson C, Seed K, Bruce FC, Callaghan WM. Pregnancy-related mortality in the United States, 2006-2010. Obstet Gynecol 2015;125(1):5-12.

[41] Callaghan WM. Overview of maternal mortality in the United States. Semin Perinatol 2012;36(1):2-6.

completed college education or higher was 1.6 times that of white women with less than a high school diploma.[42]

Maternal mortality is also significantly higher in rural areas, where obstetrical providers may not be available,[43] and delivery in rural hospitals is associated with higher rates of postpartum hemorrhage.[44] In October 2018, March of Dimes released a report showing that 5 million women live in "maternity care deserts," which are communities without a hospital offering obstetric services or providers. Each year, 150,000 babies are born to mothers living in maternity care deserts.

Of the 700 pregnancy-related deaths in the United States, approximately one-third occur during pregnancy, another third happen during delivery and up to one week afterward, and the final third come in the year following delivery.[45] The CDC estimates that up to 60 percent of these deaths are preventable.[46] For every maternal death, there are about 100 episodes of severe maternal morbidity (SMM) affecting more than 50,000 women in the United States every year.[47] Black women are 27 percent more likely to experience severe pregnancy complications than white women.[48]

According to the CDC, pregnancy-related deaths are those that occur during pregnancy or within the following year due to pregnancy complications, because of a chain of events initiated by pregnancy, or because of an unrelated condition that was aggravated by pregnancy.[49] SMM includes unexpected outcomes of labor and delivery that result in significant short or longer term consequences to a woman's health.[50]

Causes of maternal deaths include cardiovascular conditions, hypertensive disorders of pregnancy (preeclampsia/eclampsia), infection, hemorrhage, suicide and drug overdose. Identifying and treating medical conditions before, during and after pregnancy are essential to preventing maternal morbidity and maternal mortality, as part of the continuum of care for all women of childbearing age. This requires a commitment to high-quality clinical care and enhanced maternal quality improvement

---

[42] Petersen EE, Davis NL, Goodman D, et al. Racial/Ethnic Disparities in Pregnancy-Related Deaths — United States, 2007–2016. MMWR Morb Mortal Wkly Rep 2019;68:762–765. Available at: http://dx.doi.org/10.15585/mmwr.mm6835a3external.

[43] Faron, Dina. Maternal Health Care is disappearing in rural America. Scientific American, February 15, 2017.

[44] Kozhimannil KB, Thao V, Hung P, Tilden E, Caughey AB, Snowden JM. Association between hospital birth volume and maternal morbidity among low-risk pregnancies in rural, urban, and teaching hospitals in the United States. Am J Perinatol 2016 May;33(6):590-9.

[45] Petersen EE, Davis NL, Goodman D, et al. Vital Signs: Pregnancy-Related Deaths, United States, 2011–2015, and Strategies for Prevention, 13 States, 2013–2017. MMWR Morb Mortal Wkly Rep 2019;68:423–429. Available at: http://dx.doi.org/10.15585/mmwr.mm6818e1.

[46] Ibid.

[47] CDC. Severe Maternal Morbidity in the United States. Available at: https://www.cdc.gov/reproductive health/maternalinfanthealth/severematernalmorbidity.html.

[48] Leonard SA, Main EK, Scott KA, et al. Racial and ethnic disparities in severe maternal morbidity prevalence and trends. Annals of Epidemiology 2019:33:30-36. Available at https://www.sciencedirect.com/science/article/pii/S1047279718308998.

[49] CDC. Pregnancy Mortality Surveillance System. Available at: https://www.cdc.gov/reproductive health/maternalinfanthealth/pmss.html

[50] CDC. Severe Maternal Morbidity in the United States. Available at: https://www.cdc.gov/ reproductivehealth/maternalinfanthealth/severematernalmorbidity.html.

and safety initiatives in hospitals, particularly those that address disparities, structural barriers to care, differential care experienced by women of color, and provider implicit racial bias.[51]

March of Dimes supports efforts to eliminate preventable maternal mortality and SMM and the unacceptable large disparities in rates experienced by black and native women. To achieve this, March of Dimes:

- Encourages every state to have a maternal mortality review committee (MMRC) that investigates each death of a pregnant woman or new mother to understand causes and recommend interventions for the future.
- Supports efforts to improve ways to collect data on maternal mortality and SMM, research into their causes and prevention, and promotion of proven ways to keep all mothers healthy.
- Champions policies to address provider implicit bias and eliminate systemic barriers in health care that perpetuate inequities in maternal health outcomes.
- Supports ensuring access to inpatient obstetrical facilities and qualified obstetrical providers, including Certified Nurse Midwives and Certified Midwives, in underserved and rural settings.
- Supports state perinatal quality collaboratives working with hospitals to identify and review cases of SMM and implement quality improvement initiatives to improve care and promote optimal maternal health.
- Supports efforts to ensure that all women have quality, affordable health insurance and health care to include but not limited to postpartum depression screening, mental health treatment, substance use treatment, affordable contraception, including long-acting reversible contraception (LARC), and access to health care providers who understand and meet their health needs before, during and after pregnancy.
- Champions extending health insurance coverage offered to new mothers through Medicaid and the Children's Health Insurance Program (CHIP) to a full year after pregnancy.
- Supports improving the social and economic conditions and quality of health care at all stages of a woman's life.
- Encourages acceleration of policies and programs shown to provide preventive and supportive care for women during pregnancy and childbirth, including group prenatal care and coverage for doula services.

---

[51] Jain JA, Temming LA, D'Alton ME, et al. SMFM Special Report: Putting the "M" back in MFM: Reducing racial and ethnic disparities in maternal morbidity and mortality: A call to action. Am J Obstet Gynecol 2018;218(2):B9-B17.

Opportunities for Congressional Action

Last year, Congress took an important step toward addressing the nation's maternal mortality crisis by passing the *Preventing Maternal Deaths Act of 2018* (P.L. 115-344). This legislation is helping states to support MMRCs to review each instance of maternal death and develop recommendations to prevent them in the future. In FY 2019, Congress also provided $50 million in new funding to support state reviews and other activities to protect the health of pregnant women and new mothers.

Congress cannot stop now. We know that the causes of maternal mortality and SMM are diverse; they include physical health, mental health, social determinants, and much more. They can be traced back to issues in our health care system, including quality of care, systemic problems, and implicit bias. They stem from factors in our homes, our workplaces, and our communities. The effort to save women's lives can't just end with one bill. Congress must build upon its record of success by advancing a comprehensive legislative package in the 116th Congress that incorporates the principles outlined above. March of Dimes has endorsed several bills in this Congress (Table 1) that advance these important tenets.

Table 1.

MOMMA's Act (H.R. 1897/S. 916) *Rep. Robin Kelly (D-IL) Sen. Dick Durbin (D-IL)*	• Authorizes the Alliance for Innovation on Maternal Health (AIM) program and state-based perinatal quality collaboratives (PQCs). • Extends postpartum coverage for women served by Medicaid, the Children's Health Insurance Programs (CHIP), and the Special Supplemental Nutrition • Program for Women, Infants and Children (WIC). • Supports implicit bias and cultural competency training. • Improves national maternal mortality surveillance.
Quality Care for Moms and Babies Act (H.R. 1551/S. 1960) *Reps. Eliot Engel (D-NY) and Steve Stivers (R-OH)* *Sen. Debbie Stabenow (D-MI) and* *Sen. Susan Collins (R-ME)*	• Authorizes state-based PQCs. • Creates a core set of maternal care quality measures.
MOMS Act (S. 116) *Sen. Kirsten Gillibrand (D-NY)*	• Authorizes the AIM program and supports hospital implementation of best practices. • Improves national maternal mortality surveillance.
MOMMIES Act (H.R. 2602/S. 1343) *Rep. Ayanna Pressley (D-MA) Sen. Cory Booker (D-NJ)*	• Extends postpartum coverage for women served by Medicaid and CHIP. • Creates a maternity care home demonstration project. • Requires reports on access to doula care and how states are using telemedicine to increase access to maternity care.

Maternal Care Access and Reducing Emergencies (Maternal CARE) Act (S. 1600) *Sen. Kamala Harris (D-CA)*	• Support evidence-based implicit bias training. • Establishes a demonstration project for implementing pregnancy medical homes. • Directs the National Academy of Medicine to make recommendations for incorporating implicit bias • recognition in U.S. medical schools.
The Healthy Maternity and Obstetric Medicine Act (Healthy MOM Act) (H.R. 2778/S. 1481) *Rep. Bonnie Watson Coleman (D-NJ) Sen. Sherrod Brown (D-OH)*	• Establishes a special enrollment period for expectant mothers to sign up for health insurance. • Extends postpartum coverage for women served by Medicaid. • Ensures comprehensive coverage of maternity care.
Rural Maternal and Obstetric Modernization of Services (MOMS) Act (S. 2373) *Sens. Tina Smith (D-MN), Lisa Murkowski (R-AK), Doug Jones (D-AL), and Shelley Moore Capito (R-WV)*	• Establishes new rural obstetric network grants. • Integrates maternal and obstetric care into existing federal telehealth grant programs. • Creates a new rural maternal and obstetric care training program. • Improves rural maternal and obstetric care data.

We are pleased that today's hearing will focus specifically on the MOMMA's Act (H.R. 1897), the Quality Care for Moms and Babies Act (H.R. 1551), the Maternal CARE Act (H.R. 2902) and the Healthy MOMMIES Act (H.R. 2602). Each one of these bills includes proposals that are essential to address the multifaceted contributors to maternal mortality and SMM. March of Dimes thanks Reps. Robin Kelly (D-IL), Eliot Engel (D-NY), Steve Stivers (R-OH), Alma Adams (D-NC) and Ayanna Pressley (D-MA) for championing maternal health and spearheading these important bills.

March of Dimes encourages the Energy & Commerce Committee to demonstrate its commitment to healthy mothers by working in a bipartisan fashion to craft a comprehensive legislative package to address maternal mortality and SMM that incorporates proposals from H.R. 1551, H.R. 1897, H.R. 2902, H.R. 2602, and the other bills listed below. We stand ready to assist you in this effort to protect and improve the health of all women and babies.

Statement for the Record of the American College of Obstetricians and Gynecologists, Before the House Committee on Energy & Commerce, Subcommittee on Health, Regarding the Hearing, Improving Maternal Health: Legislation to Advance Prevention Efforts and Access to Care, September 10, 2019

Chairwoman Eshoo, Dr. Burgess, Chairman Pallone, Ranking Member Walden, and distinguished members of the House Energy & Commerce Subcommittee on

Health, thank you for holding today's hearing entitled "Improving Maternal Health: Legislation to Advance Prevention Efforts and Access to Care." The American College of Obstetricians and Gynecologists (ACOG), is pleased to submit this statement for the record in support of your efforts to advance bipartisan legislation to improve maternal health outcomes. ACOG, with a membership of more than 58,000, is the leading physician organization dedicated to advancing women's health. Key to that mission is our core value that all women should have access to affordable, high-quality, safe health care.

Background

As you know, the United States has a maternal mortality crisis. More than 700 women die each year in the United States from pregnancy-related or pregnancy-associated complications.[52] We have a higher maternal mortality rate than any other developed country. At a time when 157 of 183 countries in the world report decreases in maternal mortality, ours is rising.[53] Black women and Native American/Alaska Native women are two to three times more likely to experience a pregnancy-related mortality than white women.[54] For every maternal death in the United States, there are 100 women who experience severe maternal morbidity, or a "near miss." This is all unacceptable, and the time for action is now.

ACOG is committed to our goal of eliminating preventable maternal deaths, and we are eager to continue our strong partnership with this Committee and other valuable partners to achieve this important goal.

We know, and the Centers for Disease Control and Prevention (CDC) has confirmed, that over 60 percent of maternal deaths are preventable.[55] Common causes include hemorrhage, cardiovascular and coronary conditions, cardiomyopathy, and infection. Overdose and suicide, driven primarily by the opioid epidemic, are also emerging as leading causes of maternal mortality in a growing number of states.[56] If we have a clear understanding of why these deaths are occurring, and what we can do to prevent them in the future, we can save women's lives.

We applaud this Committee and your colleagues in the US Congress for taking an important first step last year in passing the Preventing Maternal Deaths Act, P.L. 115-344, to encourage states to create and expand maternal mortality review

---

[52] Building U.S. Capacity to Review and Prevent Maternal Deaths. (2018). Report from nine maternal mortality review committees. Retrieved from http://reviewtoaction.org/Report_from_Nine_MMRCs.

[53] Lu MC. Reducing Maternal Mortality in the United States. JAMA. Published online September 10, 2018. doi:10.1001/jama.2018.11652.

[54] Petersen EE, Davis NL, Goodman D, et al. Racial/Ethnic Disparities in Pregnancy-Related Deaths — United States, 2007–2016. MMWR Morb Mortal Wkly Rep 2019;68:762–765. DOI: http://dx.doi.org/10.15585/mmwr.mm6835a3.

[55] Building U.S. Capacity to Review and Prevent Maternal Deaths. (2018). Report from nine maternal mortality review committees. Retrieved from http://reviewtoaction.org/Report_from_Nine_MMRCs.

[56] Ibid.

committees (MMRCs). MMRCs are multidisciplinary groups of local experts in maternal and public health, as well as patient and community advocates, that closely examine individual maternal deaths and identify locally-relevant ways to prevent future deaths, saving mothers' lives. While traditional public health surveillance using vital statistics can tell us about trends and disparities, MMRCs are best positioned to comprehensively assess and characterize maternal deaths, to understand the causes and contributing factors and identify opportunities for prevention.

The CDC recently announced the first round of funding for the newly established Enhancing Reviews and Surveillance to Eliminate Maternal Mortality (ERASE MM) Program, supporting 25 states in their efforts to coordinate and manage MMRCs. This rapid implementation of P.L. 115-344 enables us to look ahead to how we can support states in their efforts to translate the findings of their MMRCs to meaningful action and improved maternal health outcomes.

Accelerating Evidence-Based Patient Safety Changes

Once those opportunities for prevention are identified by MMRCs, states can best target resources toward needed interventions. The Alliance for Innovation on Maternal Health, or the AIM program, is helping translate MMRC findings and recommendations into action at the state and facility levels. The AIM program is a national cross-sector, data-driven maternal safety and quality improvement initiative working in partnership with states, birthing facilities, and communities to increase adoption of evidence-based maternal safety best practices. Launched in 2014, the AIM program is funded through a cooperative agreement from the U.S. Department of Health and Human Services (HHS), Health Resources and Services Administration's (HRSA) Maternal and Child Health Bureau (MCHB). Program activities are implemented with oversight and program management from ACOG staff members.

The goal of AIM is to reduce maternal deaths and severe maternal morbidity by engaging provider organizations, state-based public health systems, consumer groups, and other stakeholders within a national partnership to assist state-based teams in implementing evidence-based maternal safety best practices. AIM's vision is to offer every pregnant woman in the US a safe birthing experience by improving the culture and delivery of maternity care services. AIM's goal is accomplished through 1) promoting safe and respectful maternal care for every US birth, 2) engaging multidisciplinary partners at the national, state and hospital levels, 3) developing and implementing evidence-based maternal safety best practices, 4) utilizing data-driven quality improvement strategies, and 5) aligning existing safety efforts and developing, collecting, and promoting the use of maternal safety resources.

To participate in the AIM program, states must have an MMRC or another state-focused initiative that collects, analyzes, and reports maternal health outcome data. Also key to the successful implementation of the AIM program are state perinatal quality collaboratives (PQCs), largely considered the implementation arm of MMRCs. The CDC provides oversight and resources to PQCs through its National Network on Perinatal Quality Collaboratives (NNPQC), which is focused on accelerating improvement efforts for both maternal and infant health outcomes. This coordinated collaboration at the federal level helps to support and enhance the ability of PQCs to adopt and implement AIM maternal safety bundles. Hospitals and health systems implementing AIM's evidence-based maternal safety best practices, such as obstetric hemorrhage, severe hypertension in pregnancy, and obstetric care for women with opioid use disorder, aren't bound by a single protocol, but instead have a standard framework for each facility to develop protocols specific to its resources and patients. Currently in the pilot phase is a maternal safety best practice tool specific to reduction of racial/ethnic disparities, with the goal of incorporating into each AIM patient-safety best practice.

Implementation of a particular program is not enough to achieve meaningful, sustained change in outcomes. AIM promotes a culture of safety and teamwork, encouraging multidisciplinary drills for obgyns, anesthesiologists, certified nurse-midwives, nurses, and laboratory staff, to ensure readiness of the team for complications that may be rare, but are life-threatening.

AIM is now in 27 states, reaching roughly 1300 birthing facilities in the US. Early indications support AIM as a critical way we as a Nation can help ensure high quality maternity care for every woman, regardless of her race, income, or location.

At the same time, we must address the rural access gap, exacerbated by the rapid rate of rural hospital closures and the shuttering of obstetric units, and its impact on adverse maternal health outcomes. ACOG is working closely with the American Academy of Family Physicians and the National Rural Health Association to ensure access to high quality maternity care for every woman, regardless of if you live in a rural, urban, or suburban community. As the Committee considers potential actions to address maternal mortality, we urge you to keep this access concern front of mind, support policies that increase the number of physicians and nurses practicing in rural communities, and ensure that no actions unintentionally exacerbate rural access gaps.

Addressing Racial Disparities

While there is an AIM bundle specific to reducing perinatal racial and ethnic disparities, we know that is just a start, providing the guidance for collection of data, utilization of a disparities dashboard in all birthing facilities and clinics, and examination of bias. We intend to incorporate mechanisms to address disparities in all AIM bundles.

To help achieve that in a meaningful way, ACOG is working with our partners at the National Birth Equity Collaborative and the California Maternal Quality Care Collaborative to eliminate preventable maternal mortality by raising up the voices and experiences of Black women through Mother's Voices Driving Birth Equity, a project funded by the Robert Wood Johnson Foundation. This work is being led by Black scholars to better understand Black women's birth experiences in different geographic regions.

Through this project, we'll be able to incorporate patient voices and lived experiences in our patient safety work. If we hope to change how care is delivered, we must ensure that the methods hospitals and clinicians use to address implicit bias and racism align with Black women's needs, values, and preferences. Black women's feedback must be a driver for quality improvement measures.

We recognize that we – and all care providers – have work to do and are committed to addressing implicit bias and increasing the provision of culturally competent care to our patients.

Extending Medicaid Coverage Postpartum

Medicaid is the largest single payer of maternity care in the US, covering 42.6% of births.[57],[58] Yet that coverage ends roughly 60-days postpartum. As MMRCs have increasingly revealed, many deaths related to pregnancy occur after this time. In fact, the CDC estimates that 33% of maternal deaths occur one week to 12 months after delivery, which is likely underestimated as the CDC assessment did not account for deaths from overdose, suicide, homicide, or unintentional injury.[59] Accordingly, a number of MMRCs have recommended extending Medicaid coverage for women to a full year postpartum.[60,61,62,63,64] Already, federal statute requires that a baby born to a mother on Medicaid is covered under Medicaid through the first year of life.

---

[57] Martin JA, Hamilton BE, Osterman MJK, Driscoll AK, and Drake P. Births: Final Data for 2016. National vital statistics reports; vol 67 no 1. Hyattsville, MD: National Center for Health Statistics. 2018. Retrieved from https://www.cdc.gov/nchs/data/nvsr/nvsr67/nvsr67_01.pdf.

[58] The percent of births financed by Medicaid is higher in certain states. For instance, based on the latest available data, Medicaid financed 58% of births in Alabama (2010) and 54% of births in Georgia (2014). Source: Vernon K. Smith, Kathleen Gifford, Eileen Ellis, and Barbara Edwards, Health Management Associates; and Robin Rudowitz, Elizabeth Hinton, Larisa Antonisse and Allison Valentine, Kaiser Commission on Medicaid and the Uninsured. Implementing Coverage and Payment Initiatives: Results from a 50-State Medicaid Budget Survey for State Fiscal Years 2016 and 2017, The Henry J. Kaiser Family Foundation, October 2016.

[59] Petersen EE, Davis NL, Goodman D, et al. Vital Signs: Pregnancy-Related Deaths, United States, 2011–2015, and Strategies for Prevention, 13 States, 2013–2017. MMWR Morb Mortal Wkly Rep 2019;68:423–429. DOI: http://dx.doi.org/10.15585/mmwr.mm6818e1.

[60] Maternal Mortality and Morbidity Task Force and Department of State Health Services Joint Biennial Report, September 2018. Retrieved from https://www.dshs.texas.gov/mch/pdf/MMMTFJoint Report2018.pdf.

[61] Illinois Maternal Morbidity and Mortality Report. Illinois Department of Public Health. (October 2018). Retrieved from http://dph.illinois.gov/sites/default/files/publications/publicationsowhmaternalmorbiditymortalityreport 112018.pdf.

[62] Maternal Mortality Report. Georgia Department of Public Health. (2014). Retrieved from https://reviewtoaction.org/sites/default/files/portal_resources/Maternal%20Mortality%20BookletGeor gia.FINAL_. hq_.pdf.

[63] Perinatal Mortality Review: Maternal Mortality in Utah 2015-2016. Utah Department of Health. (July 2018). Retrieved from https://mihp.utah.gov/wp-content/uploads/PMR-Update-0718.pdf.

As Congress explores additional ways to improve health outcomes, closing this critical gap in coverage during this incredibly vulnerable time can mean the difference between life and death for some women.

What Can Congress Do: Enact a MOMNIBUS

Thank you for enacting the Preventing Maternal Deaths Act, a critical step in our efforts to eliminate preventable maternal mortality. We urge this Committee and the Congress to build on its commitment to healthy moms and babies, and take important next steps.

As the Committee considers actions to take in the 116th Congress, ACOG urges you to prioritize four key initiatives to accelerate evidence-based patient safety changes:

1. Support the AIM program, as included in HR 1897, the MOMMA's Act, sponsored by Representative Robin Kelly (D-IL) and HR 4215, the Excellence in Maternal Health Act, sponsored by Representatives Larry Bucshon, MD (R-IN) and Andre Carson (D-IN). Help achieve AIM's vision to offer every pregnant woman in the US a safe birth by changing the culture of maternity care with authorization of the program.
2. Support state-based perinatal quality collaboratives, as included in HR 1551, the Quality Care for Moms and Babies Act, sponsored by Representatives Eliot Engel (D-NY) and Steve Stivers (R-OH), HR 1897, the MOMMA's Act, and HR 4215, the Excellence in Maternal Health Act. Collaboratives bring together local experts to accelerate adoption of best practices, including recommendations of MMRCs and AIM safety protocols. Additional federal investment would help ensure collaboratives have the resources they need to continue to spearhead state and regional quality improvement work.
3. Support efforts to end racial and ethnic disparities in maternal outcomes, as included in HR 2902, the Maternal CARE Act, sponsored by Representative Alma Adams (D-NC), HR 1897, the MOMMA's Act, and HR 4215, the Excellence in Maternal Health Act. While ACOG's work continues, we support proposals to establish implicit bias and cultural competency training programs for medical students, residents, and practicing health care professionals.
4. Extend Medicaid coverage to 12-months postpartum, as included in HR 1897, the MOMMA's Act and HR 2778, the Healthy MOM Act, sponsored by Representative Bonnie Watson Coleman (D-NJ). Notably, the CDC, in its

---

[64] Maternal Mortality Review: A Report on Maternal Deaths in Washington 2014-2015. Washington State Department of Health. (July 2017). Retrieved from https://www.doh.wa.gov/Portals/1/Documents/Pubs/140-154-MMRReport.pdf.

recent *Vital Signs* report, included extending Medicaid coverage as a strategy to prevent pregnancy-related deaths.[65]

We're extremely pleased that so many congressional leaders have recognized and are committed to this important issue, with a number of key bills supporting the initiatives listed above. Packaged together as a "MOMNIBUS," these provisions would have a meaningful impact on women and families and improve maternal health outcomes.

Thank you for the opportunity to share our work with you today. We are making significant and meaningful progress on the path to better maternal outcomes for all moms, and look forward to working together with you to achieve our goal of eliminating preventable maternal mortality.

Statement of the American Hospital Association, for the Subcommittee on Health of the Committee on Energy and Commerce of the U.S. House of Representatives, "Improving Maternal Health: Legislation to Advance Prevention Efforts and Access to Care," September 10, 2019

On behalf of our nearly 5,000 member hospitals, health systems and other health care organizations, our clinician partners – including more than 270,000 affiliated physicians, 2 million nurses and other caregivers – and the 43,000 health care leaders who belong to our professional membership groups, the American Hospital Association (AHA) commends the Committee on Energy and Commerce for its efforts to examine legislation to improve maternal health.

Maternal health is a top priority for the AHA and our member hospitals and health systems, and our initial efforts are aimed at eliminating maternal mortality and severe morbidity. The causes of maternal mortality and morbidity are complex, including a lack of consistent access to comprehensive care and persistent racial disparities in health and health care. As hospitals work to improve health outcomes, we are redoubling our efforts to improve maternal health across the continuum of care and reaching out to community partners to aid in that important effort.

The May 2019 *Vital Signs* report issued by the Centers for Disease Control and Prevention (CDC) noted that about 700 women die each year from complications related to pregnancy, and more than half of those deaths are preventable. An estimated 31% of pregnancy-related deaths occur during pregnancy, 36% during delivery or the week after, and 33% one week to one year after delivery. The CDC last week released its Morbidity and Mortality Weekly Report that showed that

[65] Petersen EE, Davis NL, Goodman D, et al. Vital Signs: Pregnancy-Related Deaths, United States, 2011–2015, and Strategies for Prevention, 13 States, 2013–2017. MMWR Morb Mortal Wkly Rep 2019;68:423–429. DOI: http://dx.doi.org/10.15585/mmwr.mm6818e1.

between 2007-2016, the pregnancy-related mortality ratio increased from 15 to 17 pregnancy-related deaths per 100,000 births and that black, American Indian and Alaska Native women were two to three times more likely to die from pregnancy-related causes than white women, and this disparity increases with age. The report also noted that racial and ethnic disparities in pregnancy-related deaths have persisted over time.

AHA Activity on Maternal Health

The AHA has been active in improving maternal health by working to reduce early-elective deliveries, unnecessary caesarian sections, obstetric hemorrhage and preeclampsia, and substance use disorders. We also partner with national organizations to safeguard mothers and babies, both before and after delivery. For example, we are a member of the Alliance for Innovation on Maternal Health (AIM), a national, data-driven maternal safety and quality initiative with proven implementation approaches to improving maternal safety and outcomes.

Within the AHA, our *Better Health for Mothers and Babies* initiative serves as the organizational framework for addressing maternal morbidity and mortality. We recognize that mothers are at risk from the first days of pregnancy through the postpartum period, and know that hospitals and their community partners want to do more to improve their care.

The AHA provides a number of resources to our members, including:

- Evidence-based tools that can be implemented by hospitals of all sizes, such as AIM patient safety bundles, California Maternal Quality Care Collaborative toolkits, the Centers for Medicare & Medicaid Services' (CMS) Maternal Opioid Misuse Model, and recommendations from maternal mortality review committees (MMRCs);
- Information for patients and families about the mental health conditions associated with pregnancy and screening recommendations, as well as initiatives from the March of Dimes and Merck for Mothers, among others; and
- Links to clinical organizations, including the CMS Strong Start for Mothers and Newborns Initiative and the Council on Patient Safety in Women's Health Care.

Recently, we developed an Action Plan and Checklist to help our members meet the goal of eliminating maternal mortality and reducing severe morbidity. They include recommendations for providers and toolkits reflecting best-practices to help hospitals and health systems evaluate and act on their data.

The Action Plan recommends that hospitals:

1. Evaluate and act on data.
2. Examine disparities.
3. Engage mothers and families.
4. Partner with clinicians and stakeholders in their community.

This Action Plan is being implemented in partnership with the AHA Physician Alliance; American Organization for Nursing Leadership; Institute for Diversity and Health Equity; the state, regional and metropolitan hospital associations; and AIM.

We also developed a Discussion Guide to help hospital-based clinicians – working with community-based providers and other stakeholders – improve access to care and reduce health inequities for expectant and new mothers. The guide is designed to facilitate discussion and information-sharing within a hospital or health system's practice and among providers across the continuum, covering prenatal care, labor and delivery, discharge protocols and the postpartum period.

Our most recent advisory to the field shares an interactive Data Visualization and Infographic that highlight racial disparities in maternal health. The Data Visualization allows hospital, health system and state, regional and metropolitan hospital association leaders to examine maternal mortality data, which is stratified by race and time of maternal death (up to 42 days and one year), by U.S., region and state.

In addition to the resources outlined above, the *Better Health for Mothers and Babies* website features podcasts, webinars and case studies focused on the field's ongoing work to improve maternal health.

Supporting Changes in Legislation and Accreditation

At the federal level, a number of legislative initiatives specific to maternal mortality have been introduced. The AHA supported legislation enacted last year, the Preventing Maternal Deaths Act, which provides funding through the CDC for states and other entities to develop MMRCs. While some states and cities already have established MMRCs, participation by all states will allow for the collection of additional data that will aid in better understanding the causes of maternal mortality and ways to improve treatment. CDC is awarding more than $45 million over five years to support MMRCs through the Enhancing Reviews and Surveillance to Eliminate Maternal Mortality program. This investment will provide about $9 million a year to 24 recipients representing 25 states. We also applaud the establishment of the Black Maternal Health Caucus, whose membership includes several members of this Committee. The Caucus is working to elevate awareness about the alarming rates of maternal morbidity and mortality affecting black women and promote evidence-based policy solutions.

Mothers and Offspring Mortality and Morbidity Awareness (MOMMA's) Act

We support provisions of Rep. Robin Kelly's MOMMA's Act (H.R. 1897), including those that would:

- Improve data collection by establishing federal initiatives to assist states with reporting comprehensive data on maternal mortality and encourage uniformity in reporting and data sharing among states;
- Disseminate best practices to hospitals, professional societies and perinatal collaboratives regarding how to prevent maternal mortality;
- Fund an AIM grant program to promote the widespread adoption of maternal safety bundles at the state level;
- Fund state-based perinatal collaboratives to improve outcomes for pregnant and postpartum women and their infants;
- Extend postpartum coverage for women enrolled in Medicaid and the Children's Health Insurance Program for up to one year, allowing providers to better coordinate services for mothers across the continuum of care;
- Address implicit bias and cultural competency by improving training for health care professionals regarding implicit bias and cultural competence; and
- Extend the Special Supplemental Nutrition Program for Women, Infants and Children (WIC) program for two years postpartum, an increase from the current standard of one year.

Quality Care for Moms and Babies Act

We support efforts to improve maternal and child health through better collection of quality data and implementation of quality collaboratives, as outlined in Rep. Eliot Engel's Quality Care for Moms and Babies Act (H.R. 1551). We would make the following recommendations should the Committee decide to advance this legislation:

- We support the goal of implementing maternity/child health quality measures for Medicaid and the Children's Health Insurance Program, given the importance of these programs in providing coverage for pregnant women and children, but believe the effort should go further. To that end, we would recommend that the Secretary of Health and Human Services be instructed to seek endorsement of the measures from a national voluntary standards setting body and engage other organizations, such as private insurers, in seeking to identify those practices and strategies that lead to better maternal outcomes and track progress as those strategies are deployed nationally;
- Rather than establishing a separate Maternity Consumer Assessment of Health Care Providers and Systems (CAHPS) survey, we would recommend the addition of questions to the Hospital CAHPS survey, starting with a screener question that asks: "Were you hospitalized to give birth?" If the person answers "yes," then they would receive a small number of questions

to answer that directly address the issues of providing care to mothers and infants; and

- Regarding the establishment of maternal and child health quality collaboratives, because CMS already employs the National Quality Improvement and Innovation Contract (NQIIC) mechanism, and a set of qualified improvement organizations are identified and ready to operate, using the NQIIC could expedite the establishment of the quality collaboratives envisioned by H.R. 1551. We suggest that the bill appropriate funding to an entity such as the CDC and instruct them to consider working with CMS's established contractors.

Healthy MOMMIES Act

We support provisions of Rep. Ayanna Pressley's Healthy MOMMIES Act (H.R. 2602), including those that would:

- Extend postpartum coverage for women enrolled in Medicaid and the Children's Health Insurance Program for up to one year, allowing providers to better coordinate services for mothers across the continuum of care; and
- Establish a maternal home demonstration program.

Maternal Care Access and Reducing Emergencies (CARE) Act

We support provisions of Rep. Alma Adams' Maternal CARE Act (H.R. 2902), including those that would:

- Establish a grant program to support implicit bias for training health care professionals; and
- Establish a maternal home demonstration program.

The AHA will continue to evaluate maternal health legislation as it is introduced.

Joint Commission

The Joint Commission, which accredits more than 21,000 U.S. health care organizations and programs, including hospitals and health systems, recently adopted standards for perinatal safety. The standards are effective as of July 1, 2020 and hospitals' compliance will be evaluated during accreditation surveys. The AHA supports the Joint Commission's focus on evidence-based procedures and responses that will ensure the most medically appropriate and effective course of treatment for women diagnosed with either maternal hemorrhage or severe hypertension/preeclampsia. In addition, we support the requirement for education of staff, and believe conducting complication-specific training and drills will better prepare providers to act effectively and efficiently when these situations arise. Further, we support standards to provide patients and their families with the necessary educational materials to recognize symptoms that require immediate care as another important safeguard in this process.

Conclusion

Thank you for the opportunity to share information regarding hospitals and health systems' efforts to address maternal morbidity and mortality. We look forward to working with partners in the health care field, policymakers – including the Committee on Energy and Commerce – and community organizations to improve outcomes and reduce health inequities for expectant and new mothers, and give their children the best possible start in life.

Statement for Hearing on "Improving Maternal Health: Legislation to Advance Prevention Efforts and Access to Care," Submitted to the House Energy and Commerce Committee, September 10, 2019

America's Health Insurance Plans (AHIP)[66] thanks the Committee for focusing on the important issue of maternal health. Despite the growing sophistication of the U.S. health care system and the increasing quality of care for women during pregnancy, childbirth, and post-partum, relative to other high-income countries, women in the United States still have the highest rate of maternal mortality. This problem is particularly acute among women of color. Recently, the Centers for Disease Control and Prevention (CDC) released data showing that African-American, Native American, and Alaska native women die of pregnancy-related causes at a rate nearly three times higher than those of white women.[67]

AHIP believes that all Americans deserve high-quality, accessible and affordable maternal, newborn and infant health care. Health insurance providers cover and improve access to maternity care and work hard to identify and address health disparities. An issue brief that AHIP released last December outlines many strategies that health insurance providers are pursuing to improve women's health.[68]

We welcome additional opportunities to work with the Committee and other key stakeholders - such as our provider partners state, federal and local governments;

---

[66] AHIP is the national association whose members provide coverage for health care and related services to millions of Americans every day. Through these offerings, we improve and protect the health and financial security of consumers, families, businesses, communities, and the nation. We are committed to market-based solutions and public-private partnerships that improve affordability, value, access, and well-being for consumers.

[67] https://www.cdc.gov/mmwr/volumes/68/wr/mm6835a3.htm?s_cid=mm6835a3_w.

[68] Health Plans' Commitment to Improving Women's Reproductive Health, Issue Brief, November 2018, AHIP https://www.ahip.org/wp-content/uploads/2018/11/IB_WomensHealth-112118-FINAL.pdf.

community partners; and our employer, government and individual customers - to tackle this important issue.

Women's Health Care Is a Priority for Health Insurance Providers

Health insurance providers cover the full continuum of health care services for women, including expectant mothers. These services encompass prevention (e.g., annual gynecological well woman exams, contraception, Human Papillomavirus (HPV) vaccine) and screening (e.g., mammography, cervical and ovarian cancer screening), prenatal care, maternity and postpartum health, mental health care, and more. Under the requirements of the Affordable Care Act (ACA), maternity and newborn care are covered as part of the Essential Health Benefits (EHB) delivered by all qualified health plans and nearly all plans offered in the group market.

In addition, health insurance providers support recommendations from the U.S. Preventive Services Task Force (USPSTF) and the CDC Advisory Council for Immunization Practices (ACIP) pertaining to pre- and post-natal care. Women, newborns, and infants receive coverage for these services with no cost sharing or co-payments, per the provisions of the ACA.

Beyond these requirements, health plans deliver a wide range of maternity-related care and case management services as outlined throughout our statement and in our Women's Health Issue Brief.

Preventive Care Is the Foundation of Good Health

Improving preventive care for women is a top priority of health insurance providers. When delivered by an in-network provider, health plans cover recommended screenings for women with no cost-sharing. For women who are pregnant or may become pregnant, these services include anemia screening; breastfeeding support and counseling; contraception; folic acid supplements; gestational diabetes screening; gonorrhea screening; Hepatitis B screening; preeclampsia prevention and screening; Rh incompatibility screening; syphilis screening; expanded tobacco intervention counseling; and urinary tract or other infection screening.

Vaccines are also an essential preventive measure that insurance providers strongly support. To promote adoption of the HPV vaccine, for example, health insurance providers communicate with clinicians to encourage the routine provision of the vaccine and to offer guidance on how they may discuss the importance of the vaccine with children and their parents; incorporate the administration of the vaccine in quality measures on which providers are measured; provide financial incentives to encourage providers to offer the vaccine; and communicate with patients about the safety, efficacy, and purpose of the vaccine, and the importance of completing the vaccine series to ensure full protection.

Despite the presence of coverage and outreach from health plans encouraging members to use preventive services and prescribers to administer these services with no cost sharing, preventive services are still underused. Health insurance providers continuously evaluate their member engagement strategies to improve the use of these preventive services and reduce disparities.

Breaking Down Social Barriers to Good Health

Health insurance providers are committed to ensuring that patients and consumers receive high-quality care during pregnancy, childbirth and after delivery. As part of that commitment, insurance providers are addressing certain social determinants of health that may lead to disparities in care. Research shows that these social factors (the conditions and environment in which people are born, grow, live, work and age) can have a tremendous impact on a person's health. Health insurance providers are increasingly developing and expanding programs to address social barriers to help American families with housing, transportation, food, and educational opportunities as complements to traditional health services.

Successfully addressing social barriers and health care disparities requires cultural competency among our health care institutions. Cultural competency reflects how clinicians, health insurance providers, and other organizations deliver health care services to meet the social, cultural, and linguistic needs of patients. Research shows that racial and ethnic minorities are often disproportionately burdened by chronic illness and disease. Health insurance providers understand that every patient has different needs, and our member companies invest in strategies and programs to reach people where they are to improve their health outcomes.

As a part of these efforts, health insurance providers are increasingly focused on racial disparities in pregnancy and birth outcomes and their implications for maternal health.[69] Our members work collaboratively with doctors and hospitals to deliver culturally competent care, and to use state of the art research and analytics to identify potentially high-risk pregnancies. Early identification and intervention in high-risk pregnancies can improve the mother's care experience, better identify comorbidities during pregnancy, and increase the chances of delivering full-term, healthy babies.

Unfortunately, at-risk expectant women often seek care later in their pregnancies, potentially missing the window for vital prenatal care. Leveraging data and predictive analytics tools, health insurance providers are able to identify high-risk pregnancies

---

[69] "Weathering" and Age Patterns of Allostatic Load Scores Among Blacks and Whites in the United States, Arline T. Geronimus, ScD, Margaret Hicken, MPH, Danya Keene, MAT, and John Bound, PhD. Am J Public Health. 2006 May; 96(5): 826–833. doi: 10.2105/AJPH.2004.060749.

early on and connect mothers-to-be with necessary clinical care, education, and social supports.

Health insurance providers are continually developing ways to engage with patients and consumers and encourage them to use maternity care effectively. Often, insurance providers leverage care management services, community health workers, and other care team members to help coordinate care. For example, several of our member health insurance providers use nurse care managers to contact expectant mothers who are experiencing a high-risk pregnancy to provide regular pre-natal coaching. The care team members follow these patients throughout their pregnancy and post-partum checkups and coordinate care with the mother's doctors. These types of approaches can improve maternal and infant outcomes.

These experts also provide support in addressing socioeconomic factors that may impact a woman's pregnancy. Care team members connect expectant mothers with resources, such as access to healthy foods, baby supplies, housing, and even mobile technologies for those who may not have reliable access to communication platforms. For example, one insurance provider launched a program to offer integrated case management, care coordination, and disease management for expectant mothers through the first year of their infants' life. As a result of this program, there has been a statistically significant improvement in delivery outcomes and a decrease in low- and very low-infant birth weights.[70]

After pregnancy and delivery, health insurance providers strive to find ways to support new moms as well as their newborns and infants. Many health insurance providers offer early childhood support services; nutritional assistance for pregnant women, mothers, and children; and case management services that can help mothers coordinate their care.

Networks Rely on Meeting Clinical Guidelines, Quality Metrics, and Accreditation Standards

To improve the birth outcomes of both mothers and their babies, maternity care must be safe, guided by sound medical evidence, and affordable. To support these goals, health insurance providers require hospitals in their networks to adhere to peer-reviewed medical guidelines for maternity care.

Clinical guidelines and quality metrics for maternal and infant care are set by independent experts, provider professional societies, government, and credentialing/accreditation entities. These include, for example, clinical guidelines promulgated by the American College of Obstetricians and Gynecologists (ACOG) and the American Academy of Pediatrics (AAP), recommended preventive services from the USPSTF, and the Joint Commission's accreditation and certification standards.

[70] Health Plans' Commitment to Improving Women's Reproductive Health, Issue Brief, November 2018, AHIP https://www.ahip.org/wp-content/uploads/2018/11/IB_WomensHealth-112118-FINAL.pdf.

To assure that mothers receive the recommended care, health insurance providers rely on quality measures, such as the rates of early elective deliveries, cesarean deliveries, and high-risk deliveries. Early elective deliveries can have serious consequences for the mother and baby. Births delivered via cesarean section have the potential to create additional surgical and health risks to the patient.

As a part of the Core Quality Measures Collaborative (CQMC) established by AHIP and the Centers for Medicare & Medicaid Services (CMS), now run by the National Quality Forum (NQF), health insurance providers, doctors, hospitals and other participants in the maternal and child health continuum collaborated on the development of a set of core measures to guide the collective assessment of the quality of care delivered to mothers and their children.

Engaging Mothers during Pre-Natal and Postpartum Care

Pre-natal care is critically important for a healthy pregnancy, and post-partum care is imperative to the health of both mother and baby. Health insurance providers recognize that early engagement and intervention can improve health outcomes for expectant mothers. Before and during a pregnancy, a woman is cared for by her doctor, who provides advice on how to ensure a healthy pregnancy. Health insurance providers play an important supporting role by reinforcing the recommendations of the doctor.

In addition, many health insurance providers offer targeted programs to engage and assist women with resources before, during and after pregnancy to improve health and identify possible risks. This may include access to nurse helplines, educational materials, referrals to prenatal classes, connections to support programs (e.g., the Special Supplemental Nutrition Program for Women, Infants, and Children (WIC)), wellness resources, health coaching, and breastfeeding support.

Additional high-touch case management services are available if factors are identified that indicate a high-risk pregnancy. In these instances, case managers may take additional steps to more proactively address maternal and infant diseases that may result from high-risk pregnancies. Some health insurance providers also offer incentives and support to women to encourage compliance with recommended prenatal care visits, tobacco cessation, provide transportation assistance, and waive co-pays for prenatal visits, for example.

Many health insurance providers have also launched digital tools and mobile applications to enhance access to education resources, recognizing that smart phones provide an easy and convenient access point for their patients. Often, these tools are based on evidence-based guidance and connected to 24/7 nurse triage lines so that expectant mothers can connect directly with clinicians as questions arise.

A Commitment to Work Together for Healthy Moms and Babies

Every woman deserves access to care that will ensure the good health of both that mother and her baby. Health insurance providers deliver on that commitment by offering access to a full continuum of pre- and post-natal care services. To do this, maternity care needs to be safe, guided by sound medical evidence, and affordable. As an industry, our members are focused on improving birth outcomes and are focused on reducing racial and ethnic disparities in care; we are continuously evaluating our approaches to providing maternal health care and look forward to collaborating with stakeholders moving forward. Together with our provider partners, health insurance providers are working hard to improve health care outcomes for all women and to deliver innovative and culturally competent approaches to improve maternity and infant care.

Thank you for the opportunity to provide these comments. We look forward to working with the Committee and other stakeholders on ways improve the health of moms and babies. Please contact us if you have questions or would like more information.

September 9, 2019

The Honorable Eliot Engel
2426 Rayburn House Office Building
Washington, DC 20515

The Honorable Steve Stivers
2234 Rayburn House Office Building
Washington, DC 20515

Dear Representatives Engel and Stivers,

On behalf of the undersigned organizations dedicated to the health of mothers, infants, and families, thank you for introducing the Quality Care for Moms and Babies Act (H.R. 1551). This legislation represents an essential next step in Congress' effort to address the nation's maternal mortality crisis, which claims the lives of 700 new moms each year. It will also address alarming recent increases in preterm birth, the leading contributor to infant death in the United States.

In late 2018, Congress passed the Preventing Maternal Deaths Act (P.L. 115-344) to support states in establishing and improving maternal mortality review committees (MMRCs). MMRCs are responsible for investigating each instance of maternal death and then making recommendations to prevent future tragedies. However, the recommendations are only meaningful if states take action to implement them.

The Quality Care for Moms and Babies Act would help states translate recommendations into action by supporting new and existing perinatal quality collaboratives. Collaboratives share best practices and lessons learned with each other, but are each operated and controlled at the state and regional level, meaning that solutions and approaches to innovation are locally relevant. By fostering these collaboratives, diverse groups of stakeholders help reduce preventable maternal mortality, severe maternal morbidity, and infant mortality by encouraging local providers through the adoption of best practices, including eliminating elective deliveries before 39 weeks, increasing breastfeeding rates, reducing cesarean sections, and much more. Improved outcomes will mean healthier moms, healthier babies, and cost savings for the entire health care system.

The Quality Care for Moms and Babies Act would also improve the quality of care for pregnant women and infants by directing the Department of Health and Human Services (HHS) to develop a core set of evidence-based perinatal quality measures to be used in Medicaid and the Children's Health Insurance Program (CHIP), improving care for pregnant women and infants enrolled in those programs. Our organizations strongly support the focus your bill brings to perinatal quality issues and care delivery. While HHS currently has a core set of quality measures for adults and a separate one for children, there is a great need for a single, recognized core set for pregnant women and their babies. Quality care and better data will lead to improved health outcomes, which in turn will reduce health expenditures for patients, the states, and the federal government.

Thank you again for your leadership and commitment to improving the care delivered to moms and babies. We look forward to working with you to pass this important legislation.

Sincerely,

American College of Nurse-Midwives
American College of Obstetricians and Gynecologists
Association of Maternal & Child Health Programs
Lamaze International
March for Moms
March of Dimes
National Partnership for Women & Families
Society for Maternal-Fetal Medicine

Statement for the Record Submitted by the Premier Inc. Healthcare Alliance, "Improving Maternal Health: Legislation to Advance Prevention Efforts and Access to Care," House Energy and Commerce Subcommittee on Health, September 10, 2019

The Premier healthcare alliance appreciates the opportunity to submit a statement for the record on the House Energy and Commerce Subcommittee on

Health hearing titled *"Improving Maternal Health: Legislation to Advance Prevention Efforts and Access to Care"* held on September 10, 2019. We applaud the leadership of Chairman Pallone and Chairwoman Eshoo, Ranking Members Walden and Burgess and members of the Subcommittee for holding this hearing to examine legislative solutions to address the factors contributing to maternal mortality.

Premier is a leading healthcare improvement company, uniting an alliance of more than 4,000 U.S. hospitals and health systems and approximately 175,000 other providers and organizations to transform healthcare. With integrated data and analytics, data-driven collaboratives, supply chain solutions, consulting and other services, Premier enables better care and outcomes at a lower cost.

Every new mother and child deserves the best beginning possible, whether they live in the suburbs, cities or in a rural setting. *Getting at the root cause and raising the performance bar on maternal health for the nation is why Premier has launched the Bundle of Joy™ campaign.* The goal for the *Bundle of Joy* campaign is to ensure mothers and babies are always at the center of care and supported by the latest evidence, the best doctors and the most successful practices. By mobilizing an alliance of 4,000+ hospitals and health systems, 100 billion data points, the expertise of our industry partners and history of proven best practices, Premier aims to build and deploy new care delivery models, ultimately scaling proven advancements across the industry.

As part of the Bundle of Joy campaign, Premier released a report on inpatient maternal mortality and morbidity based on a nationally representative sample with 25 percent of U.S. births from 2008 - 2018. The report found a 24 percent decline in deaths during in-hospital deliveries in this timeframe across 900+ hospitals. Additionally, we found that the mortality disparity gap between whites and all other races substantially narrowed, and specifically found that delivery-related deaths for black mothers decreased by 80 percent over the 10-year period.

The analysis also identified a 36 percent increase in severe maternal morbidity (SMM) rates, including a 79 percent higher SMM rate for black women than white women. SMM, as measured by the CDC, includes unexpected outcomes of labor and delivery that result in significant short- or long-term health effects, including eclampsia, cardiac arrest and sepsis. The increase in SMM rates are affected by several factors, such as changes in coding, age, race, payer, type of delivery, substance misuse, region and hospital type. Further research is needed to understand the drivers and implications of these factors on SMM rates.

Taking the Premier analysis in conjunction with the report released last week by the Centers for Disease Control and Prevention (CDC), "Racial/Ethnic Disparities in Pregnancy-Related Deaths," suggests that steps need to be taken to better integrate care delivery between the hospital and pre- and post-care services for mothers and their newborns, as well as to better manage high-risk patients. The CDC has found that black, American Indian and Alaska Native women are more than 2.5 times as likely to die from pregnancy-related causes than white women, that maternal mortality is on an overall upward trend and that many of these deaths are preventable.

Premier's analysis complements the CDC's findings because it examines one site of care within the larger birth-related mortality findings. While the CDC data pertains to all pregnancy-related deaths, Premier's analysis highlights inpatient-related maternal mortality, at the time of delivery. The Premier analysis included standardized inpatient data from 8.9 million births (approximately 25 percent of births nationally) that occurred in 903 hospitals across 45 states between 2008-2018.

To be clear, if the disparity gap is narrowing for in-hospital delivery-related mortality, but widening overall, that means we need to focus beyond the hospital to the care mothers are receiving pre- and post-delivery. This is why it is imperative that mothers get to the hospital for urgent care of pregnancy-related complications and to safely deliver their babies. We believe this also underscores *the need for new payment models and a focus on incentivizing integrated care across ambulatory and inpatient settings.*

Premier's full report, *"Bundle of Joy™ Maternal & Infant Health Trends"* is attached.

Premier will be conducting additional analysis on our *extensive data on maternal death rates and maternal health trends.* We look forward to continuing to share these data and findings with the Subcommittee to help develop evidence-based policy solutions to improve the quality, safety and cost of care for mothers and infants.

In closing, the Premier healthcare alliance appreciates the opportunity to submit a statement for the record on the House Energy and Commerce Subcommittee on Health hearing on maternal health. Premier is available as a resource and looks forward to working with Congress as it considers policy options to address this very important issue.

STATEMENT FOR THE RECORD OF GAUSS SURGICAL, INC., TO THE U.S. HOUSE OF REPRESENTATIVES, COMMITTEE ON ENERGY AND COMMERCE, SUBCOMMITTEE ON HEALTH

Gauss Surgical appreciates the opportunity to provide testimony to the U.S. House of Representatives Committee on Energy and Commerce for the hearing on "Improving Maternal Health: Legislation to Advance Prevention Efforts and Access to Care" and to offer our perspective on the important issue of reducing pregnancy-related morbidity and mortality.

We believe that the Federal Government should strongly explore and consider supporting the adoption of adjunct technologies to improve perinatal safety. In this statement, we highlight a proven Artificial Intelligence (AI) enabled mobile technology solution that is playing a meaningful role in improving detection and treatment of Postpartum Hemorrhage, the leading preventable cause of maternal mortality in the United States.

Hemorrhage Is the Leading Preventable Cause of Maternal Mortality in the United States

The United States has the highest maternal mortality rate in the developed world [1]. According to the Centers for Disease Control and Prevention, 60% of pregnancy-related deaths are preventable [2]. Postpartum hemorrhage is a leading cause of preventable maternal morbidity and mortality [3]. To address this problem, organizations such as the American College of Obstetrics and Gynecology and the California Maternal Quality Care Collaborative recommend use of standardized hemorrhage management protocols to facilitate appropriate care of patients suffering from postpartum bleeding [4, 5].

On August 21, 2019, The Joint Commission, the body that accredits approximately 77% of hospitals in the United States, announced a perinatal safety guideline [6] that requires accredited hospitals to "develop written, evidence-based procedures for stage-based management of pregnant and postpartum patients who experience maternal hemorrhage" incorporating "the use of an evidence-based tool that includes an algorithm for identification and treatment of hemorrhage" This new standard will go into effect July 1, 2020.

Ineffective Blood Loss Monitoring Hinders Hemorrhage Management

Widely accepted clinical protocols for hemorrhage detection and response rely on the ongoing, quantitative evaluation of cumulative blood loss as the lynchpin for triggering interventions to manage bleeding at predetermined levels or "stages" of blood loss [7].

However, traditional approaches to assessing blood loss, such as visual estimation and manual weighing of blood-soaked sponges, are known to be unreliably subjective, inaccurate, labor-intensive, and confounded by the presence of fluids other than blood (e.g., irrigation, amniotic fluid) [8-11]. These difficulties have severely limited providers' ability to recognize and respond to hemorrhage in a timely manner [12].

As Laura Ungar reported in a July 2018 USA TODAY investigation [13],

> "In July, a USA TODAY investigation revealed that thousands of women in the U.S. suffer life-changing injuries or die during childbirth because hospitals, doctors and nurses ignore basic best practices known to head off disaster. Experts say half of those women's lives could be saved if doctors and nurses took simple steps, including measuring blood loss during and after delivery and giving timely treatment for high blood pressure."

Artificial Intelligence (AI) Enabled Technology Can Significantly Improve Hemorrhage Recognition and Response

Gauss Surgical, Inc., a leading healthcare Artificial Intelligence (AI) company based in Menlo Park, California, has developed an actionable solution that leverages cost-effective mobile technology and recent advances in AI to accurately estimate blood loss during both vaginal and cesarean deliveries. The company's Triton technology is a mobile application for the iPad that enables providers to assess blood loss in a way that is objective, accurate, and available in real-time during or after a delivery. The Triton App is FDA cleared as a Class II medical device, and is currently used by leading U.S. hospitals performing approximately 250,000 deliveries per year.

The Triton mobile application uses computer vision and machine learning algorithms to accurately estimate blood loss from digital images of blood-soaked sponges captured by the iPad as part of the routine sponge counting process. Similarly, the mobile application captures and processes images of the suction canister using sophisticated algorithms. As each new sponge or canister is scanned, the cumulative blood loss for the patient is displayed, providing doctors and nurses with clear insight into a critical aspect of the patient's condition. The technology seamlessly integrates into the busy workflow of a delivery room, operating room, or patient care unit.

Clinical Evidence Suggests Substantial Improvement in Hemorrhage Recognition and Response with the use of Technology

Several clinical studies have documented the accuracy [14, 15, 16] of the Triton mobile application as well as its ability to improve hemorrhage recognition, affect transfusion decision-making, and appropriately implement hemorrhage response protocols during both cesarean and vaginal deliveries [17, 18].

Earlier this year, researchers at Mount Sinai Hospital in New York published an independent 7,600-patient study in *The International Journal of Obstetric Anesthesia* comparing Triton with visual estimation of blood loss. The use of Triton to support implementation of a stage-based hemorrhage protocol was associated with (i) a nearly four-fold improvement in hemorrhage recognition, (ii) a 34% reduction in delayed interventions to control bleeding in vaginal deliveries, a reduced transfusion dose in cesarean deliveries, and (iv) significant cost savings yielding a 152% return on investment to the hospital [18].

Triton provides additional benefits; each hospital's Hemorrhage Protocol can be loaded into the mobile application to alert the care team to hemorrhage stages in real time. This makes it significantly easier for providers to rapidly and correctly implement the proper treatments to improve outcomes, by placing evidence-based protocols at their fingertips based on objective data on the patient's blood loss.

Quantification of Blood Loss with Technology Should be a Required Standard of Care in US Hospitals

Leading maternal health organizations have recommended use of stage-based hemorrhage protocols, and the use of objective, cumulative, quantitative blood loss. However, most hospitals and providers lack accurate, objective data needed to detect and respond to hemorrhage in time to improve maternal health outcomes.

Given that user-friendly and cost-effective mobile medical technology is now available to simplify, streamline, and objectively provide accurate and timely blood loss information, we believe that quantification of blood loss (QBL) should be a required standard of care in US hospitals for every delivery. The Federal Government should also strongly consider supporting the adoption of technology for quantifying blood loss and digital hemorrhage protocols through Medicaid reimbursement incentives and through grant programs to under-resourced hospitals.

Conclusion

Gauss Surgical sincerely thanks the Committee for this hearing and for your commitment to addressing the problem of maternal morbidity and mortality. We deeply support your efforts and welcome the opportunity to work with the Committee and Congress to draft legislation to improve maternal outcomes.

Respectfully yours,

Robert L. Thurer, MD
Medical Director (Consulting)
Gauss Surgical, Inc.

Fmr. Associate Professor of Surgery
Harvard Medical School

Brendan Carvalho, MBBCh, FRCA, MDCH
Medical Director (Consulting)
Gauss Surgical, Inc.

Chief, Obstetric Anesthesia
Professor of Anesthesiology
Stanford University Medical Center

Past President
Society for Obstetric Anesthesia and Perinatology

Griffeth W. Tully, MD
Chief Medical Officer
Gauss Surgical, Inc.

Siddarth Satish
Founder and Chief Executive Officer
Gauss Surgical, Inc.

References

[1] Kassebaum NJ, Barber RM, Bhutta ZA, et al; GBD 2015 Maternal Mortality Collaborators. *Global, regional, and national levels of maternal mortality, 1990-2015: a systematic analysis for the Global Burden of Disease Study 2015.* Lancet. 2016; 388(10053):1775-1812.

[2] Petersen EE, Davis NL, Goodman D, et al. Vital signs: pregnancy-related deaths, United States, 2011-2015, and strategies for prevention, 13 states, 2013-2017. *MMWR Morb Mortal Wkly Rep* 2019; 68:423–9.

[3] Main EK, McCain CL, Morton CH, et al. Pregnancy-related mortality in California. Obstet Gynecol 2015; 125:938–47.

[4] Practice Bulletin No. 183 Summary: Postpartum Hemorrhage. *Obstet Gynecol.* 2017; 130:923-925.

[5] Lyndon A, Lagrew D, Shields L, et al. *Improving Health Care Response to Obstetric Hemorrhage. (California Maternal Quality Care Collaborative Toolkit to Transform Maternity Care) Developed under contract #11-10006 with the California Department of Public Health; Maternal, Child and Adolescent Health Division; Published by the California Maternal Quality Care Collaborative*, 3/17/15.

[6] *New Standards for Perinatal Safety, PC.06.01.01,* The Joint Commission https://www.jointcommission.org/assets/1/6/New_Perinatal_Standards_Prepub_Report.pdf.

[7] Quantification of blood loss: AWHONN practice brief number 1. *J Obstet Gynecol Neonatal Nurs* 2015; 44:158-60.

[8] Bose P, Regan F, Paterson-Brown S. Improving the accuracy of estimated blood loss at obstetric haemorrhage using clinical reconstructions. *BJOG* 2006;113:919-924.

[9] Schorn MN. Measurement of blood loss: review of the literature. *J Midwifery Women's Health* 2010;55:20-27.

[10] Johar R, Smith R. Assessing gravimetric estimation of intraoperative blood loss. *J Gynecol Surg* 1993; 9:151.

[11] Lilley G, Burkett-St-Laurent D, Precious E, et al. Measurement of blood loss during postpartum haemorrhage. *Int J Obstet Anesth* 2015; 24:8-14.

[12] Bingham D, Scheich B, Byfield R, et al. Postpartum hemorrhage preparedness elements vary among hospitals in New Jersey and Georgia. *J Obstet Gynecol Neonatal Nurs*. 2016; 45:227-38.

[13] Ungar, L. What states aren't doing to save new mothers' lives. *USA TODAY*, September 19, 2018 https://www.usatoday.com/in-depth/news/investigations/deadly-deliveries/2018/09/19/maternal-death-rate-state-medical-deadly-deliveries/547050002/.

[14] Konig G, Holmes AA, Garcia R, et al; In vitro evaluation of a novel system for monitoring surgical hemoglobin loss. *Anesth Analg*. 2014; 119:595-600.

[15] Konig G, Waters JH, Hsieh E, et al. In vitro evaluation of a novel image processing device to estimate surgical blood loss in suction canisters. *Anesth Analg*. 2018; 126:621-628.

[16] Doctorvaladan S, et al. "Accuracy of Blood Loss Measurement During Cesarean Section" *Am J Perinatol Rep* 2017;7(2):e93-e100.

[17] Rubenstein, Zamudio S, Al-Khan A, et al. Clinical experience with the implementation of accurate measurement of blood loss during cesarean delivery: influences on hemorrhage recognition and allogeneic transfusion. *Amer J Perinatol* 2018; 35: 655-659.

[18] Katz, D., Wang, R., O'Neil, L., et al. The association between the introduction of quantitative assessment of postpartum blood loss and institutional changes in clinical practice: an observational study. *Int J Obstet Anesth*. 2019 May 13. pii: S0959-289X(19)30070-6. doi: 10.1016/j.ijoa.2019.05.006. [Epub ahead of print].

BANDLE OF JOY™, MATERNAL & INFANT HEALTH TRENDS

About the Bundle of Joy™ Campaign

In April 2019, Premier® launched the *Bundle of Joy* campaign to test and scale measurable improvement in the quality, safety and cost of care for mothers and babies in the United States. The campaign builds on Premier alliance's long-standing commitment to providing safe care to help ensure healthy mothers and babies across its network of more than 4,000 hospitals, provider collaboratives and partnerships with employers and other industry organizations.

Bundle of Joy is organized to tackle issues that data prove continue to be associated with maternal and infant healthcare. With data from 45 percent of all U.S. hospital discharges, Premier can analyze standardized data to gain meaningful insights for providers and the industry. This data includes more than 1.2 million annual hospital births, as of 2018. These research and analytic capabilities provide a source of truth that enables stakeholders across the industry to identify, target and monitor critical quality and safety improvement opportunities.

Premier provides the following resources for healthcare organizations to join its campaign to improve maternal and infant health. To learn more, please contact us by visiting the *Bundle of Joy* website.

- *Data-driven Insights:* The maternal and infant health trends analysis leverages the Premier Healthcare Database and is used to help hospitals and the nation better understand and target solutions to this national problem. Premier's analytic capabilities and data assets are used to study specific therapeutic interventions and assess clinical efficacy over time to implement new solutions for unmet medical needs. This is the first of several analyses on maternal and infant health trends.
- *Maternal & Infant Outcomes Dashboard:* The industry's only integrated analytics dashboard enables a comprehensive analysis of an organization's select perinatal and neonatal data sets, including peer-level and regional benchmarks and individualized reports assessing quality and outcomes. Premier continues to develop innovative analytics solutions to enable hospitals and health systems to benchmark and assess performance against its comprehensive maternal and infant database.
- *Performance Improvement Services:* Premier provides one-to-one consulting support as well as collaborative initiatives to advance and scale national efforts to improve maternal and infant health. In July 2019, Premier announced it is working with 10 leading hospitals on a Perinatal Collaborative designed to reach zero preventable maternal and neonatal harm and deaths. Learnings from the collaborative will be shared nationally. In January 2020, the QUEST® quality improvement collaborative will launch a new perinatal specialty network to further test and adopt evidence-based strategies to improve care and the overall experience for women, infants and their families.
- *New Payment Models and Policy:* Premier is working with private and public organizations to test and scale new payment models and reforms to improve maternal healthcare.

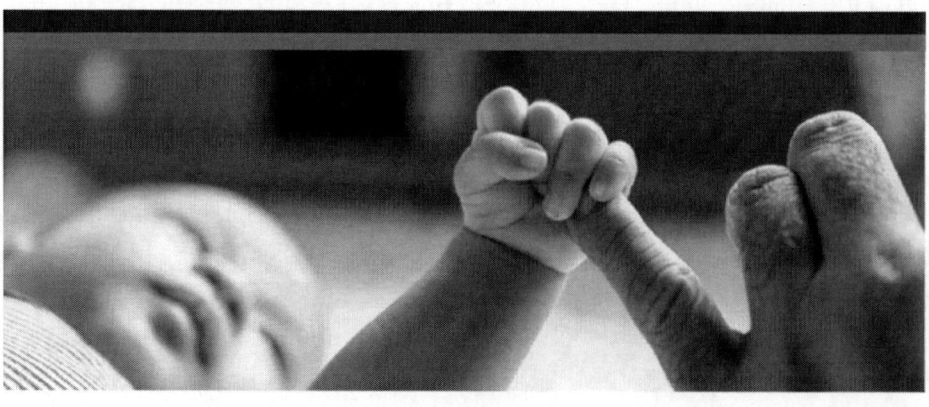

Premier Maternal & Infant Analysis: Key Findings

In July 2019, Premier conducted a national trend analysis to explore maternal and infant health outcomes in the hospital, at the time of delivery. The analysis leveraged the nationally representative Premier Healthcare Database and included standardized inpatient data from 8.9 million births that occurred in 903 hospitals across 45 states between 2008-2018. The data in the Premier analysis represent approximately 25 percent of all U.S. in-hospital births and were comparable in patient and hospital demographics to the data used by the Centers for Disease Control and Prevention (CDC) in its *Vital Signs* report on pregnancy-related deaths.

Comprised of nearly 20 years of de-identified inpatient data, Premier's best-in-class database is more current and standardized than the CDC's data. Therefore, Premier data can help provide policymakers and clinicians with additional insights into hospital performance on maternal health. This is Premier's first analysis of maternal and infant mortality and morbidity, with additional analyses forthcoming.

Patient demographics and clinical outcomes were measured using the CDC's methodology for severe maternal morbidity (SMM), which includes the birth admission definition as the denominator and the numerator, as well as additional standardized national methodologies.

Note that as hospitals switched from ICD-9 to ICD-10 mid-way through 2015, changes in documentation and coding may have affected year 2015 trending in comparison with previous years.

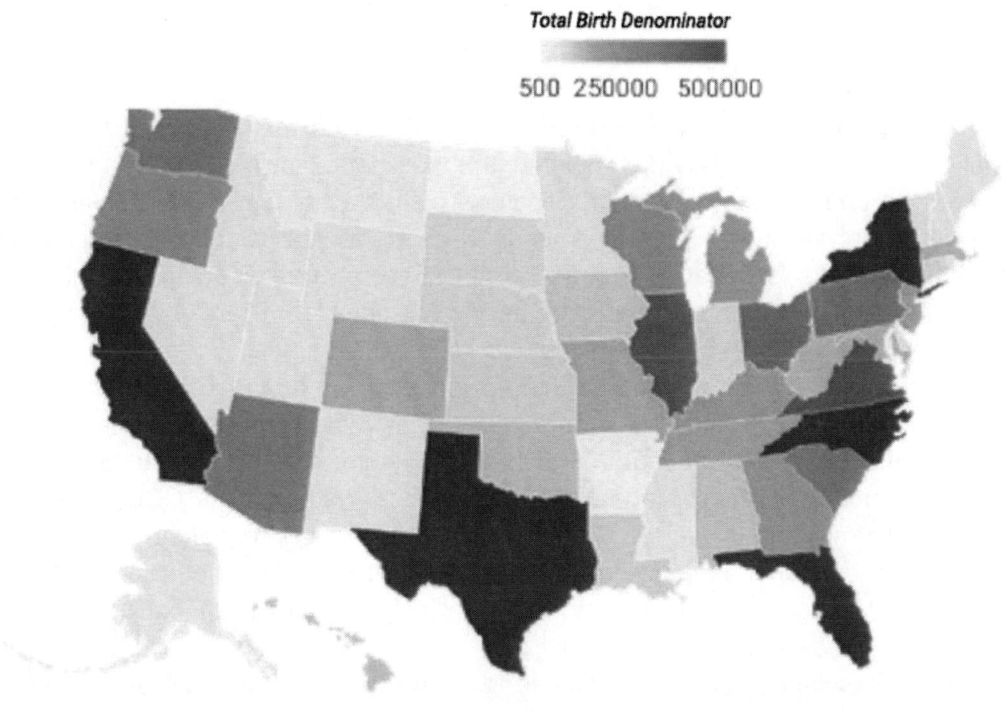

Figure 4. Total Inpatient Birth Volume by State.

U.S. Hospitals Are Demonstrating a Dramatic Decrease in Delivery-Related Maternal Deaths

Overall, Premier found that U.S. hospitals showed a 24 percent decrease in delivery-related maternal deaths between 2008-2018 (Figure 5).

This trend suggests that progress is being made in the hospital at the time of delivery. However, the analysis did not explore maternal deaths occurring outside of delivery in the hospital or preventability of these deaths. Additional occurrences of maternal mortality across the continuum of pregnancy will be explored in a later analysis.

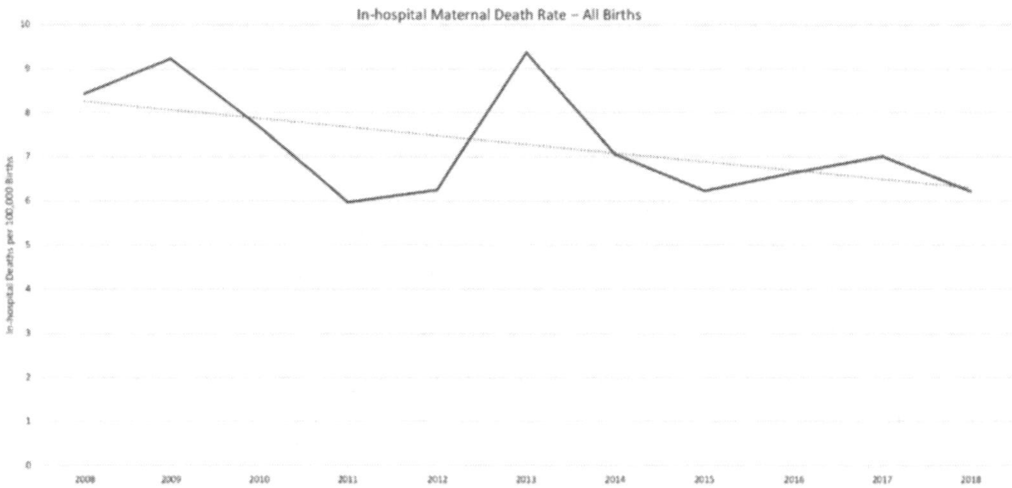

Figure 5. In-Hospital, Delivery-Related Death Rate Trend.

Premier worked closely with the CDC to ensure the methodology used in this analysis was aligned with and complemented their data. However, there are several differences and details in Premier's findings compared to the CDC. For instance, Premier's analysis shows a reduction in delivery-rated maternal mortality rates within the hospital. This is because Premier's data is more current, going through 2018 while the CDC's most recent mortality trends end in 2015. Premier's analysis was also conducted using standardized inpatient data, which allows for greater specificity when exploring trends happening within the hospital, at the time of delivery. These insights, however, are based only on inpatient stays. In comparison, the CDC uses mortality data from the National Vital Statistics System, death certificates from each state and the Pregnancy Mortality Surveillance System. The CDC defines a pregnancy-related death as the death of a woman during pregnancy or within one year of the end of pregnancy from a pregnancy complication, a chain of events initiated by pregnancy, or the aggravation of an unrelated condition by the physiologic effects of pregnancy.

While Premier's analysis was limited to delivery-related hospitalizations and the CDC tracks maternal death outside of the hospital, the CDC has stated that "errors in reported pregnancy status on death certificates have been described, potentially leading to overestimation of the number of pregnancy-related deaths." Premier's in-hospital measure provides a more consistent assessment of facility performance.

When comparing women who had a cesarean versus a vaginal delivery, Premier identified a slight increase in delivery-related maternal mortalities for vaginal deliveries (Figures 6 & 7).

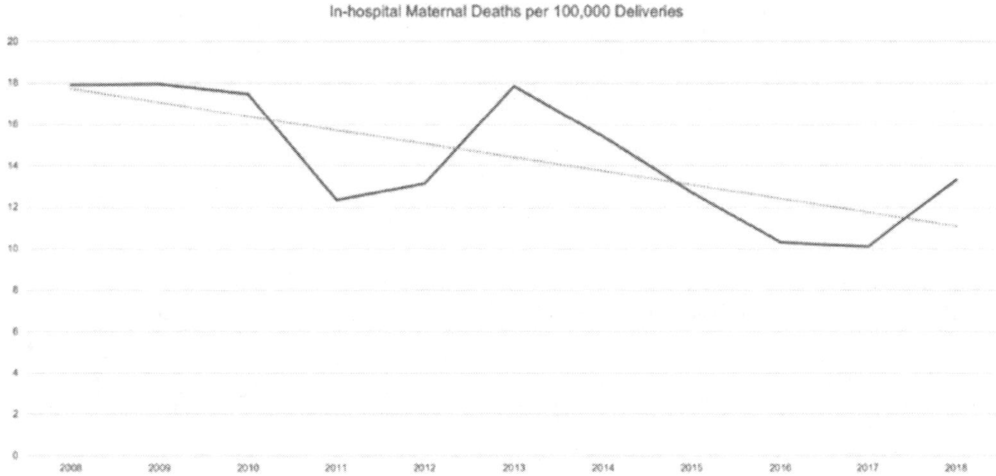

Figure 6. Inpatient Maternal Death Rate for Cesarean Delivery.

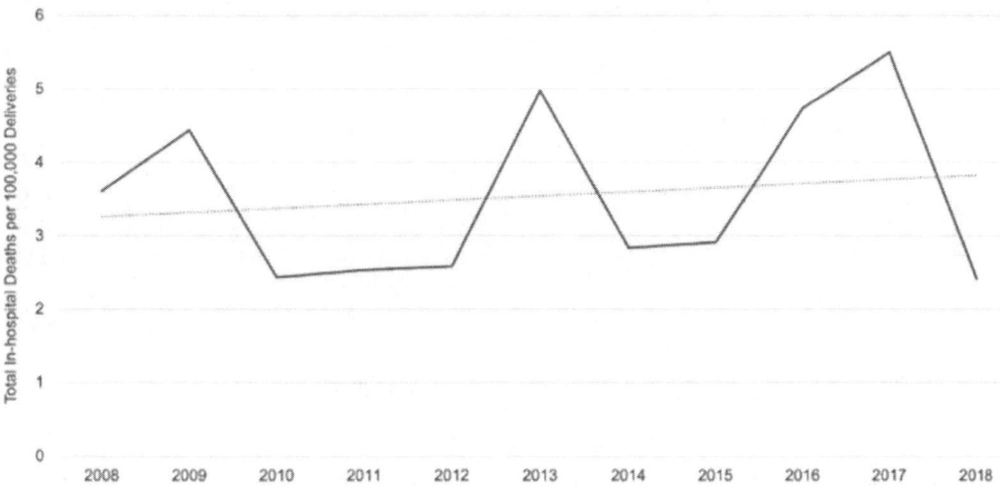

Figure 7. Inpatient Maternal Death Rate for Vaginal Delivery.

Notably, the disparity gap between black women and all other races for inpatient delivery-related deaths has substantially declined. Premier identified an 80 percent decrease in maternal mortality for black women between 2008-2018 (Figures 8 & 9).

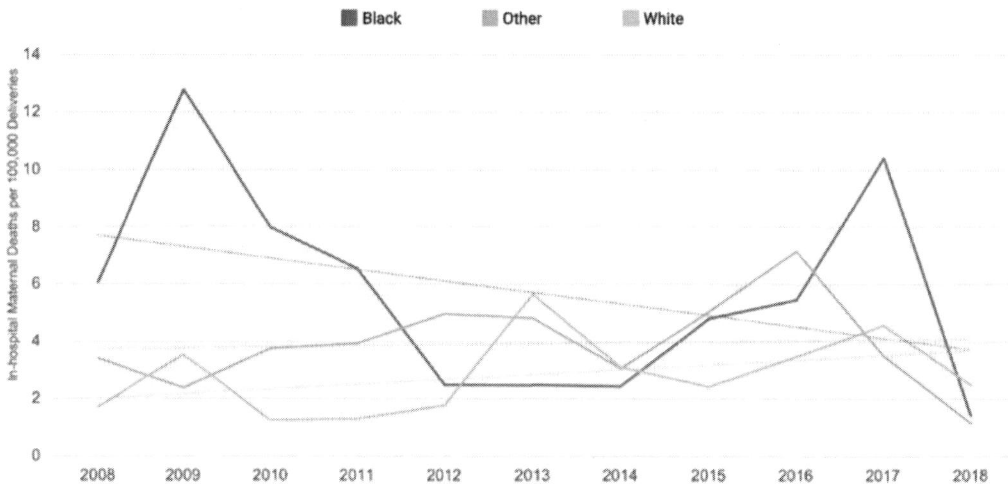

Figure 8. Inpatient Maternal Death Rate After/During Vaginal Delivery by Race.

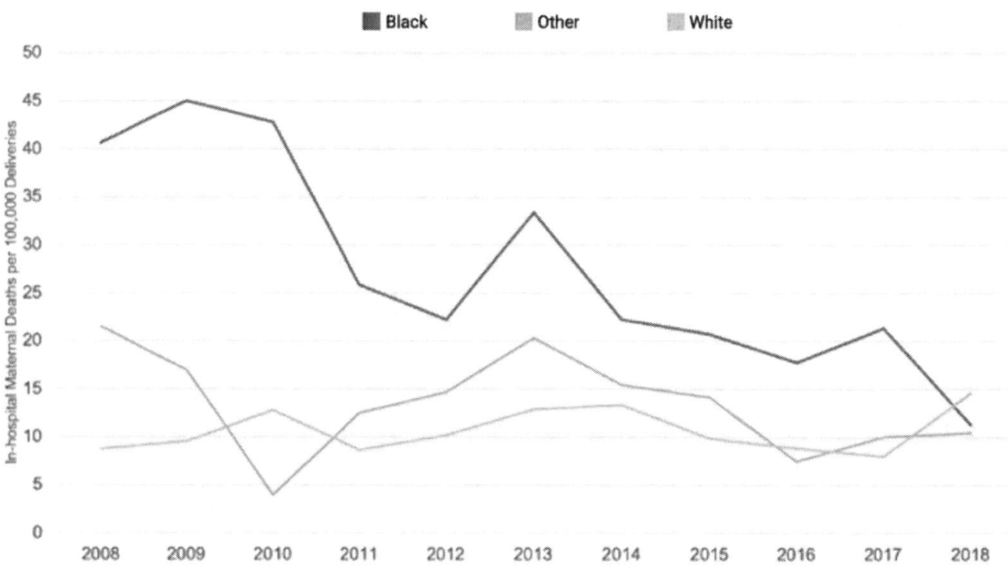

Figure 9. Inpatient Maternal Death Rate for Cesarean Delivery by Race.

Severe Maternal Morbidity Has Increased

While inpatient maternal mortality has decreased, the analysis showed an increase of 36 percent in severe maternal morbidity (SMM) between 2008-2018, and a 14 percent increase from 2015 through the end of 2018 (Figure 10). SMM includes unexpected outcomes of labor and delivery that result in significant short-or long-term health effects, including eclampsia, cardiac arrest and sepsis.

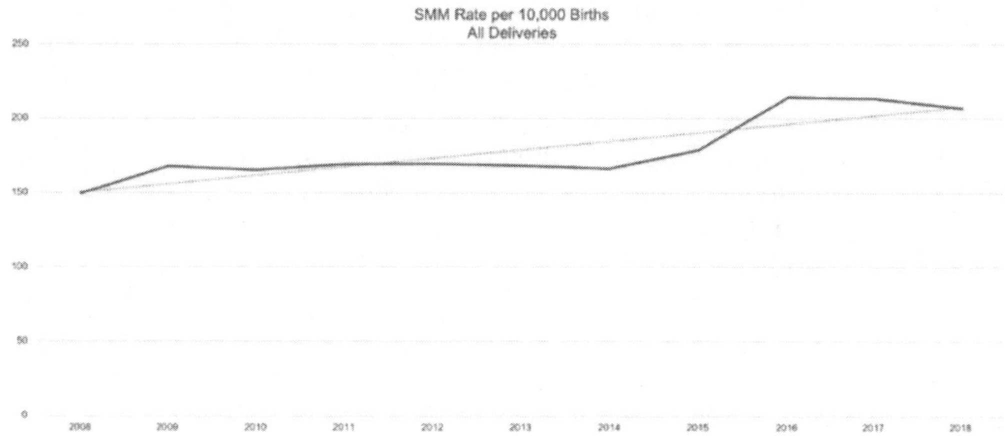

Figure 10. Overall SMM Rate.

The increase in SMM rates could be due to several factors outlined below, including changes in coding, age, race, payer, type of delivery, substance use, region, hospital type and other factors.

As illustrated in Figure 8, the change from ICD-9 to ICD-10 may have affected the accuracy of SMM rates in year 2015. In other words, part of the increase may be attributable to coding and documentation changes. However, the Premier analysis showed a higher SMM rate than what was reported by the CDC for the same time period. This suggests that there may have been an increase in SMM rates regardless of the transition to ICD-10.

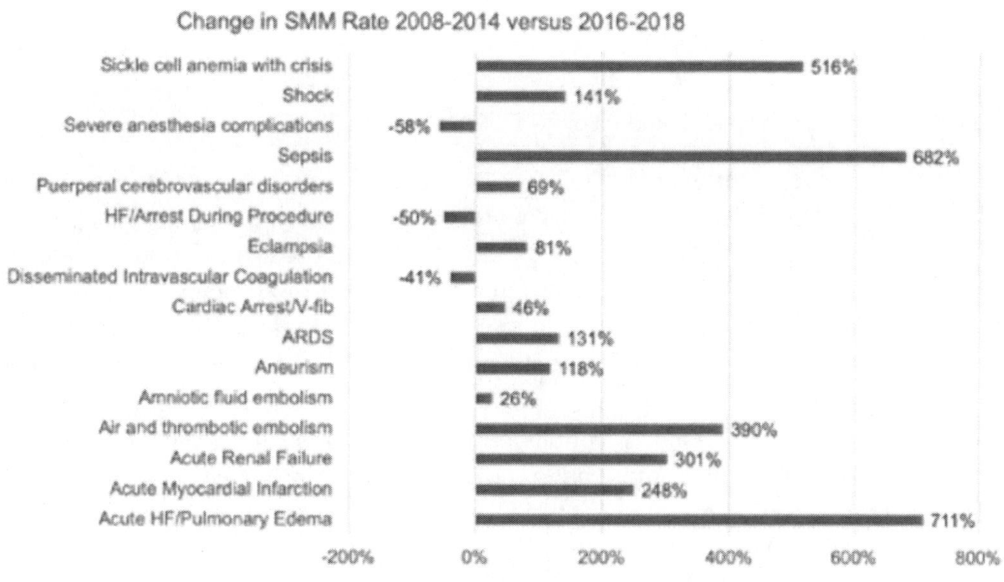

Figure 11. SMM Rate Change: ICD-9 versus ICD-10.

Viewing by year, SMM rates increased by 14 percent between 2008-2012, then remained flat or even slightly decreased in 2013 and 2014. As illustrated in Figure 12, these findings are closely aligned with the CDC's findings over this same time period. However, the CDC's SMM data is only available through 2014. In contrast, Premier's analysis shows a slightly higher rate post ICD-10 implementation (2015) than what was observed by the CDC. Of note is the large increase in SMM rate in 2016 (19 percent) and the decrease in SMM rate (3 percent) in 2018.

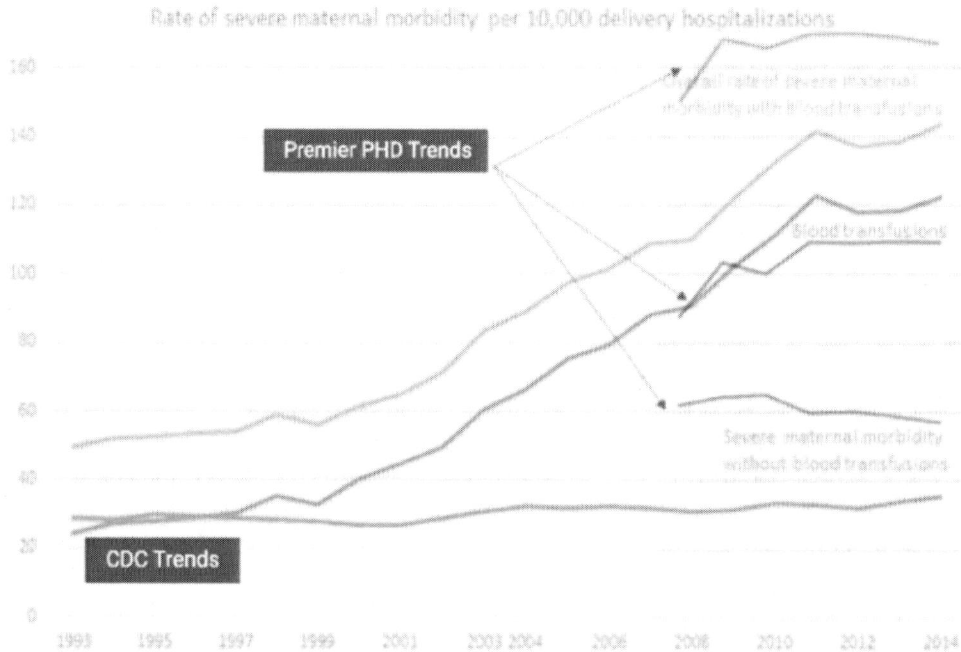

Figure 12. Overall SMM Rate Comparison to CDC Data.

Overall, blood transfusions, disseminated intravascular coagulation, hysterectomy, heart failure and sepsis were the top factors associated in patients who experienced a SMM as defined by the CDC (Figure 13). Blood transfusion incidence in this analysis is 34 percent higher compared to all other conditions and complications that constitute SMM. It is well recognized that blood transfusions are associated with women who have a higher risk of SMM and mortality. Transfusions are often used as a lifesaving measure in obstetrical hemorrhaging patients and other critical events. The clinical conditions triggering these transfusions and direct relationship to clinical outcomes have not been well described and provide an opportunity for further study.

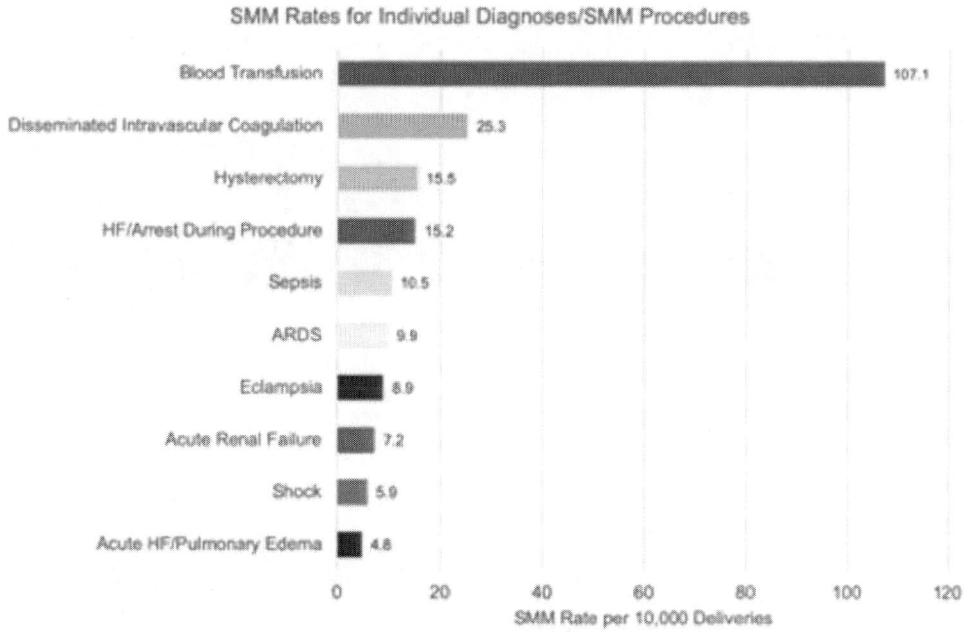

Figure 13. Top 10 Diagnoses and Procedures Associated with SMM.

Premier's analysis also identified the proportion of maternal complications attributable to various direct causes of SMM, which include cardiovascular conditions (21.3 percent), obstetric hemorrhage (24.6 percent), hypertensive disorders (11.4 percent), sepsis (6.4 percent), stroke (2.1 percent) and embolism (4.5 percent). Further study to determine indirect causes, such as preexisting conditions, maternal mental health and substance use, will be conducted in later Premier analysis.

The Race Disparity Gap Remains Open for SMM

Black women had a 79 percent higher SMM rate than white women (Figure 14). Specifically, black women had higher SMM rates for heart failure, acute respiratory distress syndrome, eclampsia, acute renal failure and sepsis. Black women also have a 94 percent higher rate of blood transfusions than white women.

Disparities among black women compared to all other populations is evident. More research is needed to understand the specific attributes affecting the variation in hospital performance and SMM rates associated with these disparities.

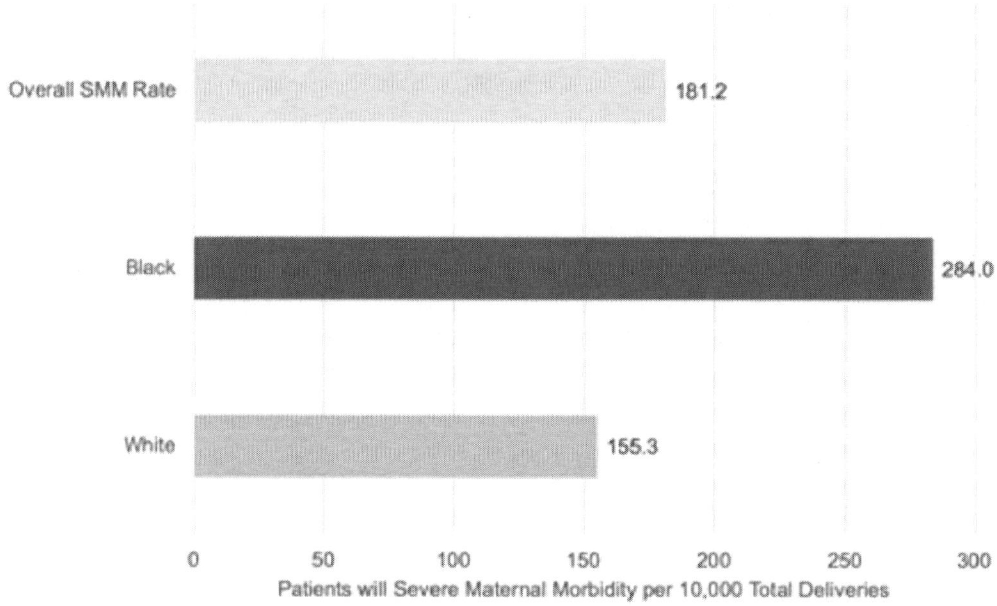

Figure 14. Overall SMM Rate by Maternal Race.

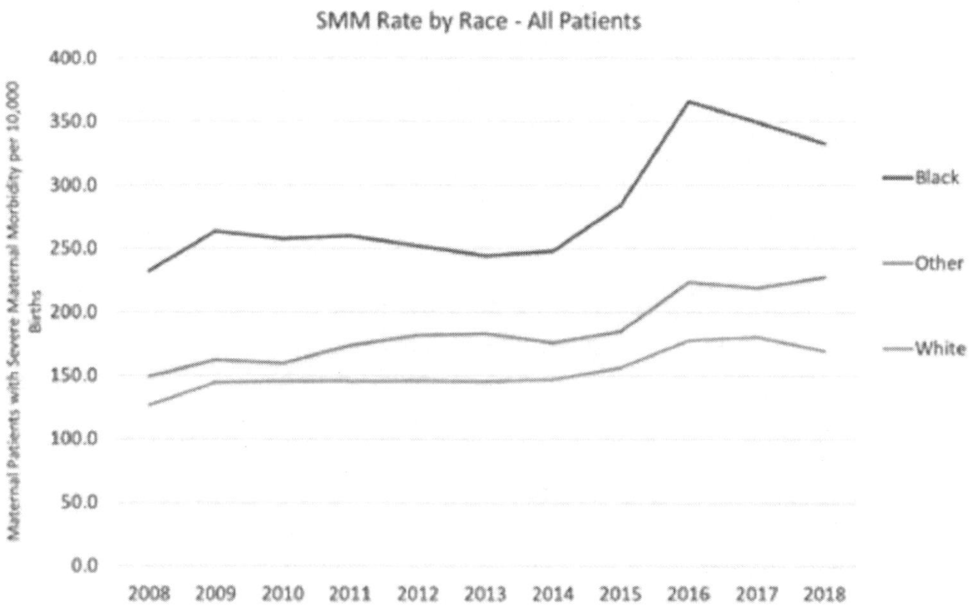

Figure 15. Overall SMM Rate by Maternal Race.

The Maternal Population Is Aging

Another consistent trend in the analysis is the aging of the U.S. maternal population. The percent of women giving birth who are older than 35 years of age increased by 24 percent and by 12 percent for mothers 25-35. Women giving birth under the age of 25 decreased by 29 percent (Figure 16).

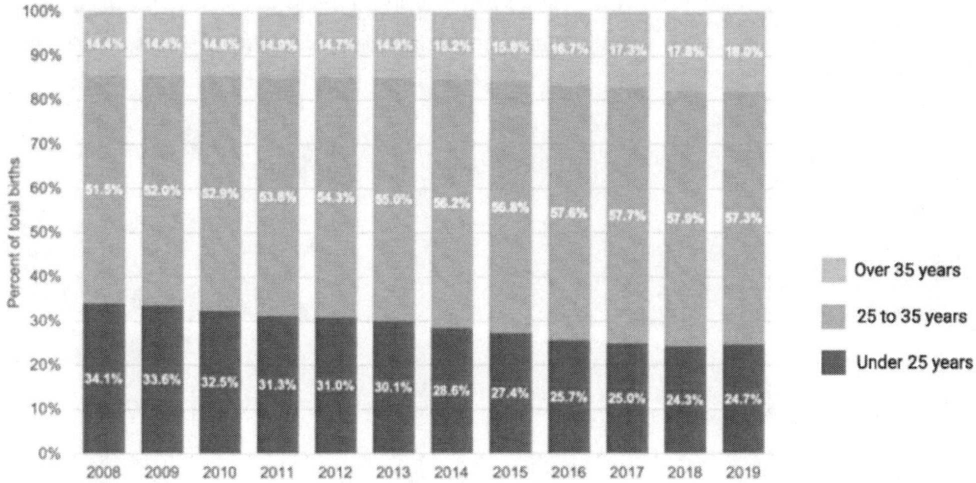

Figure 16. Overall Inpatient Maternal Age Distribution.

Mothers older than 35 tend to have a higher rate of cesarean sections as illustrated in Figure 17. Cesarean deliveries, which can increase the risk of complications, are 41 percent more common for women older than 35 as compared to women younger than 35.

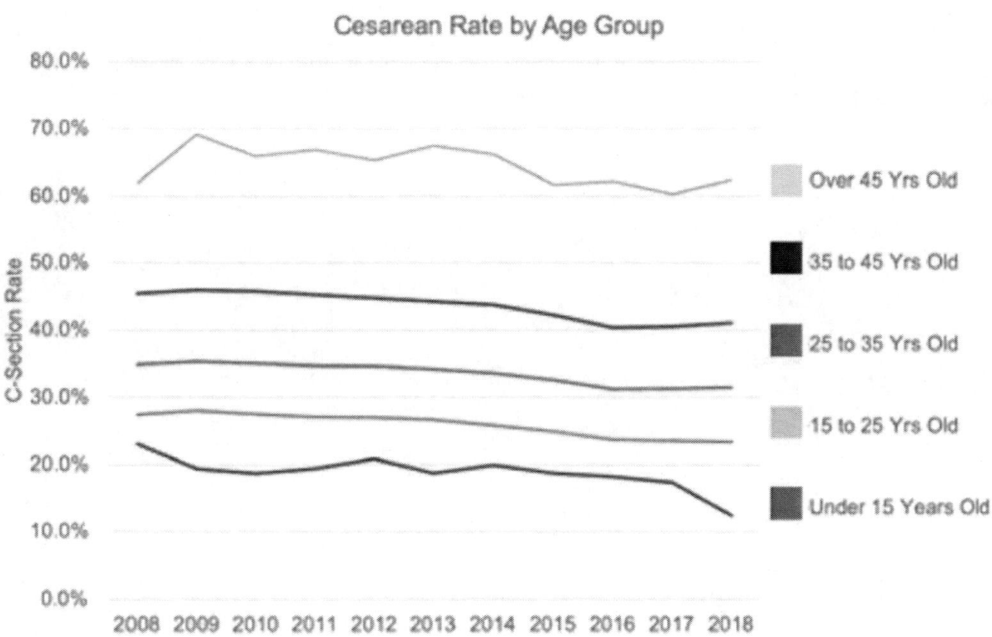

Figure 17. Cesarean Deliveries by Age Group.

Overall, the SMM rate for patients aged 35 and older is 32 percent higher than those younger than 35. Although mothers older than 45 years demonstrate the highest risk for SMM, women between the ages of 15 – 24 experienced the greatest increases in SMM rates with a 51 percent increase, followed by those 25 – 34 at 35 percent, and a 28 percent increase for mothers ages 35 – 44. Those under the age of 15 demonstrated a 13 percent decrease in SMM (Figure 18).

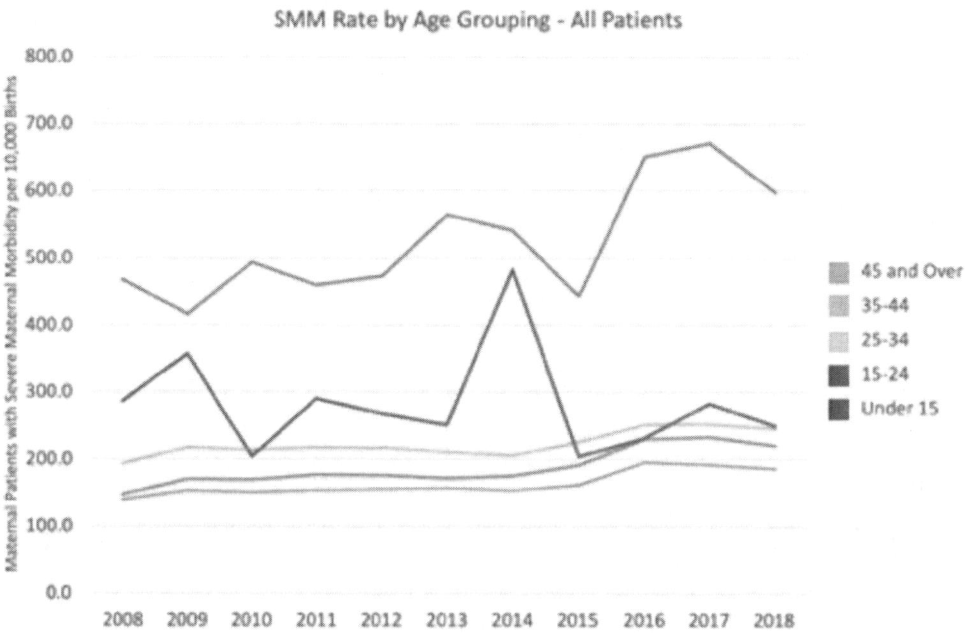

Figure 18. Overall SMM Rate by Maternal Age Group.

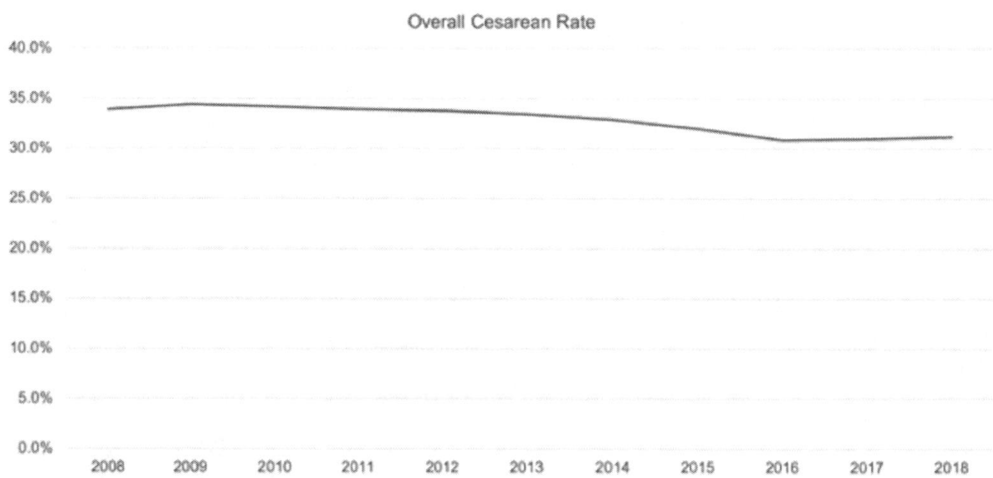

Figure 19. Overall Cesarean Rate Trend.

Premier's analysis confirmed that SMM rates for cesareans are higher than for vaginal deliveries. However, SMM rates for vaginal deliveries have increased by 67 percent since 2015 (Figure 19). Note that much of this increase could be attributed to coding changes. The actual SMM rate decreased in 2017 and 2018 over 2016, after three full years of ICD-10.

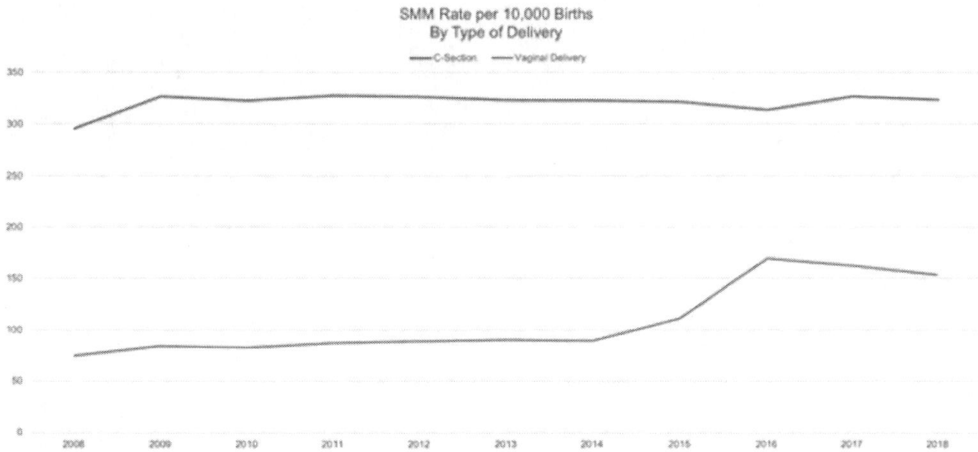

Figure 20. Overall SMM Rate by Type of Delivery.

Due to the differences between Premier's and the CDC's findings for SMM trends, additional analyses and research are needed to identify how coding changes may contribute to the SMM trend. For example, the changes in coding may demonstrate an enhanced capability to identify complications and SMM at a greater level of accuracy, thus enabling a better understanding of preventable harm and complications associated with pregnancy.

Patients with Commercial Insurance Have the Lowest SMM Rates

Women with commercial insurance had the lowest SMM rates. Mothers with charity/indigent coverage had the highest SMM rates – a 71 percent higher SMM rate than commercial insurance carriers. Mothers with Medicaid had the second highest SMM rate – 32 percent higher than commercial carriers (Figure 21). In Premier's analysis, 42 percent of women were covered by Medicaid and 50 percent by commercial insurance. The remaining 8 percent were covered through charity, indigent or other payment sources.

Comparing rural to urban hospitals, SMM rates remained relatively the same, with a 50 percent increase for rural and 39 percent increase for urban hospitals from 2008 – 2018 (Figure 22).

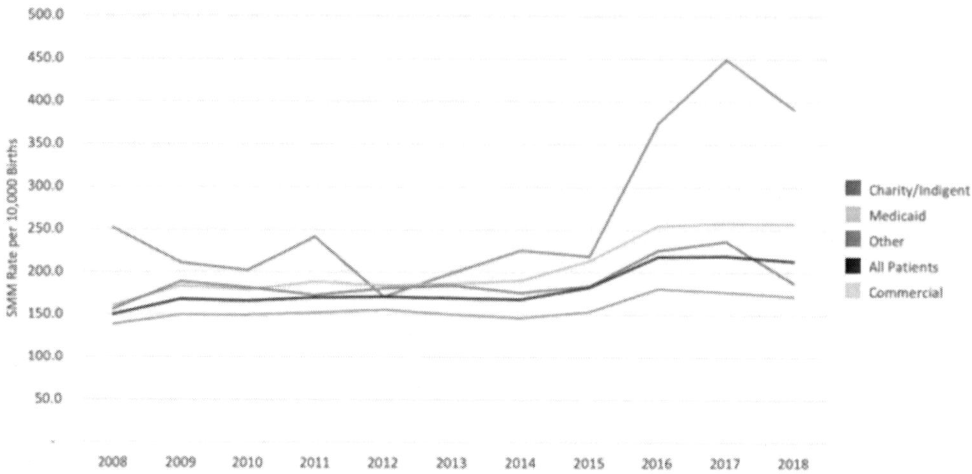

Figure 21. Overall SMM Rate by Type of Payer.

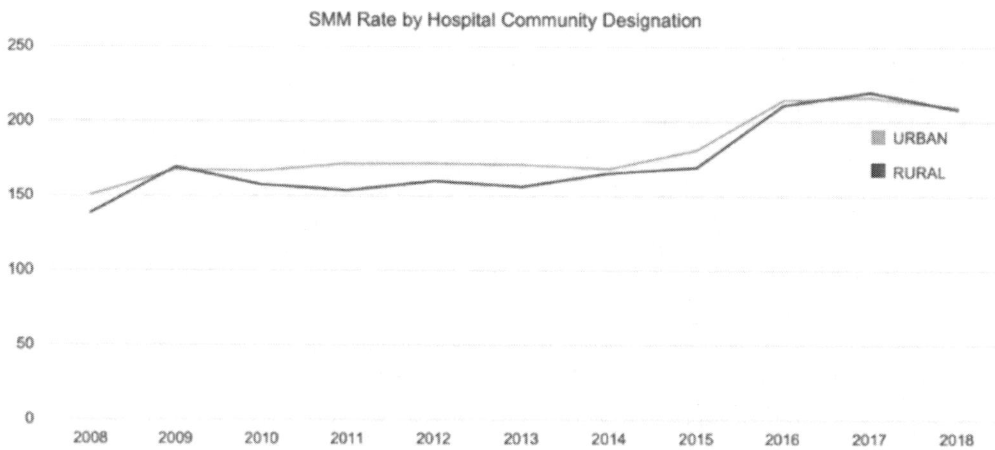

Figure 22. SMM Rates for Rural VS Urban Hospitals.

Comparing SMM rate by census region, hospitals in the Mid-Atlantic region had the highest SMM rates over the past four years. Hospitals in the Mountain region had the lowest rates over the past four years (Figure 23).

There are several other factors that could have influenced the increase in SMM rates. Premier plans to perform follow-up analyses to identify the key drivers, as well as how age, race, payer, type of delivery, region, hospital type, substance use and other key factors may be influencing SMM rates.

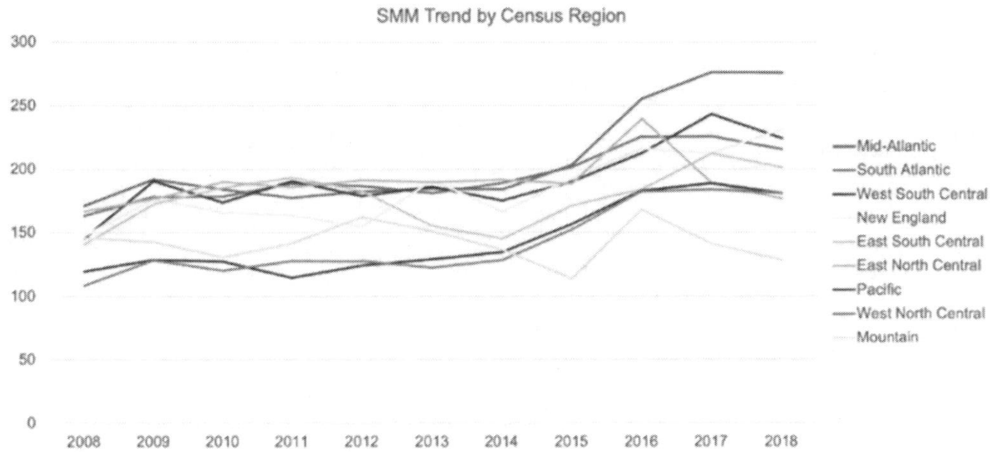

Figure 23. SMM Rates by Census Region.

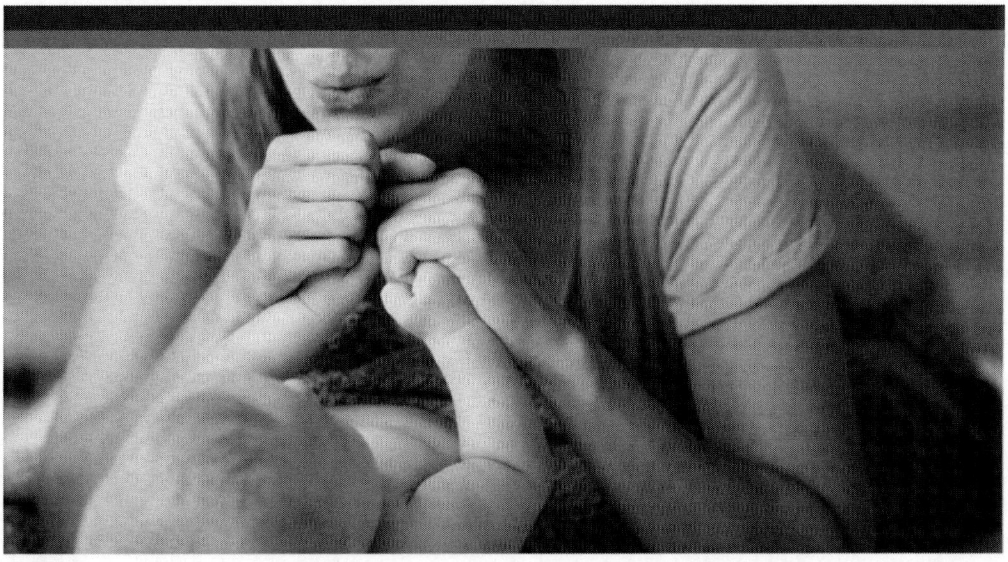

Maternal Substance Use and Neonatal Abstinence Syndrome

Alarmingly, the rate of infants born with neonatal abstinence syndrome (NAS) has increased by 140 percent since 2008 (Figure 24).

The increasing rate of NAS aligned closely with an increased trend for birth mothers with documented substance use, which has increased by 153 percent since 2008 overall. Additionally, these mothers are 221 percent more likely to experience a SMM (Figure 25).

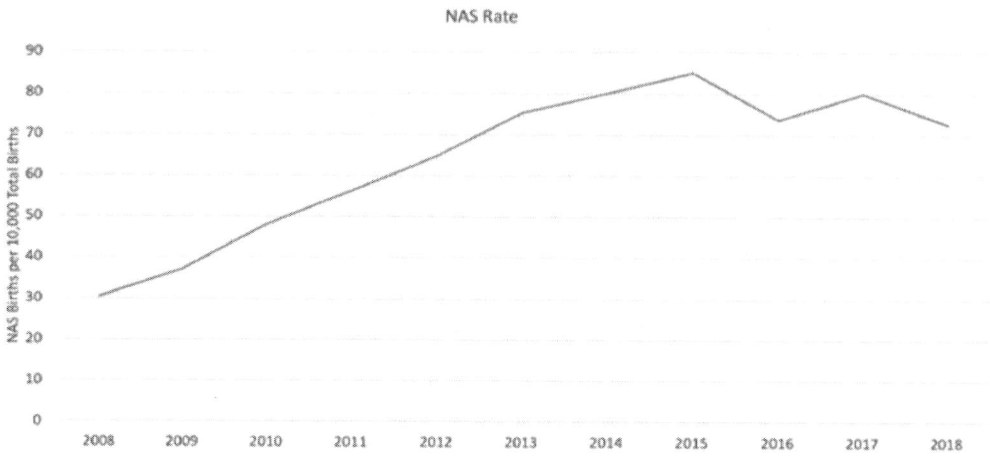

Figure 24. Rate of Babies born with Neonatal Abstinence Syndrome in the Hospital.

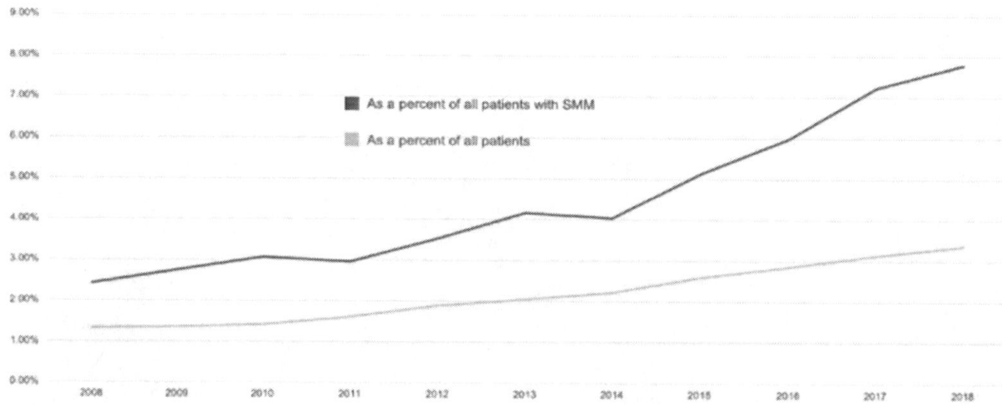

Figure 25. Inpatient Birth Mothers with Documented Substance Use.

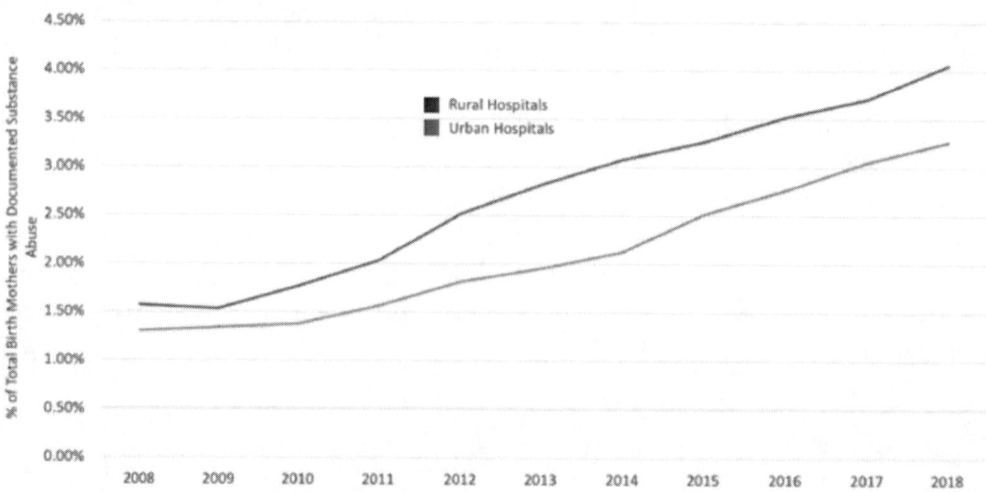

Figure 26. Rate of Substance Use by Hospital Location.

When comparing rural to urban hospitals, rural hospitals had a 34 percent higher rate of maternal patients with substance misuse (Figure 26).

Conclusion

In the United States, we have a limited understanding of why women are dying, or nearly dying, during pregnancy and childbirth. Unfortunately, state departments of health have limited sources of consistent, detailed data required to conduct accurate population-level analyses of maternal and infant health outcomes.

Premier's analysis showed that hospitals are making progress in reducing maternal deaths. It also showed that the disparity gap has been narrowed for maternal mortality among black women at the time of delivery, in the hospital setting. However, SMM rates have increased, likely a result of multifactorial causes that will require additional detailed analyses. This will include deeper study of the migration to ICD-10 and how that change affected the calculation of quality measures. The disparity gap for SMM remains wide when comparing black women to all other races. Additionally, the maternal population is aging and demonstrating a higher rate of cesarean sections and complications. Caesarean delivery rates are decreasing, although they continue to have higher associated SMM rates than vaginal deliveries.

Substance misuse remains a serious public health concern, and has been linked to harmful maternal and infant outcomes. Premier's analysis demonstrates substantial increases in substance use among women who are pregnant, and subsequently an alarming increase in the number of babies born with NAS. The analysis confirmed SMM is significantly higher among women with substance use disorders.

There are several factors that occur outside of the hospital during pre- and post-natal care that could be influencing overall maternal mortality and morbidity trends identified in Premier's analysis. The U.S. healthcare system continues to be fragmented in the way it cares for pregnant women, new mothers and infants. A more integrated approach to the care expectant and new mothers receive before, during and after delivery is needed in order to improve overall maternal and infant health in the United States.

Comprised of nearly 20 years of de-identified inpatient data, Premier's database is best-in-class and provides focused insights and are more specific than what has been reported by the CDC. Premier will continue to leverage the scale and depth of its database, which offers healthcare providers, patients, policymakers and industry organizations authoritative guidance on improving the quality, safety and efficiency of care delivered across the continuum.

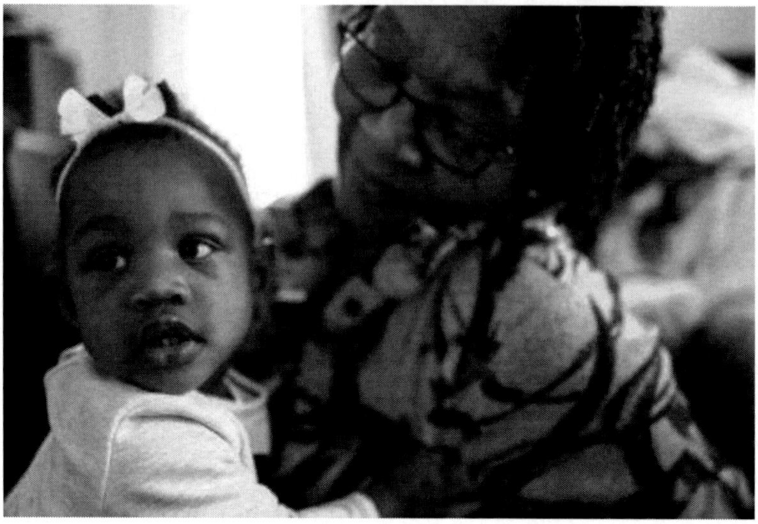

Figure 27. Soleil Irving "just lights up a room when she smiles," Wanda Irving, her grandmother, says. (Sheila Pree Bright for ProPublica).

Lost Mothers: Nothing Protects Black Women from Dying in Pregnancy and Childbirth

Not education. Not income. Not even being an expert on racial disparities in health care. By Nina Martin, ProPublica, and Renee Montagne, NPR News

This story was co-published with NPR.

On a melancholy Saturday this past February, Shalon Irving's "village" — the friends and family she had assembled to support her as a single mother — gathered at a funeral home in a prosperous black neighborhood in southwest Atlanta to say goodbye and send her home. The afternoon light was gray but bright, flooding through tall arched windows and pouring past white columns, illuminating the flag that covered her casket. Sprays of callas and roses dotted the room like giant corsages, flanking photos from happier times: Shalon in a slinky maternity dress, sprawled across her couch with her puppy; Shalon, sleepy-eyed and cradling the tiny head of her newborn daughter, Soleil. In one portrait Shalon wore a vibrant smile and the crisp uniform of the Commissioned Corps of the U.S. Public Health Service, where she had been a lieutenant commander. Many of the mourners were similarly attired. Shalon's father, Samuel, surveyed the rows of somber faces from the lectern. "I've never been in a room with so many doctors," he marveled. "… I've never seen so many PhDs."

At 36, Shalon had been part of their elite ranks — an epidemiologist at the Centers for Disease Control and Prevention, the preeminent public health institution in the U.S. There she had focused on trying to understand how structural inequality, trauma and violence made people sick. "She wanted to expose how peoples' limited health options were leading to poor health outcomes. To kind of uncover and undo the victim blaming that sometimes happens where it's like, 'Poor people don't care about their health,'" said Rashid Njai, her mentor at the agency. Her Twitter bio declared: "I see inequity wherever it exists, call it by name, and work to eliminate it."

Much of Shalon's research had focused on how childhood experiences affect health over a lifetime. Her discovery in mid-2016 that she was pregnant with her first child had been unexpected and thrilling.

Then the unthinkable had happened. Three weeks after giving birth, Shalon had collapsed and died.

The sadness in the chapel was crushing. Shalon's long-divorced parents had already buried both their sons; she had been their last remaining child. Wanda Irving had been especially close to her daughter —role model, traveling companion, emotional touchstone. She sat in the front row in a black suit and veiled hat, her face a portrait of unfathomable grief. Sometimes she held Soleil, fussing with her pink blanket. Sometimes Samuel held her, or one of Shalon's friends.

A few of Shalon's villagers rose to pay tribute; others sat quietly, poring through their funeral programs. Daniel Sellers, Shalon's cousin from Ohio and the baby's godfather, spoke for all of them when he promised Wanda that she would not have to raise her only grandchild alone. "People say to me, 'She won't know her mother.' That's not true," Sellers said. "Her mother is in each and every one of you, each and every one of us. ... This child is a gift to us. When you remember this child, you remember the love that God has pushed down through her for all of us. Soleil is our gift."

Underneath the numb despair was a profound sense of failure — and an acute understanding of what Shalon's death represented. The researcher working to eradicate disparities in health access and outcomes had become a symbol of one of the most troublesome health disparities facing black women in the U.S. today, disproportionately high rates of maternal mortality. The main federal agency seeking to understand why so many American women — especially black women — die and nearly die from complications of pregnancy and childbirth had lost one of its own. Even Shalon's many advantages — her B.A. in sociology, her two master's degrees and dual-subject PhD, her gold-plated insurance and rock-solid support system — had not been enough to ensure her survival. If a village this powerful hadn't been able to protect her, was any black woman safe?

The memorial service drew to a close, the bugle strains of "Taps" as plaintive as a howl. Two members of the U.S. Honor Guard removed the flag from Shalon's coffin and held it aloft. Then they folded it into a precise triangle small enough for Wanda and Samuel to hold next to their hearts.

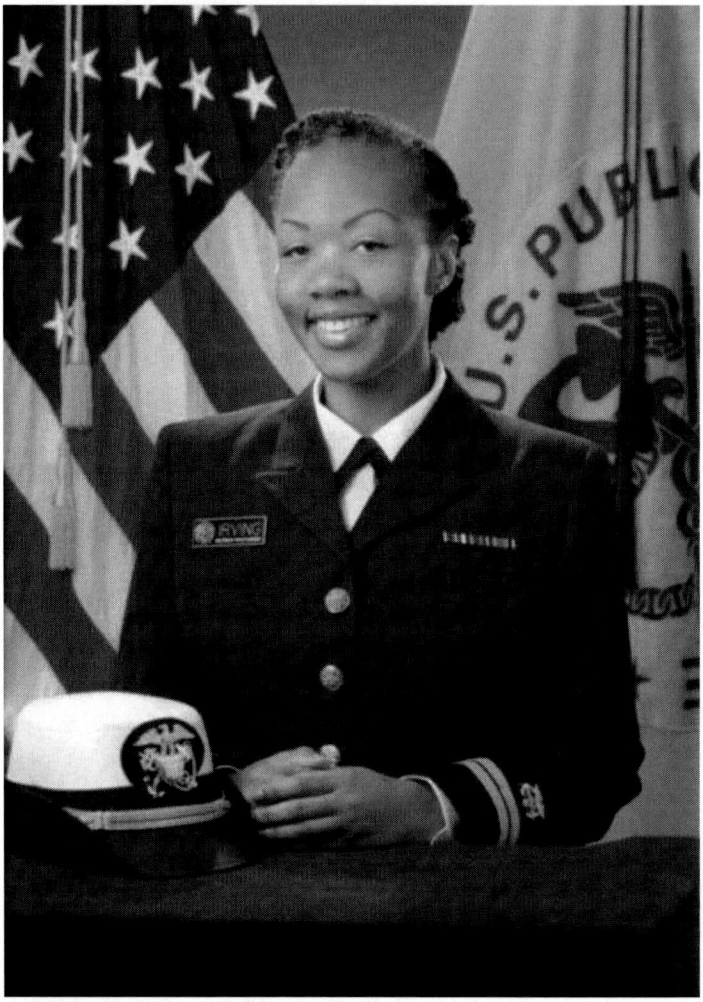

Figure 28. Shalon MauRene Irving was a lieutenant commander in the uniformed ranks of the U.S. Public Health Service. (Courtesy of Wanda Irving).

In recent years, as high rates of maternal mortality in the U.S. have alarmed researchers, one statistic has been especially concerning. According to the CDC, black mothers in the U.S. die at three to four times the rate of white mothers, one of the widest of all racial disparities in women's health. Put another way, a black woman is 22 percent more likely to die from heart disease than a white woman, 71 percent more likely to perish from cervical cancer, but 243 percent more likely to die from pregnancy- or childbirth-related causes. In a national study of five medical complications that are common causes of maternal death and injury, black women were two to three times more likely to die than white women who had the same condition.

That imbalance has persisted for decades, and in some places, it continues to grow. In New York City, for example, black mothers are 12 times more likely to die than white mothers, according to the most recent data; from 2001 to 2005, their risk of death was seven times higher. Researchers say that widening gap reflects a dramatic improvement for white women but not for blacks.

The disproportionate toll on African Americans is the main reason the U.S. maternal mortality rate is so much higher than that of other affluent countries. Black expectant and new mothers in the U.S. die at about the same rate as women in countries such as Mexico and Uzbekistan, the World Health Organization estimates.

What's more, even relatively well-off black women like Shalon Irving die or nearly die at higher rates than whites. Again, New York City offers a startling example: A 2016 analysis of five years of data found that black college-educated mothers who gave birth in local hospitals were more likely to suffer severe complications of pregnancy or childbirth than white women who never graduated from high school.

The fact that someone with Shalon's social and economic advantages is at higher risk highlights how profound the inequities really are, said Raegan McDonald-Mosley, the chief medical officer for Planned Parenthood Federation of America, who met her in graduate school at Johns Hopkins University and was one of her closest friends. "It tells you that you can't educate your way out of this problem. You can't health-care-access your way out of this problem. There's something inherently wrong with the system that's not valuing the lives of black women equally to white women."

For much of American history, these types of disparities were largely blamed on blacks' supposed innate susceptibility to illness — their "mass of imperfections," as one doctor wrote in 1903 — and their own behavior. But now many social scientists and medical researchers agree, the problem isn't race but racism.

The systemic problems start with the type of social inequities that Shalon studied — differential access to healthy food and clean drinking water, safe neighborhoods and good schools, decent jobs and reliable transportation. Black women are more likely to be uninsured outside of pregnancy, when Medicaid kicks in, and thus more likely to start prenatal care later and to lose coverage in the postpartum period. They are more likely to have chronic conditions such as obesity, diabetes, and hypertension that make having a baby more dangerous. The hospitals where they give birth are often the products of historical segregation, lower in quality than those where white mothers deliver, with significantly higher rates of life-threatening complications.

Those problems are amplified by unconscious biases that are embedded throughout the medical system, affecting quality of care in stark and subtle ways. In the more than 200 stories of African-American mothers that ProPublica and NPR have collected over the past year, the feeling of being devalued and disrespected by medical providers was a constant theme. The young Florida mother-to-be whose breathing problems were blamed on obesity when in fact her lungs were filling with fluid and her heart was failing. The Arizona mother whose anesthesiologist assumed she smoked marijuana because of the way she did her hair. The Chicago-area businesswoman with a high-risk pregnancy who was so upset at her doctor's attitude that she changed OB-GYNs in her seventh month, only to suffer a fatal postpartum stroke.

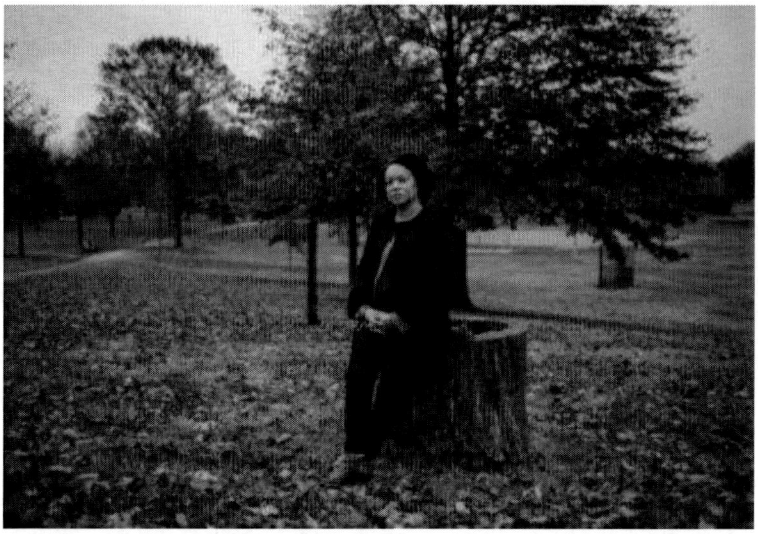

Figure 29. Looking over Shalon's medical records, her friend Raegan McDonald-Mosley saw many missed opportunities "at multiple parts of the health care system." (Ariel Zambelich for ProPublica).

Over and over, black women told of medical providers who equated being African American with being poor, uneducated, noncompliant and unworthy. "Sometimes you just know in your bones when someone feels contempt for you based on your race," said one Brooklyn woman who took to bringing her white husband or in-laws to every prenatal visit.

Hakima Tafunzi Payne, a mother of nine in Kansas City, Missouri, who used to be a labor-and-delivery nurse and still attends births as a student midwife, has seen this cultural divide as both patient and caregiver. "The nursing culture is white, middle-class, and female, so is largely built around that identity. Anything that doesn't fit that identity is suspect," she said. Payne, who is also a nurse educator lecturing on unconscious bias for professional organizations, recalled "the conversations that took place behind the nurse's station that just made assumptions — a lot of victim blaming, 'If those people would only do blah, blah, blah, things would be different.'"

Black expectant and new mothers frequently told us that doctors and nurses didn't take their pain seriously — a phenomenon borne out by numerous studies that show pain is often undertreated in black patients for conditions from appendicitis to cancer. When Patrisse Cullors, a cofounder of the Black Lives Matters movement who has become an activist to improve black maternal care, had an emergency C-section in Los Angeles in March 2016, the surgeon "never explained what he was doing to me," she said. The pain medication didn't work: "My mother basically had to scream at the doctors to give me the proper pain meds." When white people advocate for themselves or their family members, she said, providers "think they're acting reasonably. When black people are advocating for our family members, we're complaining, we're being uppity, we don't know what we're talking about, we're exaggerating."

Limited diversity in the medical profession contributes to the black mothers' sense of alienation. Blacks make up 6 percent of doctors (though 11 percent of OB-GYNs), 3 percent of medical school faculty and less than 2 percent of National Institutes of Health-funded principal investigators. "That's a real problem that across the spectrum that [black women] are not feeling listened to and respected—that's a structural problem," said Monica McLemore, a nursing professor at the University of California, San Francisco, who has conducted focus groups with dozens of mothers as part of a $50 million initiative to reduce preterm births. "The health sector doesn't want to admit how much of this is about us."

But it's the discrimination that black women experience in the rest of their lives — the double-whammy of race and gender — that may ultimately be the most significant factor in poor maternal outcomes. An expanding field of research shows that the stress of being a black woman in American society can take a significant physical toll during pregnancy and childbirth.

Watch the Video

The U.S. medical system is still haunted by slavery.

"It's chronic stress that just happens all the time — there is never a period where there's rest from it, it's everywhere, it's in the air, it's just affecting everything," said Fleda Mask Jackson, an Atlanta researcher and member of the Black Mamas Matter Alliance who studies disparities in birth outcomes.

It's a type of stress from which education and class provide no protection. "When you interview these doctors and lawyers and business executives, when you interview African-American college graduates, it's not like their lives have been a walk in the park," said Michael Lu, a longtime disparities researcher and former head of the Maternal and Child Health Bureau of the Health Resources and Services Administration, the main federal agency funding programs for mothers and infants. "It's the experience of having to work harder than anybody else just to get equal pay and equal respect. It's being followed around when you're shopping at a nice store, or being stopped by the police when you're driving in a nice neighborhood."

Arline Geronimus, a professor at the University of Michigan School of Public Health, coined the term "weathering" for how this continuous stress wears away at the body. Weathering "causes a lot of different health vulnerabilities and increases susceptibility to infection," she said, "but also early onset of chronic diseases, in particular, hypertension and diabetes" — conditions that disproportionately affect blacks at much younger ages than whites. It accelerates aging at the cellular level; in a 2010 study, Geronimus and colleagues found that the telomeres (chromosomal markers of aging) of black women in their 40s and 50s appeared 7 1/2 years older on average than those of whites.

Weathering can have particularly serious repercussions in pregnancy and childbirth, the most physiologically complex time in a woman's life. Stress has been linked to one of the most common and consequential pregnancy complications, preterm birth. Black women are 49 percent more likely than whites to deliver prematurely (and, closely related, black infants are twice as likely as white babies to die before their first birthday). Here again, income and education aren't protective.

The effects on the mother's health may also be far-reaching. Maternal age is an important risk factor for many severe pregnancy-related complications, as well as for chronic diseases that can affect pregnancy, like hypertension. "As women get older, birth outcomes get worse," Lu said. "If that happens in the 40s for white women, it actually starts to happen for African-American women in their 30s."

This means that for black women, the risks for pregnancy likely start at an earlier age than many clinicians — and women— realize, and the effects on their bodies may be much greater than for white women. This doesn't mean that pregnancy should be thought of as inherently scary or dangerous for black women (or anyone). It does mean, in Geronimus' view, that "a black woman of any social class, as early as her mid-20s, should be attended to differently" — with greater awareness of the potential challenges ahead.

That's a paradigm shift that professional organizations and providers have barely begun to wrap their heads around. "There may be individual doctors or hospitals that are doing it [accounting for the higher risk of black women], but ... there's not much of that going on," Lu said. Should doctors and clinicians be taking into consideration this added layer of vulnerability?

"Yeah," Lu said. "I truly think they should."

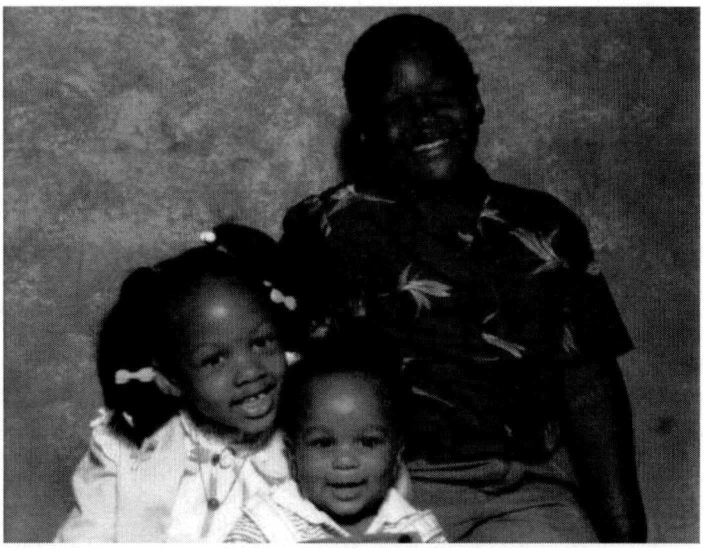

Figure 30. Shalon, her baby brother Simone and her older brother Sam III, in a photo taken in the mid-1980s (Courtesy of Wanda Irving).

Shalon Irving's history is almost a textbook example of the kinds of strains and stresses that make high-achieving black women vulnerable. The child of two Dartmouth graduates, she grew up in Portland, Oregon, where her father's father was pastor of a black church. Even in its current liberal incarnation, Portland is one of the whitest large cities in the U.S.

Thirty years ago, Portland was a much more uncomfortable place to be black. African-American life there was often characterized by social isolation, which Geronimus' research suggests can be especially stressful. Samuel Irving spent years working as a railroad engineer; he got a law degree and later ran a city agency, but felt his prospects were still constrained by his race. Wanda held various jobs in marketing and communications, including at the U.S. Forest Service. In elementary school, Shalon was sometimes the only African-American kid in her class. "There were many mornings where she would stand outside banging on the door wanting to come back into the house because she didn't want to go to school," her mother recently recalled.

Shalon's strategy for fitting in was to be smarter than everyone else. She read voraciously, wrote a column for a black-owned weekly newspaper and skipped a grade. Books and writing helped her cope with trauma and sorrow — first the death of her 20-month-old brother Simone in a car accident when she was six, then the fracturing of her parents' marriage, then the diagnosis of her beloved older brother, Sam III, with a virulent form of early-onset multiple sclerosis when he was 17. Amid all the family troubles, Shalon was funny and driven, with a fierce sense of loyalty and "a moral compass that was amazing," her mother said. She was also overweight and often anxious, given to daydreaming (as she later put it) about "alternative realities where people hadn't died and things had not been lost." When it came time to go away to college, she chose the historically black Hampton University in Virginia. "She wanted to feel that nurturing environment," Wanda said. "She had had enough."

By then, Shalon had noticed that many of her relatives — her mother's mother, her aunts, her far-flung cousins — died in their 30s and 40s. Her brother, Sam III, sardonically joked that the family had a "death gene," but Shalon didn't think that was funny. "She didn't understand why there was such a disparity with other families that had all these long lives," Wanda said. Shalon nagged her father to stop smoking and her mother to lose weight. She set an example, shedding nearly 100 pounds while managing to graduate summa cum laude. At the start of graduate school at Purdue University, she was a svelte 138 pounds, "very classy and elegant, a lot like her mom," said Bianca Pryor, a master's student in consumer behavior who became one of what Shalon called her cherished circle of "sister friends."

They were all bearing the same burden. "There's this feeling that we're carrying the expectations of generations, the first ones trying to climb the corporate ladder, trying to climb in academe," said Pryor, now a marketing executive in New York City. "There is this idea that we have to work twice as hard as everyone else. But there's also, 'I'm first-generation, I don't know the ropes, I don't how to use my social capital.' There's a bit of shame in that ... this constant checking in with yourself — am I doing this right?"

Shalon set the bar especially high: She was pursuing a double Ph.D. in sociology and gerontology, focusing on themes she would return to often — the long-term effects of early childhood trauma and maltreatment, the impact of the parent-child relationship on lifelong health. She finished in under five years, once again with top honors — "one of the best writers I've had in my academic career," her adviser, sociologist Kenneth Ferraro, said.

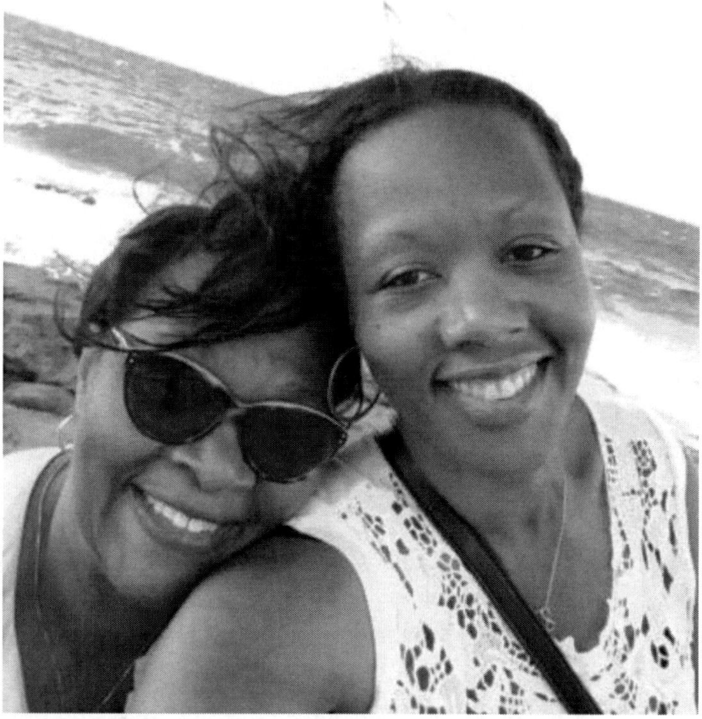

Figure 31. Wanda and Shalon were so close, "they were like the 'Gilmore Girls,'" one friend said. (Courtesy of Wanda Irving).

She tried teaching, then decided to pursue a second master's degree, this time from Johns Hopkins. She was also juggling family responsibilities. Wanda had followed Shalon around the country, earning her own master's degree and working in nonprofit management. "They were like the 'Gilmore Girls,'" Pryor said. In 2008, Sam III joined them in Baltimore to take part in a study on an experimental MS therapy. With his family's support, he'd managed to finish college and run a poetry-slam nonprofit for kids. His next goal was to walk across the stage to receive his diploma instead of using his wheelchair. In February 2009, while he was doing physical rehab to regain strength in his legs, a blood clot traveled to his lung, killing him at the age of 32. Afterward, Wanda and Shalon clung to each other more tightly than ever.

In 2011 came what Ferraro called Shalon's "change-the-world opportunity" — a consulting gig at the CDC with Michelle Obama's "Let's Move!" initiative. Soon she joined the agency's prestigious Epidemic Intelligence Service, a training program in applied epidemiology — in her case, with a focus on community health — whose members served as first responders in health emergencies. As part of the uniformed ranks of the U.S. Public Health Service, she could eventually discharge her student debt — more than $165,000 for Hopkins alone — travel, buy a house. "The permanence was very appealing," Pryor said.

What Shalon wasn't prepared for was how unfulfilled she was. After Johns Hopkins, she had worked on the frontlines helping at-risk infants, teenage girls and mothers with HIV/AIDS. She was passionate about improving food and housing security to reduce people's risk for high blood pressure and other cardiovascular problems, but felt like much of her CDC research ended up sitting on a shelf. It bothered her that she rarely met the people behind the data she was analyzing. "She might see the numbers, but I don't think she actually saw that little girl or little boy have a healthier lunch," Pryor said.

The stress and frustration triggered the old corrosive self-doubts. But gradually, Shalon saw a way out of the box. She joined the CDC's Division of Violence Prevention, refocusing on issues around trauma and domestic abuse— a mission she saw as "liberating" for African-American women, Wanda said. She started a coaching business called Inclusivity Standard to advise young people from disadvantaged backgrounds who wanted to get into college or grad school, as well as organizations seeking to become more diverse. She enlisted her mother, now working as a consultant, and Pryor to join her team. And she decided to write a self-help book, on the theory that many people in the communities she cared about couldn't afford psychotherapy or didn't trust it. "She was one of those people — one thing is just not enough," said her coauthor Habiba Tran, a therapist and life coach with a multicultural clientele. "One modality is just not enough. One way of [reaching people] is just not enough."

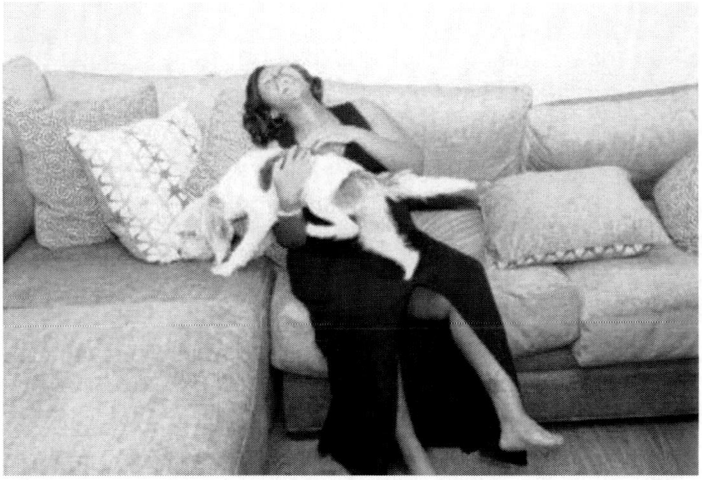

Figure 32. "No words have been created to adequately capture the fear and love and excitement that I feel right now," Shalon, shown here with her puppy Lady Day, wrote to her daughter. (Courtesy of Wanda Irving).

Shalon couldn't remember a time when she didn't want to be a mother. But her romantic life had been a "20-year dating debacle," she admitted in the manuscript of her self-help book, in part because "I am deathly scared of heartbreak and disappointment, and letting people in comes with the very real risk of both."

In 2014, when Shalon was 34, medical problems forced the issue. For years she'd been suffering from uterine fibroids — non-malignant tumors that affect up to 80 percent of black women, leading to heavy menstrual bleeding, anemia and pelvic pain. No one knows what causes fibroids or why blacks are so susceptible. What is known is that the tumors can interfere with fertility — indeed, black women are nearly twice as likely to have infertility problems as whites, and when they undergo treatment, there's much less likelihood that the treatments will succeed. Surgery bought her a little time, but her OB-GYN urged her not to delay getting pregnant much longer.

Shalon had spent her adult years defying stereotypes about black women; now she wrestled with the reality that by embracing single motherhood, she could become one. The financial risk was substantial — she'd just purchased a town house in the quiet Sandy Springs area north of Atlanta, and her CDC insurance only covered artificial insemination for wives using their husbands' sperm. In Portland, no one would have blinked an eye at an unmarried professional woman having a child on her own, but in Atlanta, "there is very much a vibe there that things should happen in a certain order," Pryor said. "And Shalon was not having that at all. She was like, 'Nope, this is what it is.'"

The gamble — funded with her parents' help — ended in a series of devastating failures. In September 2015, in the midst of one unsuccessful insemination treatment, Shalon was alarmed to discover that her right arm had become swollen and hard. Doctors found a blood clot and diagnosed her with Factor V Leiden, a genetic mutation that makes blood prone to abnormal clumping. Suddenly a part of the family's medical mystery was solved. Wanda's mother had died of a pulmonary embolism, so had Sam III, so had other members of their extended family. But no one had been tested for the mutation, which is primarily associated with European ancestry. Had they known they carried it, maybe Sam's deadly blood clot could have been prevented. It was a what-if too painful to dwell on.

By April 2016, Shalon had given up. She had a new boyfriend and she was on her way to Puerto Rico to help with the CDC'S Zika response, working to prevent the spread of the virus to expectant mothers and their unborn babies. There she discovered she'd gotten pregnant by accident. Her excitement was tempered by fear that the baby might have contracted Zika, which can cause microcephaly and other birth defects. But a barrage of medical tests confirmed all was well.

More good news: A few weeks later Pryor learned she was pregnant, too. "All right," she told Shalon, "let's finally go after our rainbows and unicorns! Because for so long it was just dark clouds and rain."

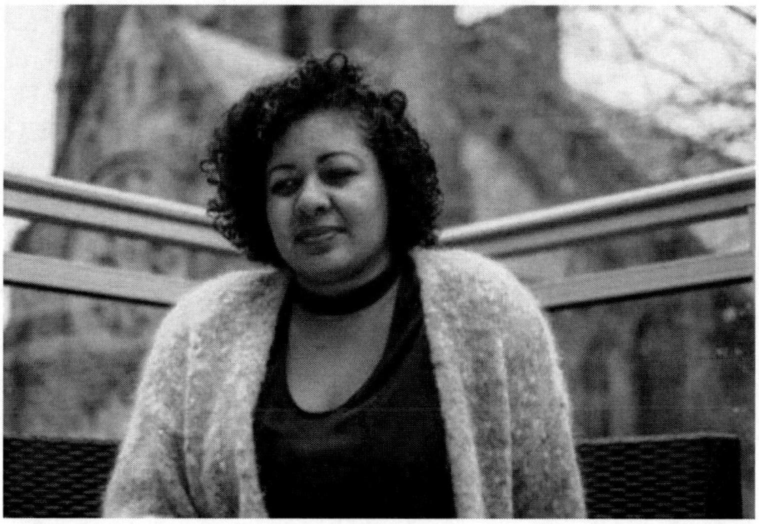

Figure 33. A worried Bianca Pryor quizzed her best friend from grad school: “Are you getting out of the house? Are you going for your walks?” (Melissa Bunni Elian for ProPublica).

In reality, Shalon’s many risk factors — including her clotting disorder, her fibroid surgery, the 36 years of wear and tear on her telomeres, her weight — boded a challenging nine months. She also had a history of high blood pressure, though it was now under control without medication. “If I was the doctor taking care of her, I'd be like, ‘Oh, this is going to be a tough one,’” her OB-GYN friend Raegan McDonald-Mosley said.

Shalon got though the physical challenges surprisingly well. Her team at Emory University, one of the premier health systems in the South, had no trouble managing her clotting disorder with the blood thinner Lovenox. They worried that scarring from the fibroid surgery could result in a rupture if her uterus stretched too much, so they scheduled a C-section at 37 weeks. At several points, Shalon’s blood pressure did spike, Wanda said, but doctors ruled out preeclampsia (pregnancy-induced hypertension) and the numbers always fell back to normal.

Wanda blamed stress. There was the painful end to Shalon’s romance with her baby’s father and her dashed hopes of raising their child together. There were worries about money and panic attacks about the difficulties of being a black single mother in the South in the era of Trayvon Martin and Tamir Rice. Shalon told everyone she was hoping for a girl.

Steeped in research about how social support could buffer against stress and adversity, Shalon joined online groups for single moms and assembled a stalwart community she could quickly deploy for help. “She was all about the village,” Rashid Njai said. “She’d say, ‘I’m making sure that when I have my baby, the village is activated and ready to go.’”

She poured more of her anxious energy into finishing the first draft of the book. She sent Tran the manuscript on Jan. 2, the day before the planned C-section, then typed one last note to her child. Boy or girl, its nickname would be Sunny, in honor of her brother Sam, her “sunshine.”

"You will always be my most important accomplishment," she wrote. "No words have been created to adequately capture the fear and love and excitement that I feel right now."

Until recently, much of the discussion about maternal mortality has focused on pregnancy and childbirth. But according to the most recent CDC data, more than half of maternal deaths occur in the postpartum period, and one-third happen seven or more days after delivery. For American women in general, postpartum care can be dangerously inadequate — often no more than a single appointment four to six weeks after going home. "If you've had a cesarean delivery, if you've had preeclampsia, if you've had gestational diabetes or diabetes, if you go home on an anticoagulant — all those women need to be seen significantly sooner than six weeks," said Haywood Brown, a professor at Duke University medical school. Brown has made reforming postpartum care one of his main initiatives as president of the American Congress of Obstetricians and Gynecologists.

The dangers of sporadic postpartum care may be particularly great for black mothers. African Americans have higher rates of C-section and are more than twice as likely to be readmitted to the hospital in the month following the surgery. They have disproportionate rates of preeclampsia and peripartum cardiomyopathy (a type of heart failure), two leading killers in the days and weeks after delivery. They're twice as likely as white women to have postpartum depression, which contributes to poor outcomes, but they are much less likely to receive mental health treatment. If they experience discrimination or disrespect during pregnancy or childbirth, they may be more likely to skip postpartum visits to check on their own health (they do keep pediatrician appointments for their babies). Lack of paid maternity leave and childcare can create additional hurdles. In one study published earlier this year, two-thirds of low-income black women never made it to their doctor visit.

Meanwhile, many providers wrongly assume that the risks end when the baby is born — and that women who came through pregnancy and delivery without problems will stay healthy. In the case of black women, providers may not understand their true biological risks or evaluate those risks in a big-picture way. "The maternal experience isn't over right at delivery. All of the due diligence that gets applied during the prenatal period needs to continue into the postpartum period," said Eleni Tsigas, executive director of the Preeclampsia Foundation.

It's not just doctors and nurses who need to think differently. Like a lot of expectant mothers, Shalon had an elaborate plan for how she wanted to give birth, even including what she wanted her surgical team to talk about (nothing political) and who would announce the baby's gender (her mother, not a doctor or nurse). But like most pregnant women, she didn't have a postpartum care plan for herself. "It was just trusting in the system that things were gonna go okay," Wanda said. "And that if something came up, she'd be able to handle it."

The birth was "a beautiful time," Wanda said. Shalon did so well that she convinced her doctor to let her and Soleil — French for "sun" — leave the hospital after two nights (three or four nights are more typical). Then at home, "things got real," Pryor said. "It was Shalon and her mom trying to figure things out, and the late nights, and trying to get baby on schedule. Shalon was very honest. She told me, 'Friend, this is hard.'"

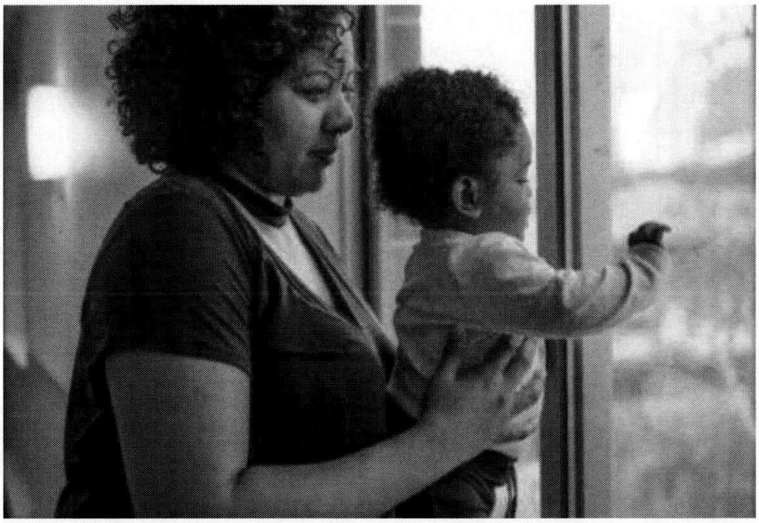

Figure 34. When Pryor found she was pregnant, too, with her son Everton, she told Shalon, "Let's finally go after our rainbows and unicorns!" (Melissa Bunni Elian for ProPublica).

C-sections have much higher complication rates than vaginal births. In Shalon's case, the trouble — a painful lump on her incision — emerged a few days after she went home. The first doctor she saw, on Jan. 12, said it was nothing, but as she and her mother were leaving his office, they ran into her longtime OB-GYN, Elizabeth Collins. Collins took a look and diagnosed a hematoma — blood trapped in layers of healing skin, something that happens in about 1 percent of C-sections. The OB-GYN drained the "fluctuant mass" (as her notes described it), and "copious bloody non-purulent material" poured out from the one-inch incision. Collins also arranged for a visiting nurse to come by the house every other day to change the dressing. Collins didn't respond to a request for comment.

Over the next two weeks, Shalon's records show three more visits to Emory and two nursing visits at home. She feared that the incision wasn't healing fast enough, perhaps because the blood thinners she was taking to prevent an embolism — another C-section risk — were hampering coagulation. But a wound specialist said everything looked OK. Shalon was worried about Soleil, too: Breastfeeding was harder than expected, and she'd stopped taking narcotic painkillers because she thought they were making the baby groggy. But less powerful painkillers weren't working; between the pain and the anxiety, she was hardly sleeping. "Patient has poor endurance," the visiting nurse noted on Jan. 16. "Leaving the home is a TAXING and CONSIDERABLE effort."

What troubled the nurse most, though, was Shalon's blood pressure. On Jan. 16 it was 158/100, high enough to raise concerns about postpartum preeclampsia, which can lead to seizures and stroke. But Shalon didn't have other symptoms, such as headache or blurred vision. She made an appointment to see the OB-GYN for the next day, then ended up being too overwhelmed to go, the visiting nurse noted on Jan. 18. In that same record, the nurse wrote that Shalon had to change the dressing on her wound "sometimes several times a day due to large amounts of red drainage. This is adding to her stress as a new mom." Her pain was 5 on a scale of 10, preventing her from "sleeping/relaxing." Overall, Shalon told the nurse, "it just doesn't feel right." When the nurse measured her blood pressure on the cuff Shalon kept at home, the reading was 158/112. On the nurse's equipment, the reading was 174/118.

"We provide caring and compassionate care to all of our patients," the Visiting Nurse Health System said in an email. "She was in our care for less than four days but we gave the very best care we could."

Under current ACOG guidelines, blood pressure readings that high should trigger more aggressive action, such as an immediate trip to the doctor for further evaluation, possibly medication and more careful monitoring. A history of hypertension and multiple other risks should raise more red flags, Tsigas said. "We need to look holistically at the risk factors irrespective of whether or not she had a diagnosis of preeclampsia," she said. "If somebody has a whole plateful of risk factors, how are you treating them differently?" High blood pressure in the postpartum period should always be considered an emergency, she said.

"It would have made sense to admit her to the hospital for a complete work-up, including chest xray, an echocardiogram to evaluate for heart failure, and titration of her medication (both pain meds and hypertension meds) to sort out what she needed to feel OK and get [her] blood pressure out of the severe range," wrote one doctor, a leading expert on postpartum care, who agreed to look at Shalon's records at ProPublica's request, but asked not to be identified. "Education on signs / symptoms of stroke seems insufficient — we don't want to wait until someone is having a stroke to get their BP treated. A next-day follow-up for a BP of 174/118 seems questionable for a postpartum woman. Same-day assessment in her provider's office, or in the ER, would have been very much within the bounds of common practice."

Instead, Shalon was given an appointment for the following day, Jan. 19, with an OB-GYN at Women's Center at Emory St. Joseph's, which handled her primary care. By then, Shalon's blood pressure had fallen, and there were "no symptoms concerning for postpartum [preeclampsia]," the doctor wrote in his notes. He wrote that Shalon was healing "appropriately" and thought her jumps in blood pressure were likely related to "poor pain control." Wanda and Shalon left feeling more frustrated than ever.

At home over the next couple of days, Wanda noticed that one of Shalon's legs was larger than the other. "She said, 'Yeah, I know, Mom, and my knee hurts, I can't bend it."

When McDonald-Mosley looked over the voluminous medical records a few months later, what jumped out at her was the sense that Shalon's caregivers didn't seem to think of her as a patient who needed a heightened level of attention, despite the complexity of her pregnancy.

"She had all these risk factors. If you're gonna pick someone who's going to have a problem, it's gonna be her. ... She needs to be treated with caution." The fact that her symptoms defied easy categorization was all the more reason to be vigilant, McDonald-Mosley said. "There were all these opportunities to identify that something was going wrong. To act on them sooner and they were missed. At multiple levels. At multiple parts of the health care system. They were missed."

Shalon's other friends were growing uneasy, too. Back in New York, Bianca Pryor had her own pregnancy emergency — her son was born very prematurely, at 24 weeks — so she couldn't be in Atlanta. But she and Shalon talked often by phone. "She knew so much about her body one would think she was an M.D. and not a Ph.D. To hear her be concerned about her legs — that worried me." Pryor encouraged her, "'Friend, are you getting out of the house? Are you going for your walks? She told me, 'No, I'm on my chaise lounge, and that's about as much as I can do.'"

Habiba Tran was so upset at Shalon's condition that she took her frustrations out on her friend. "I was cussing her out. 'Go to the f— ing doctor.' She's like, 'I called them. I talked to them. I went to see them. Get off my back.'"

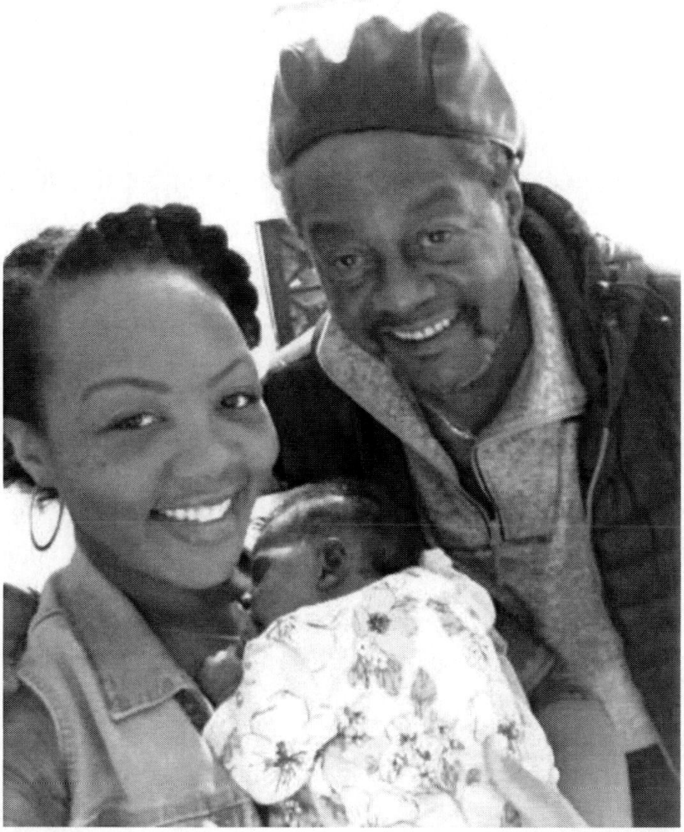

Figure 35. Shalon took this selfie with her dad, Samuel, and her newborn daughter on the morning of Jan. 24, 2017. Twelve hours later, she collapsed. (Courtesy of Wanda Irving).

On the morning of Tuesday, Jan. 24, Shalon took a selfie with her father, who'd been visiting for a week, then sent him to the airport to catch a flight back to Portland. Towards noon, she and Wanda and the baby drove to the Emory Women's Center one more time. This time, Shalon saw a nurse practitioner. "We said, 'Look, there's something wrong here, she's not feeling well,'" Wanda recalled. "'One leg is larger than the other, she's still gaining weight'— nine pounds in 10 days — 'the blood pressure is still up, there's gotta be something wrong."

The nurse's records confirmed Shalon had swelling in both legs, with more swelling in the right one. She noted that Shalon had complained of "some mild headaches" and her blood pressure was back up to 163/99, but she didn't have other preeclampsia signs, like blurred vision. She checked the incision — "warm dry no [sign/symptom] of infection" — and noted Shalon's mental state ("cooperative, appropriate mood & affect, normal judgment"). She ordered an ultrasound to check the legs for blood clots, as well as preeclampsia screening.

Both tests came back negative. As Wanda remembers it, Shalon was insistent: "There *is* something wrong, I know my body. I don't feel well, my legs are swollen, I'm gaining weight. I'm not voiding. I'm drinking a lot of water, but I'm retaining the water." Before sending Shalon home, the nurse gave her a prescription for the blood pressure medication nifedipine, which is often used to treat pregnancy-related hypertension.

Emory Healthcare "is dedicated to the highest quality patient care," it said in an email. It declined to answer questions about Shalon's care, citing patient confidentiality.

Shalon and Wanda stopped at the pharmacy, then decided to go out to dinner with the baby. While they ate, they talked about a trip Shalon had planned for the three of them to take in just a few weeks. Ever since Sam III had died, Wanda and Shalon made a point of traveling someplace special on painful anniversaries. To mark his 40th birthday and the eighth anniversary of his death, Shalon had gotten the idea of going to Dubai. ("It's cheap," Shalon had told Wanda. "The money is worth so much more there. It's supposed to be beautiful.") She had long ago purchased their tickets and ordered the baby's passport. Now Wanda was worried — would she be feeling well enough to make such a big trip with an infant? Shalon wasn't willing to give up hope just yet. Wanda recalls her saying, "I'll be fine, I'll be fine."

They got home and sat in Shalon's bedroom for a while, laughing and playing with the baby. Around 8:30 p.m., Shalon suddenly declared, "I just don't know, Mom, I just don't feel well." She took one of the blood pressure pills. An hour later, while she and Wanda were chatting, Shalon clutched her heart, gasped and passed out.

Paramedics arrived to find Shalon on the floor near the foot of her bed "pulseless and not breathing..." They tried to stabilize her, then rushed her to Atlanta's Northside Hospital, just a couple of miles from her home. In the emergency room, doctors discovered that the breathing tube had been "incorrectly placed," according to the ambulance service report — into her esophagus instead of her lungs. She never regained consciousness. Four days later, on Jan. 28, Wanda and Samuel withdrew life support and she died.

The news spread quickly among her colleagues at the CDC. William Callaghan, chief of the maternal and infant health branch, recalled in March that his boss, who had visited Shalon at the hospital, called to let him know. “It was a chilling phone call,” said Callaghan, one of the nation’s leading researchers on maternal mortality. “It certainly takes, in that moment, what I do, it made it very, very, very concrete. ... This was not about data, this was not about whether it was going up or it was going down. It was about this tragic event that happened to this woman, her family.”

Northside declined to do an autopsy, telling Wanda and Samuel that none was required, they recalled. (The hospital declined to comment.) So Wanda paid $4,500 for an autopsy by the medical examiners in neighboring DeKalb County. The report came back three months later. Noting that Shalon’s heart showed signs of damage consistent with hypertension, it attributed her death to complications of high blood pressure.

Wanda always knew she would be spending a lot of time caring for her granddaughter. She and Shalon loved the idea of the three of them making their way in the world together, trying to change it for the better.

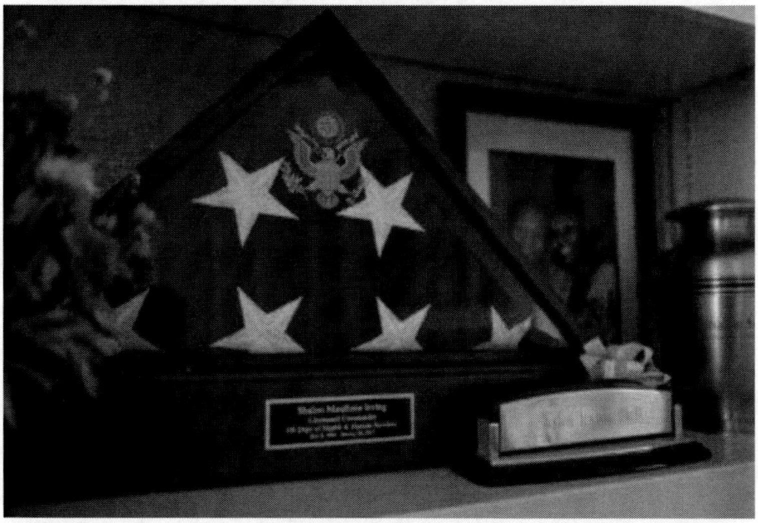

Figure 36. The flag that covered Shalon’s casket is now in a memorial case with other mementos and photos (Sheila Pree Bright for ProPublica).

Instead, Wanda has had to find a way to go on without her daughter and best friend. She took a break from her consultant work and moved into Shalon’s cozy townhouse, now crowded with baby books and gear, to assume her new role. Soleil was colicky, prone to gastric problems that kept both of them up all night. Shalon’s villagers stopped by often to help, but much of the time Wanda was on her own. Her grief was most acute at nights, but she couldn’t let it interfere with her duties to Soleil.

Eventually the colic went away and Soleil thrived. In June, Wanda and her five-month-old granddaughter went to Chattanooga for the annual meeting of U.S. Public Health Service scientists. A new honor — the Shalon Irving Memorial (Junior) Scientist Officer of the Year Award — had been created to celebrate Shalon’s legacy, and Wanda had been asked to say a few words. She handed the baby to one of Shalon's CDC colleagues and took the small stage.

"Striving for excellence is a choice," she told the audience through barely suppressed tears. "It is a commitment. ... It's a struggle to become the person you want to be. It's harder than you want. It takes longer than you want. And it takes more out of you than you expected it should."

Shalon personified excellence, Wanda said. "I don't know if Shalon became the woman that she ultimately wanted to be. But I do know that she wanted to be the woman she was."

She also knew how Shalon wanted to raise her daughter, and she was determined to do the same: reading to her, traveling with her, taking her to gymnastic and music classes. "She wanted Soleil to go to Montessori school, so I'm looking for a Montessori school for her," Wanda said. "She wanted her to be christened, we got her christened." Wanda and Soleil have developed a routine: Every morning they say hello to the photos of Shalon on the living room walls. Every evening they say goodnight. Sometimes Wanda shows Soleil the flag from her mother's casket, now encased in a wooden frame. She set aside other mementos for later — the academic writings, the certificates and awards, the manuscript of her book with Tran. If all goes according to plan, it will be published early next year.

One Saturday afternoon in October, Wanda received another book, this one compiled by Shalon's friends from the Epidemic Intelligence Service and entitled "Letters to Soleil." She put the baby on her lap and said, "I'm gonna read you some letters about your mom." One thing Wanda has tried never to do is cry in front of Soleil. But as she began reading aloud, she was sobbing. "And Soleil just kept looking at me — she couldn't understand what was going on. And about a minute later she took my glasses off with her hands and put them down and then laid her head right on my chest and started patting me. Which made me cry all the more."

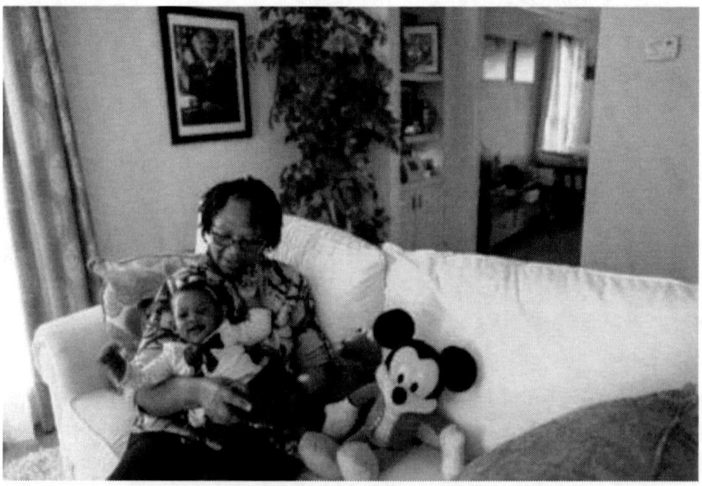

Figure 37. Wanda in the living room of the town house she shares with Soleil. A photo of Shalon is in the background. (Sheila Pree Bright for ProPublica).

Shalon was a letter-writer too. One day not long after the funeral, Wanda found a note that her daughter had written to her two years earlier, around the sixth anniversary of Sam III's death. Shalon had left it among the other important items in her computer, trusting that if something ever happened to her, Wanda would find it. The letter reads like a premonition of her own death: Shalon wasn't afraid for herself, but agonized over how it would affect her mother.

Read More: The New U.S. Maternal Mortality Rate Fails to Capture Many Deaths

Since 2007, the government had held off on releasing an official estimate of expectant and new mothers who died from causes related to pregnancy and childbirth. It waited for the data to get better. But the new, long-anticipated number falls short.

> I am sorry that I have left you. On the particular day that I am writing this I have no idea how that may have occurred but know that I would never choose to leave.
>
> I know it seems impossible right now, but please do not let this break you. I want you to be happy and smile. I want you to know that I am being watched after by my brothers and grandma and that we are all watching you. Please try not to cry. Use your energy instead to feel my love through time and space. Nothing can break the bond we have and you will forever be my mommy and I your baby girl!

Now 11 months old, Soleil has her mother's precociousness, energy and headstrong yet sweet disposition. Like the sun she was named for, "she just lights up a room when she smiles," Wanda said. She comes into Wanda's bed every night and wakes her early to play. "She'll bite my nose and kick me — 'Nana, time to get up! Time to get up!'" And so Wanda does.

Do you know someone who died in pregnancy, childbirth or the postpartum period? Please tell us your story. If you want to reach out to us directly, email us at Maternal@propublica.org.

Correction, Dec. 8, 2017: An earlier version of this story said that black women are 300 percent more likely to die of pregnancy- or childbirth-related causes than black women. In fact, according to CDC data from 2011-2013, black women nationally are 243 percent more likely to die than white women.

Nina Martin was a reporter covering sex and gender issues. She joined ProPublica in 2013 and is based in Berkeley, California.

ADDITIONAL QUESTIONS FOR THE RECORD, SUBCOMMITTEE ON HEALTH, HEARING ON "IMPROVING MATERNAL HEALTH: LEGISLATION TO ADVANCE PREVENTION EFFORTS AND ACCESS TO CARE," SEPTEMBER 10, 2019, PATRICE HARRIS, M.D., M.A. PRESIDENT, BOARD OF TRUSTEES, AMERICAN MEDICAL ASSOCIATION

The Honorable Nanette Diaz Barragan <D-CA)

Question 1: Our country is in a crisis when it comes to maternal health and maternal mortality. The United States has the worst rate of maternal deaths in the entire developed world. This should not be happening, not in the richest country in the history of mankind. This failure in our nation's health care system must be solved, so women stop dying needlessly, when in other countries they do not. What's worse, women of color disproportionately face a higher level of pregnancy related death. For instance, the Centers for Disease Control and Prevention found that black woman are 3.3 times more likely than white women to suffer a pregnancy related death.

This is an incredibly important issue for me, as my district is nearly 90 percent African American and Hispanic. I believe that one way to help solve the crisis of maternal mortality among people of color is by getting more people of color into the medical workforce. I saw a study that found that only 11.1 percent of OB-GYNs are African American and 6. 7 percent are Hispanic. It was also found that these doctors are more likely to practice in medically underserved areas.

1. Can you discuss the importance of a diverse medical workforce, how that can help reduce the rates of maternal mortality, and what can Congress be doing to incentivize more people of color to enter the medical workforce?

Response 1: It is critically important to have a diverse health care workforce, well equipped to support the health and well-being of minority and underserved populations. Our nation is rapidly growing, aging, and becoming increasingly diverse. Through loans, loan guarantees, and scholarships to students and faculty, as well as grants and contracts to academic institutions and nonprofit organizations, Title VII health professions workforce development programs ensure the nation is equipped with a workforce that reflects the population it serves, while providing well-coordinated, quality care and improving access to care for all populations today and tomorrow. No other federally funded programs exist that improve the supply, distribution, and diversity of the physician workforce. We urge Members of Congress to work together in a bipartisan manner to secure sustained, meaningful funding for the Title VII health professions workforce development programs. We also urge Congress and the Administration to work together to pass Labor-HHS appropriations for FY 2020, ensuring that patients who benefit from these programs are not negatively impacted by a lapse in funding. Additionally, we urge Congress to avoid any proposals that eliminate the Health Careers and Opportunity Program (HCOP). It is our understanding that just last year, HCOP recruited nearly 3,000 students from disadvantaged backgrounds who are more likely to practice in rural and other underserved localities as health professionals.

Question 2: An important step to ensure that we are reducing the rate of maternal mortality is to guarantee that everyone has access to affordable quality health insurance. That is why crucial programs like Medicaid must be protected and strengthened. A report from the Georgetown university Center for Children and Families found that expanding access to Medicaid under the Affordable Care Act was associated with 1. 6 fewer maternal deaths per 100,000 women compared with states that did not expand. Additionally, a study published in the American Journal of Public Health found the mortality rate among African-American infants declined by 14.5% from 2010 to 2015 in expansion states, which was more than twice the decline in states that didn't expand Medicaid.

2. Can you talk about the importance that access to Medicaid has on reducing maternal mortality, and the impact to women's health if Medicaid were cut?

Response 2: The AMA agrees that access to Medicaid plays a significant role in maternal health. We strongly supported the expansion of Medicaid under the ACA. According to research by Georgetown University's Center for Children and Families (Georgetown CCF), states that expand Medicaid improve the health of women of childbearing age by increasing access to preventive care, reducing maternal mortality rates, and reducing adverse health outcomes before, during, and after pregnancies. In addition, a recent report by Georgetown CCF concluded that Medicaid expansion is an important step in addressing persistent racial disparities in maternal health and maternal mortality. Further, as noted by MACPAC, Medicaid has long played an important role in providing maternity-related services for pregnant women, paying for nearly half of all births in the United States. In its 2018 Issue Brief, MACPAC stated that "because Medicaid eligibility for many women with low incomes is tied to pregnancy, their source of insurance coverage may be unstable, affected by their pregnancy status, income, and state eligibility rules. As a result, they may experience interrupted care and delayed access to services." Additionally, because pregnancy-related deaths occurred during pregnancy, delivery, and up to a year postpartum, the AMA strongly supports the expansion of Medicaid coverage for one-year post-partum, which is a prime feature ofH.R. 1897, the Mothers and Offspring Mortality and Morbidity Act (the MOMMA Act), which the AMA supports.

Question 3: An issue that must be addressed in the fight to reduce the rate of maternal mortality is eliminating doctor's implicit biases, as well as having doctors more effectively listening to patient's concerns. The National Partnership for Women and Families conducted a survey and issued a report entitled Listening to Latina Mothers in California. One finding that stood out to me was almost one-third of Latina mothers reported that they did not feel that the delivery room staff encouraged them to make decisions about how they wanted their births to progress, while only 21 percent of white women said they felt this way.

3. How can we ensure that doctors more effectively listen to their patients, and take their patient's concerns to heart?

Response 3: Medical education curriculum incorporates teaching and training on implicit and explicit biases, to provide tools and build skills to recognize and eliminate bias, and integrate structural competency education, which as described by Dr. Jonathan Metzl "is a framework for conceptualizing and addressing health-related social justice issues that emphasizes diagnostic recognition of economic and political conditions producing and racializing inequalities in health." Although the AMA's Center for Health Equity is just getting up and running, there is great potential to enter this space and conduct an assessment of medical schools to find out which institutions offer and/or require implicit bias and other structural competency trainings.

There also may be an opportunity to advance criteria on what needs to be included in the training as well as a list of organizations or individuals who could offer robust training in this area. We urge Congress to establish a program through the Administration to award grants to accredited schools of allopathic medicine, osteopathic medicine, and nursing, and other health professional training programs for the training of health care professionals to reduce and prevent discrimination (including training related to implicit biases) specifically related to the provision of health care services related to prenatal care, labor care, birthing, and postpartum care.

In addition, in 2019, the AMA announced its Reimaging Residency Initiative, designed to transform residency training to best address the workforce needs of our current and future health care system. Many of the applications to the graduate medical education initiative have included health systems science training in their proposals.

For practicing physicians, the AMA launched STEPSforward TM an interactive practice transformation series offering innovative strategies that will allow physicians and their staff to thrive in the evolving health care environment by working smarter, not harder. This series includes a continuing medical education module on "Addressing Social Determinants of Health: Beyond the Clinic Walls." The interactive module helps physicians identify how to best understand the needs of their community, define a plan to begin addressing social determinants of health, and explains the tools available to screen patients and link them to resources.

Question 4: The California state Department of Public Health calculates that between 2006 and 2013, California lowered its maternal mortality rate by 55 percent. To do this, they created a-pregnancy-related mortality review board to examine the causes of every death, and developed comprehensive "how to" manuals detailing the best practices to address specific medical complications. While other states have implemented similar programs, they haven't had the same success as California.

4. Based off California's success, what can be done to help other states be as effective in reducing their rates of maternal mortality?

Response 4: It is our understanding that currently the U.S. Centers for Disease Control and Prevention (CDC) operates a voluntary Pregnancy Mortality Surveillance System by which the 50 states, New York City and Washington, DC voluntarily send copies of death certificates for all women who died during pregnancy or within one year of pregnancy, and copies of the matching birth or fetal death certificates, if they have the ability to perform such record links. We urge the development of a national maternal morbidity and mortality data collection strategy so that states gather data in a consistent manner-a necessary step to developing strategies to address a problem is to first identify what the specific problems are. Additionally, it is our understanding that a total of fourteen Maternal Mortality Review Committees (MMRCs) voluntarily shared 2008-2017 data with CDC through the Maternal Mortality Review Information Application (MMRIA). Among 1,347 deaths to women during or within a year of pregnancy, a pregnancy-relatedness determination was made for 1,260 (93.5%). Among these, 454 (36.0%) were determined by the fourteen MMRCs to be pregnancy-related. As you know, MMRCs study local maternal death cases to identify how to make pregnancies safer and prevent tragic outcomes. We believe every state should have a MMRC, unfortunately however, only about thirty-three states have one. We are encouraged that the establishment ofMMRCs are gaining momentum, but they remain in varying stages of formation. Congress can help improve the health and safety of pregnant women, and save families from devastating losses, by investing in local MMRCs. In addition, there should be a national system for state MMRCs to communicate/share findings and share strategies/educational materials developed to address problems. We also urge Congress to increase funding for State perinatal quality collaboratives (PQCs)-state or multi-state networks of teams working to improve the quality of care for mothers and babies. Many states currently have active collaboratives, and others are in development.

The Honorable Michael C. Burgess (R-TX)

Question 1: What has perplexed and disturbed me in a number of stories, including that of Dr. Irving, is that the issues patients present with have been communicated up the chain of command in the health care facilities, but have been dismissed or stalled. For the doctors on our panel has there been any decrease in physician involvement in delivery and post-partum care over the course of time?

Question 1a: Follow-up: Are there improvements in elements of the electronic health record or any other parts of the provider-to-provider communication system that could address this issue?

Response to 1 and 1a: While we do not have the qualitative data that encapsulates trends of physician involvement in a woman's post-partum care and her birthing experience, there are myriad disturbing anecdotes similar to Dr. Shalon Irving's experience, as you have noted. These cases suggest that somewhere along the care continuum, clinical decisions are sometimes made-or not made--without the fullest consideration of the patient's voice. This could be a result of clinical protocol, in which case a refinement in policy and practice could result in institutional changes. Or, it could be something more insidious and sensitive to acknowledge, but nonetheless very real in consequence: implicit bias. Whether racial, gender, socioeconomic, or otherwise based, implicit bias plays a role in clinical decision-making. The AMA, under the direction of our new Center for Health Equity, is committed to engaging this issue at the clinical, research, and policy levels.

With respect to the utility of electronic health records (ERRs), we believe that a key improvement in its elements would be to decouple federal reporting programs from EHR design. Removing reporting requirements would free EHR developers to focus on innovative ways to ensure that physicians have the most important and relevant information on a patient at any given time, presenting physicians with a clearer window into a patient's health concerns-such as having a high-risk pregnancy or blood clots-without navigating through data unnecessarily captured for secondary and tertiary requirements.

Instead of focusing on EHRs as a tool for measuring physician actions, the EHR should improve physicians' clinical decision making. For example, more clarity is needed on whether the EHR was able to use the summary of care document without burdening the physician, whether the EHR was able to provide the physician with usable and actionable clinical information in a format that supports clinical decision making, and if the EHR enabled a closed-loop referral. Essentially, more needs to be done to understand how EHRs actually function and should function in the real world. This type and level of information is far more meaningful and valuable to physicians and the federal government, and should be what federal EHR reporting programs promote. Analyzing this information would expose the usefulness of the EHR, if the EHR could accommodate the needs of the physician, whether the EHR contributed to or detracted from patient care, and whether the EHR supported the goal of health information exchange. Knowing this will also help EHR vendors build better products. Opportunely, because EHRs already track what functionalities are used to perform tasks, EHR vendors should directly provide such information to the federal government.

CMS rebranded the Meaningful Use (MU) program as the Promoting Interoperability (PI) program. While it has changed names several times, the burden associated with EHR compliance remains the same. There are still requirements which force physicians to capture, document, and report on their interactions with the EHR that are unrelated to patient care. As an immediate first step, CMS should create broad categories of Promoting Interoperability (PI) objectives allowing physicians to attest "yes/no" to the use of certified EHRs to achieve those categories. This will provide flexibility for patients and physicians to efficiently test new uses of technology- identifying what does and does not work while encouraging the use ofEHRs. Removing the burden of PI compliance and reporting will also help alleviate physician burnout related to EHR use. Continuing to require prescriptive PI measurement will detract from clinical relevance, add burden, and focus PI participation on documentation, reporting, and compliance rather than patient care, patient access, and interoperability.

More needs to be done to remove the unnecessary "noise" that's added in their notes simply to justify federal reporting requirements. This noise hides important clinical facts and detracts from patients and their care coordination. It is well documented that EHRs add cognitive burden and contribute to physician burnout. This is in large part due to the continued demands on physicians to document or capture information to accommodate measurement purposes, rather than recording clinically relevant information. Medicine is a data intensive field, but data capture and documentation comes at high cost in terms of time and loss of productivity.

Furthermore, technology continues to evolve, and current PI measures are likely to become quickly outdated or fail to promote innovative uses of digital health tools. Said another way, even the proposed 2020 MIPS PI measures are tied to the legacy of Meaningful Use. Given the Administration's focus on Patients over Paperwork and emphasis on reducing physician burden, measures that track and monitor physicians' use ofEHRs should be abandoned allowing physicians to focus on providing care.

We appreciate your support in preventing MU requirements from becoming more stringent over time and believe that more must be done to limit demands on physicians' time including focusing federal reporting requirements the functionality ofEHRs, allowing for EHR vendors to directly provide such information to the federal government, and allowing physicians to "yes/no" attest to the use of certified EHRs.

The Honorable Gus M. Bilirakis (R-FL)

Question 1: Because CMS already utilizes the National Quality Improvement Innovation Contract mechanism and there's already a set of qualified improvement organizations identified and ready to operate, couldn't we just appropriate to an entity like CDC and instruct them to work with CMS's established contractors in order to expedite the establishment of the quality collaboratives envisioned by HR 1551 -why or why not?

Response 1: Providing educational information and assistance to providers and physicians on the issue is essential to tackling the issue. Collaboratives allow organizations to share learnings and best practices. Tt is premature to move forward with developing quality measures as we must first study the issue to determine the root cause before mandating in legislation a quality program. It is also a conflict of interest to have the voluntary consensus standard-setting organizations to be involved in the development of quality measures. The Department of Health and Human Services is currently under contract with an outside entity that endorses measures, identifies measure development priorities, and measure gaps pursuant to section 1890 of the Social Security Act (42 US.C. § 1395aaa). To maintain the integrity of any quality program and avoid potential, real, or perceived conflicts of interest, the AMA believes that any entities receiving funding for measure development should not be involved in endorsing quality measures. Measure evaluation and endorsement should remain impartial and kept completely separate from measure development. This ensures the integrity of the measure endorsement process and avoids the concern of having a single entity responsible for implementing all domains of the quality agenda, from measure development to measure endorsement Such a construct would inhibit engagement by other stakeholders, including physicians. In addition, it might limit access to a wide range of ideas, clinical and practical perspectives, and discourage the innovation that is truly needed for a successful program.

Currently, there is a private sector led initiative addressing measure alignment between CMS and private health insurance plans. Mandating such activity and involving the federal government would stifle progress, innovation and engagement

Question la: Along the same lines, rather than establishing a separate Maternity Consumer Assessment of Health Care Providers and Systems survey, couldn't we simply add questions to the Hospital CAHPS survey why or why not?

Response I a: Tying a measure and score related to CAHPS to publicly reported ratings and accountability can be problematic, as CAHPS often depends more on patient perceptions than on good medicine. Tt also may not be appropriate to have a single survey that measures maternity care across all settings and most likely may need a separate survey for each provider type. For example, CMS uses hospital-CARPS to measure the hospital experience and CG-CAHPS to measure the primary care/internal medicine experience. There is even a separate CAHPS survey that measures surgical specialties. In addition, we believe CAHPS survey administration protocols are outdated and a need exists to allow for measures that use multiple modes of data collection. Allowing physicians to collect the information in the office through a tablet while the patient is in the waiting room, via smartphone app, for example, is needed. The broader patient population physicians can reach, the more likely they are to receive good response rates.

CMS also needs to also look outside of CAHPS to measure patient experience, such as the CollaboRATE tool/measure. CollaboRATE is a patient-reported measure of shared decision making which contains three brief questions that patients, their parents, or their representatives complete following a clinical encounter. The CollaboRATE measure provides a performance score representing the percentage of adults 18 years of age and older who experience a high level of shared decision making.

Additional Questions for the Record, Subcommittee on Health, Hearing on "Improving Maternal Health: Legislation to Advance Prevention Efforts and Access to Care," September 10, 2019, Elizabeth Howell, M.D., M.P.P., Director, Blavatnik Family Women's Health Research Institute, Icahn School of Medicine at Mount Sinai

The Honorable Robin L. Kelly (D-IL)

Question 1: The MOMMAs Act includes funding for a grant program to build up perinatal quality collaboratives. Dr. Howell, can you provide some insight on how important these collaboratives are addressing the underlying causes of maternal mortality?

Response 1: Perinatal quality collaboratives are state or multi-state networks of teams working to improve quality of care for mothers and babies. Members of perinatal quality collaboratives work together to identify health care processes that need to be improved and use the best available methods to make changes as quickly as possible. They facilitate change in the delivery of maternity care, improve the health of mothers and babies, and bend the maternity care cost curve. By accelerating adoption of best practices, collaboratives help eliminate elective inductions before 39 weeks, increase breast feeding rates, improve treatment of and reduce the costs associated with neonatal abstinence syndrome, and much more.

An important aspect of perinatal quality collaboratives is their ability to streamline innovative ways to develop and distribute information to improve outcomes and reduce health care costs beyond just one city or hospital system. They do this by sharing best practices and lessons learned with providers and hospitals that may not typically have access to that type of information including those in small, rural communities.

Successful state and regionally based quality improvement collaboratives in places such as California, Maryland, Ohio, Illinois and Michigan have supported increased use of evidence- based guidelines, led to reductions in costly medical interventions, and improved linkages between hospital and community-based medicine. These locally responsive mechanisms for improving maternity care quality through the spread of best practices should be encouraged and expanded.

The Honorable Nanette Diaz Barragan (D-CA)

Question 1: An important step to ensure that we are reducing the rate of maternal mortality is to guarantee that everyone has access to affordable quality health insurance. That is why crucial programs like Medicaid must be protected and strengthened. A report from the Georgetown university Center for Children and Families found that expanding access to Medicaid under the Affordable Care Act was associated with 1.6 fewer maternal deaths per I 00,000 women compared with states that did not expand. Additionally, a study published in the American Journal of Public Health found the mortality rate among African-American infants declined by 14.5% from 2010 to 2015 in expansion states, which was more than twice the decline in states that didn't expand Medicaid.

1. Can you talk about the importance that access to Medicaid has on reducing maternal mortality, and the impact to women's health if Medicaid were cut?

Response 1: Medicaid is the largest single payer of maternity care in the US, covering 43% of births and playing a critical role in ensuring healthy moms and healthy babies through access to pregnancy-related care. Many state Medicaid programs also provide comprehensive well-woman care, including primary care services such as cancer and domestic violence screenings.

The ACA Medicaid expansion ensures a public safety net for no-income and low-income, non- pregnant women. This means that many women who otherwise would not qualify for coverage until becoming pregnant, or could not afford coverage offered to them, now have access to primary and preventive care, and an opportunity to optimize their health pre-pregnancy. Instead of rolling back Medicaid expansion, all states should be encouraged to expand their programs.

Currently, Medicaid coverage for pregnant women ends roughly 60-days postpartum. As Maternal Mortality Review Committees (MMRC) have increasingly revealed, many deaths related to pregnancy occur after this time. In fact, the CDC estimates that 33% of maternal deaths occur one week to 12 months after delivery, which is likely underestimated as the CDC assessment did not account for deaths from overdose, suicide, homicide, or unintentional injury. Accordingly, a number ofMMRCs have recommended extending Medicaid coverage for women to a full year postpartum. Already, federal statute requires that a baby born to a mother on Medicaid is covered under Medicaid through the first year of life. As Congress explores additional ways to improve health outcomes, closing this critical gap in coverage during this incredibly vulnerable time can mean the difference between life and death for some women.

Question 2: An issue that is eliminating doctor's implicit biases, as well as having doctors more effectively listening to patient's concerns. The National Partnership for Women and Families conducted a survey and issued a report entitled Listening to Latina Mothers in California. One finding that stood out to me was almost one-third of Latina mothers reported that they did not feel that the delivery room staff encouraged them to make decisions about how they wanted their births to progress, while only 21 percent of white women said they felt this way.

2. How can we ensure that doctors more effectively listen to their patients, and take their patient's concerns to heart?

Response 2: This is an important question. We must listen to our patients and take their concerns to heart. There is a growing focus across the US on implicit bias training. Some medical schools, including my institution, have rolled out implicit bias trainings for physicians, nurses, and trainees in an effort to help clinicians recognize their own unconscious biases and take steps to address them. While this is one needed step to address communication failures, there are a number of other important trainings that that can help to optimize patient doctor communication. In the Alliance for Innovation on Maternal Health Peripartum Disparities Reduction Bundle there are a number of resources listed to help hospitals and health systems take steps to improve communication. For example, shared decision-making is an important aspect of the physician patient relationship and AHRQ has a tool called the Share Approach which is a five-step process for shared decision-making that explores and compares the benefits, harms, and risks of each option through dialogue about what matters most to the patient. This is just one example of many tools that can be utilized to enhance communication.

Improvements in medical education can also help to improve patient doctor communication. Medical schools should ensure that best practice curricula for communication is utilized in pre- clerkship years (years l and 2 of medical school) to make sure that medical students are learning the right listening/ communication skills.

Question 3: The California state Department of Public Health calculates that between 2006 and 2013, California lowered its maternal mortality rate by 55 percent. To do this, they created a-pregnancy-related mortality review board to examine the causes of every death, and developed comprehensive "how to" manuals detailing the best practices to address specific medical complications. While other states have implemented similar programs, they haven't had the same success as California.

3. Based off California's success, what can be done to help other states be as effective in reducing their rates of maternal mortality?

Response 3: California has been a leader in the effort to reduce maternal mortality. In addition to their pregnancy-related mortality review board that aims to examine causes of every maternal death, the California Maternal Quality Care Collaborative was formed as a public-private partnership to lead maternal quality improvement activities. They have undertaken a number of key steps that other states could adopt: 1) linking public health surveillance to actions, 2) mobilizing a broad range of public and private partners, 3) developing a rapid-cycle Maternal Data Center to support and sustain quality improvement initiatives, and 4) implementing a series of data-driven large-scale quality improvement projects. California uses findings from their pregnancy-mortality review board to drive quality improvement. They have a robust data infrastructure that provides hospitals across the state with quality metrics (e.g., low risk cesarean rates, elective delivery rates, severe maternal morbidity rates) and they stratify the results by race and ethnicity so hospitals know how well they are performing on important maternal health parameters for the patients they serve.

A crucial part of our fight to reduce maternal mortality and severe maternal morbidity relies on data and measurement. California has the most robust infrastructure for data and measurement. Providing resources to insure that states across the country have access to data on performance is a critical step in our effort to reduce maternal mortality and severe maternal morbidity.

The other very important step that California has taken is the implementation of quality improvement activities targeting causes of maternal death. They have implemented maternal safety bundles in hospitals and these tools target some of the most preventable causes of a maternal death (e.g., hemorrhage, hypertension, venous thromboembolic disease). This model is currently being implemented across the United States in a program entitled the Alliance for Innovation on Maternal Health (AIM). This program currently reaches 30 states but more resources are needed to ensure adequate implementation of maternal safety bundles in hospitals and health systems across the United States.

The Honorable Michael C. Burgess (R-TX)

Question 1: What has perplexed and disturbed me in a number of stories, including that of Dr. Irving, is that the issues patients present with have been communicated up the chain of command in the health care facilities, but have been dismissed or stalled. For the doctors on our panel -has there been any decrease in physician involvement in delivery and post-partum care over the course of time?

Question 1a. Follow-up: Are there improvements in elements of the electronic health record or any other parts of the provider-to-provider communication system that could address this issue?

Response to 1 and 1a: EHRs are not designed to document many women's health conditions. For instance, there are no discrete elements to describe the following symptoms/complications: high blood pressure, pre-eclampsia, eclampsia, gestational diabetes mellitus, organ failure, prior pre-term birth, prior pregnancy complications, mental health conditions, lifestyle factors (i.e., drug/opioid dependence, tobacco use disorder).

As a result, many common conditions are buried in the problem list and may not be easily identified by the attending physician. Further, EHRs may not be designed to alert physicians to potentially problematic vital signs or test results in pregnant and postpartum women. For instance, the threshold for a problematic high blood pressure may be lower in a postpartum woman than an average patient.

Additionally, interoperability between inpatient and outpatient EHRs should be improved. Physicians should be able to access and easily interpret records from an inpatient stay during subsequent outpatient visits. Currently, the amount of information in the inpatient record often makes it difficult for a provider to find what they are looking for. EHRs could ameliorate this by allowing for the filtering of information.

The Honorable Gus M. Bilirakis (R-FL)

Question 2: Are there concerns within the research community regarding the integrity of the data being collected in states, and, if so, what are those concerns and how might they be addressed?

Response 2: The best way for us to collect data on maternal death is through state Maternal Mortality Review Committees (MMRC). These committees include a group oflocal, interdisciplinary, maternal health stakeholders - ob-gyns, nurses, social workers, epidemiologists, and patient advocates - who review individual maternal deaths and recommend solutions to prevent future deaths and complications to their State Department of Health. They utilize a variety of data sources to ascertain whether a pregnancy-related death occurred, review contributing factors, and determine whether the death was preventable. MMRCs help develop local solutions to local problems, informing national solutions to save mothers' lives.

While vital statistics-based surveillance systems can be useful for monitoring trends they often under report pregnancy-related deaths. State and local maternal mortality review committees (MMRCs) are best positioned to both comprehensively assess deaths to women during pregnancy and the year after the end of pregnancy, and identify opportunities for prevention.

MMRCs use vital records data and medical and social service records to understand the factors that influence maternal deaths. It is from MMRCs that we have learned that over half of pregnancy-related deaths in the United States are preventable. In addition to assessing preventability, MMRCs are able to make jurisdiction-specific recommendations and promote strategies to prevent future deaths. Examples of data-driven actions from MMRCs include: the development of urgent bulletins to providers on the dangers of placental disorders and peripartum cardiomyopathy, efforts to increase knowledge of maternal deaths related to substance use and suicide, efforts to address gaps in services for women related to mental health and substance use, and obstetric emergency simulation trainings to prepare hospitals to address hemorrhage, cardiomyopathy, and preeclampsia.

Additional Questions for the Record, Subcommittee on Health, Hearing on "Improving Maternal Health: Legislation to Advance Prevention Efforts and Access to Care," September 10, 2019

David B. Nelson, MD FACOG
Assistant Professor of Obstetrics and Gynecology
Division of Maternal-Fetal Medicine
University of Texas Southwestern Medical Center

October 12, 2019

Dr. Nelson - Introduction: Distinguished members of the Energy and Commerce Subcommittee on Health, thank you again for the opportunity to speak on behalf of Parkland Hospital and the University of Texas Southwestern Medical Center at the September l0, 2019, hearing entitled, "Maternal Health: Legislation to Advance Prevention Efforts and Access to Care." The following contains the questions and my responses in the format requested from each member:

The Honorable Nanette Diaz Barragan (D-CA)

Question 1. An issue that must be addressed in the fight to reduce the rate of maternal mortality is eliminating doctor's implicit biases, as well as having doctors more effectively listening to patient's concerns. The National Partnership for Women and Families conducted a survey and issued a report entitled Listening to Latina Mothers in California. One finding that stood out to me was almost one-third of Latina mothers reported that they did not feel that the delivery room staff encouraged them to make decisions about how they wanted their births to progress, while only 21 percent of white women said they felt this way.

1. How can we ensure that doctors more effectively listen to their patients, and take their patient's concerns to heart?

Response 1: There is a growing body ofliterature that validates the public health impact of racial bias, implicit and explicit, on the lives and health of people of color.[71] Moreover, evidence suggests that factors such as stereotyping and implicit bias on the part of the healthcare providers may contribute to racial and ethnic disparities in health 2 Addressing such implicit bias is one of the priorities in advancing maternal care in the United States. At a national level, for example, the American College of Obstetricians and Gynecologists are taking a leadership role in addressing this issue.[72]

At both Parkland Hospital and UT Southwestern Medical Center, we have recognized these disparities and have developed a number oflocal programs to address such bias. This includes organizational commitments to bias training and cultural competency to eliminate such bias and advance health equity. For example, at Parkland Hospital, there is a Diversity, Inclusion, and Health Equity Department with a director that uses a blueprint from the National Culture and Linguistically Appropriate Services to foster an inclusive workplace and advance health equity. There is also a no-cost instructor-led series offered once per month to Parkland Hospital employees to educate and coach on culturally-sensitive practices and to review the impact of unconscious bias and stereotypes. For our Latina mothers, a

---

[71] J. American College of Obstetricians and Gynecologist. Statement of Policy. ACOG Statement of policy on racial bias. Issued by the Executive Board of the American College of Obstetricians and Gynecologists and the American Congress of Obstetricians and Gynecologists. February 2017.

[72] Racial and ethnic disparities in obstetrics and gynecology. Committee Opinion No. 649. American College of Obstetricians and Gynecologists. Obstet Gynecol2015; 126:el30-4.

robust Language Services department provides access to translation services in an effort to ensure effective communication in shared decision-making for our non-English speaking patients is performed in an environment without barriers. In fact, more than 1 million patient interpretations were provided by Parkland Language Services last year.

This commitment to addressing bias is a cornerstone of our maternity service. On June 13, 2018, as part of the Obstetric Performance Improvement Committee meeting-the hallmark meeting of quality assurance and performance improvement for the Parkland Obstetric service--patient experience was a dedicated discussion for our team of physicians, nurses, and advance practice providers. This effort dovetailed one of the hospital-wide strategic priorities to create an inspiring and supportive environment and culture. The ultimate goal of this effort is to foster high quality and compassionate care through focus on the patient and employee experience. Indeed, several of our mother-baby ward units were chosen as the models of care last year within the organization with initiatives to include "Knock and Pause," "Leader Rounds," and "Commit to Sit" by the mother-baby nursing staff to enhance patient experience. We are proud to report that this effort has been a sustained success for the organization and emphasize its importance because culturally derived mistrust of the health care system can decrease adherence to clinical recommendations[2] Although more should be done, there is some evidence that these efforts are impactful. For the most recent patient satisfaction report for Parkland Hospital (Press Ganey Report, 4/l/2019-6/30/20 19), that included 53% of respondents that were non-white and 34% in Spanish-language, Parkland Hospital was reported as the 99th percentile (highest) for safety net hospitals for "explanations about what would happen during tests and treatments" and 94tl1 percentile for safety net hospitals for the patient reported metric of perceived "Physician's concern for your questions and worries." Moreover, for Press Ganey surveys returned from June 2019 to August 2019, Parkland Hospital is in the 9P' percentile in the country (for all hospitals in the Press Ganey Database, 2,784 hospitals) and also 91 st percentile for all University Health Systems (teaching hospitals in the Press Ganey Database, 252 hospitals) and in the 96th percentile for government hospitals with 300 beds or more. These are a tangible metrics to characterize the organizational effort to hear every one of our patients. UT Southwestern has similar results with obstetrics and gynecology patients ranking their providers in "MD Communication" at the 99 percentile for the past 3 years. While collectively more is needed across all areas of medicine, these local programs show potential in reaching our patients and hearing their voice.

Question 2: The California state Department of Public Health calculates that between 2006 and 2013, California lowered its maternal mortality rate by 55 percent. To do this, they created a-pregnancy-related mortality review board to examine the causes of every death, and developed comprehensive "how to" manuals detailing the best practices to address specific medical complications. While other states have implemented similar programs, they haven't had the same success as California.

2. Based off California's success, what can be done to help other states be as effective in reducing their rates of maternal mortality?

Response 2: The recent reports of maternal mortality trends in California offer promise. From the outset, the initiatives within California had a strong partnership with the American College of Obstetricians and Gynecologists (ACOG, District IX), that included obstetricians and maternal- fetal medicine specialists from all over California, and also involved nurses, midwives, anesthesiologists, emergency physicians, cardiologists and social scientists. Commitment-ie., "buy in"-from all of these groups is an essential first step to ensure that maternal deaths are both correctly identified as pregnancy-related as well as documentation of associated conditions for future preventability. As noted by Dr. Elliot Main from California, "The early goals were not only to identify the causes and demographics of these tragedies, but also to drill down in the medical records and see where there were opportunities to improve care." These findings became the basis for many of the recommendations in the California Maternal Quality Care Collaborative (CMQCC) Quality Improvement Toolkits for Obstetric Hemorrhage and Hypertension. Thereafter, Quality Improvement Collaboratives followed the toolkits in 20 I 0, and there is now a state-wide Quality Improvement project with over 125 hospitals engaged. California, however, is not alone. A similar program from New York inspired the National Partnership for Maternal Safety and the National Safety Bundles.

These efforts share similar principles with the ongoing work in Texas, such as the newly formed regionalization program known as "Maternal Levels of Care" as well as the Alliance for Innovation on Maternal Health (AIM) Plus program. Specifically, the AIM collaborative in Texas includes participation among the Texas Hospital Association, Department of State Health, and now includes more than 200 (95%) hospitals in Texas that provide birthing services (Figure). Indeed, more than 80% of the hospitals have joined the Texas AIM Plus program.

Collectively, these programs in states like California, New York, and Texas all share a common theme. Fundamentally, these initiatives represent an effort to standardize care with specific recognition and response to various obstetric conditions placing the mother at risk for death. In essence, these programs are attempting to refine the content of obstetric care. That is, to reduce maternal mortality, the care delivered must be both accessible and also consistent and of good quality. This is exemplified by the incorporation of "checklists," "bundles," and "protocols."

At a local level, our program at Parkland Hospital represents a unique model to demonstrate the significance of standardized care quality- i.e., content- in a Medicaid-funded population. Recall, Parkland Hospital represents a public hospital serving almost exclusively medically-indigent women. Of the 12,671 women delivered last year, 90% were Medicaid-funded. Thus, the Parkland Obstetrics model can be viewed as a system potentially generalizable to the nearly 2 million government-funded (Medicaid-funded) deliveries in our country every year. This is a system of care with administrative and medical oversight that is highly integrated.

The same prenatal protocols are used by nurse practitioners at all 10 prenatal clinic sites within the Parkland system to guarantee consistent, protocol-based care that includes standardized referrals of high-risk women to a centrally-located prenatal clinic specifically designed for women with high-risk pregnancy complications. The strength of the Parkland Obstetrics system of care is that there is uniform access with cohesive care plans across the more than 900 square miles of Dallas County for all of our patients. This avoids wastage by providing consistent care delivery, care coordination, and uniform treatment plans using evidenced-based practices.

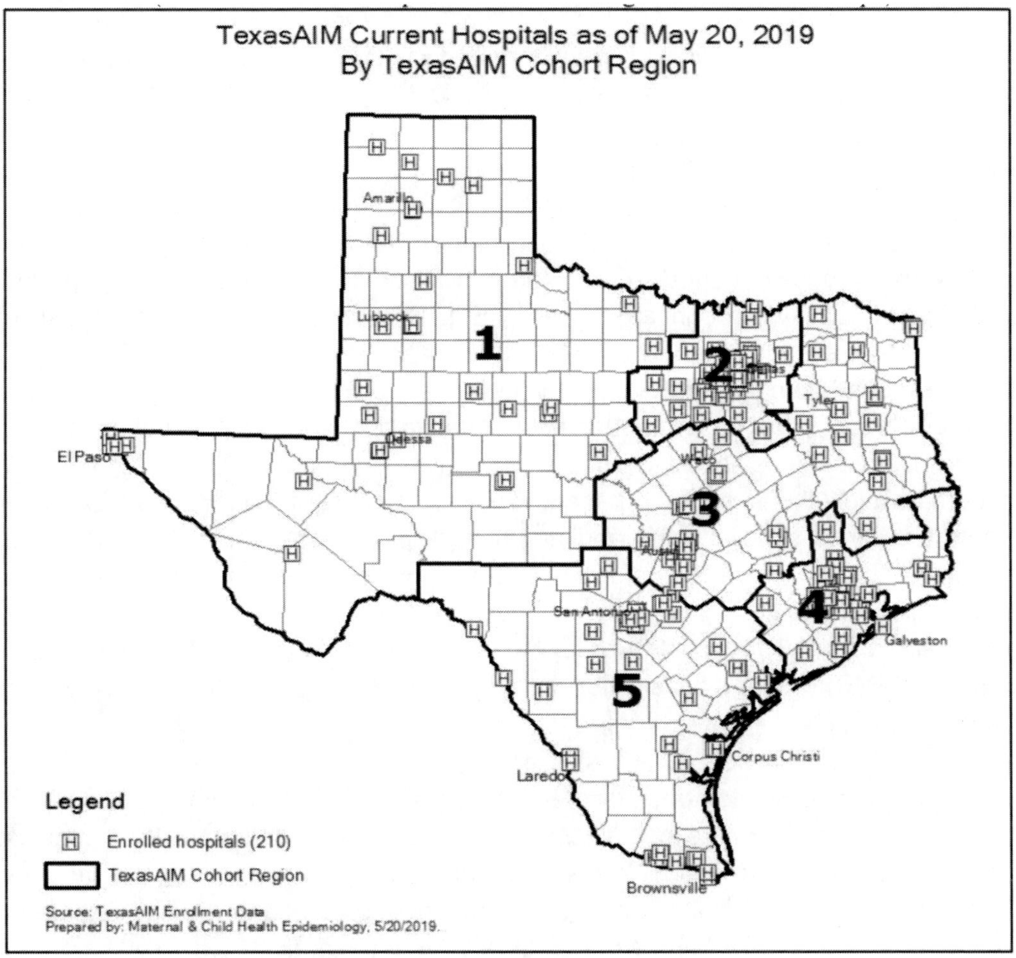

Figure 38. Texas AIM participation of hospitals in Texas as of May 20, 2019. (data available from: https://www.dshs.texas.gov/mchffexasAIM.aspx).

The Honorable Michael C. Burgess (R-TX)

Question 1: What has perplexed and disturbed me in a number of stories, including that of Dr. Irving, is that the issues patients present with have been communicated up the chain of command in the health care facilities, but have been dismissed or stalled. For the doctors on our panel has there been any decrease in physician involvement in delivery and post-partum care over the course of time?

Response 1: To address maternal mortality, engagement and involvement by medical staff is vital. There are four domains wherein such involvement can be identified to have an impact on the delivery of care. This begins with physician involvement in addressing barriers to care. A recent example is the Healthcare Effectiveness Data and Information Set (HEDIS) measure for postpartum care. HEDIS is a widely used set of performance measures in the managed care industry, developed and maintained by the National Committee for Quality Assurance (NCQA). Previously, for postpartum women the target time point for women to receive a postpartum visit was between 21-56 days after delivery. Those seen outside of this window were viewed as not meeting the measure. The unintended consequence of this measure was that physician leaders were forced to advocate for patient postpartum appointments when deemed medically appropriate despite failing the HEDIS measure. For example, our practice for women with hypertension after delivery was to see them for a visit at 7 days following delivery. Thus, physicians championed access to care despite external pressures not to do so. We are grateful that it was recently announced that this HEDIS measure for postpartum care is changing thanks in large part to physician advocacy.

The second domain of physician involvement is clinical leadership. The "chain of command" must have a clinical leader to orchestrate the increasingly complex care needs of our patients. Although this seems intuitive, physicians serving in clinical leadership roles should be encouraged. In Texas, the recent Maternal Levels of Care program outlines specific roles and responsibilities for both the medical staff and leaders (Table). This is a directive, endorsed by the state, to ensure physician alignment with specific clinical duties and expectations. Taken further, the Texas Maternal Levels of Care Level IV programs must have a dedicated "Maternal Medical Director" (MMD) who is a physician with the following credentials and responsibilities to include:

1. is a board certified obstetrics and gynecology physician with expertise in the area of critical care obstetrics; or a board certified maternal fetal medicine physician, both with privileges in maternal care;
2. demonstrates administrative skills and oversight of the Quality Assurance and Performance Improvement (QAPI) Program; and
3. has completed annual continuing education specific to maternal care, including complicated conditions.

Unfortunately, the availability of such physician leaders is limited. First, there a limited number of experienced clinicians with such credentials. Second, there are significant workforce shortages within obstetrics and gynecology altogether. Indeed, the workforce is aging, the average number of work hours are declining, and increasing numbers of obstetricians and gynecologists are retiring from obstetrics altogether. More than 15,000 of the nearly 40,000 actively practicing obstetricians and gynecologists will likely retire in the next 10 years. Importantly, the number of obstetricians and gynecologists retiring will soon equal the number of resident graduates. The demand for obstetricians and gynecologists by 2020 in Texas is projected to be among the highest in any state, and nationally there is expected to be a shortage between 3,000-9,000 obstetrician-gynecologist physicians by 2030. With projections of relatively fewer general internists and family physicians, more women will be in need of health care. Thus, the strain on the obstetric workforce will likely heighten. This is sobering when considering that approximately half (49%) of the 3107 United States counties currently lack an obstetrician-gynecologist physician.

Table 2. Texas Maternal Levels of Care designation requirements for Medical Staff and Maternal Medical Director (MMD) as outlined in Texas Administrative Code Title 25, Part I, Chapter 133 Subchapter K

133.205.c	Medical Staff. The facility shall have an organized maternal progran1 that is recognized bv the medical staff and approved bv the facilitv's governing bodv.
133.205.c.l	The crcdentialing of the maternal medical staff shall include a process for the delineation of privileges for maternal care.
133.205.c.2	The maternal medical staff will participate in ongoing staff and team based education and training in the care of the maternal patient.
133.205.d	Medical Director. There shall be an identified Maternal Medical Director (MMD) and/or Transport Medical Director (TMD) as appropriate, responsible for the provision of maternal care serYices and credentialed by the facility for the treatment of maternal patients. The responsibilities and authority of the MMD and/or TMD shall include:
133.205.d.l	Examining qualifications of medical staff requesting maternal privileges and making recommendations to the appropriate committee for such privileges:
133.205.d.2	assuring maternal medical staff competency in managing obstetrical emergencies, complications and resuscitation techniques:
133.205.d.3	monitoring maternal patient care from transport if applicable, to admission, stabilization, operative interYcntion(s) if applicable, through discharge, and inclusive of the QAPI Program;
133.205.d.4	participating in ongoing maternal staff and tean1 based education and training in the care of the maternal patient:
133.205.d.5	overseeing the inter-facilitv maternal transport:
133.205.d.6	collaborating with the MPM in areas to include: developing and/or revising policies, procedures and guidelines, assuring medical staff and personnel competency, education and training: and the QAPI Program;
133.205.d.7	frequently leading and participating in the maternal QAPI meetings;
133.205.d.8	ensuring that the QAPI Program is specific to maternal and fetal care, is ongoing, data driven and outcome based;
133.205.d.9	participating as a clinically active and practicing physician in maternal care at the facilitv where medical director scrYices arc provided:
133.205.d.10	maintaining active staff privileges as defined in the facility's medical staffby1aws; and
133.205.d.11	developing collaborative relationships with other MMD(s) of designated facilities within the applicable Perinatal Care Region.

What are possible solutions to this shortage in the physician workforce for maternal care? Without sufficient funding for graduate medical education, residency programs will not grow, and may decline, further overwhelming the service needs of our patients. Our goals should be to improve practice efficiency, and increase the use of health information technology to further expand the medical care reach. We should also encourage more medical students to pursue careers in women's health by recognizing the physician work-lifestyle balance and support loan repayment programs to attract obstetricians and gynecologists to provider shortage areas. Lastly, and most importantly, our efforts should promote collaborative models with certified nurse midwives, certified nurse practitioners, and physician assistants to establish "teams" led by obstetrician-gynecologist physicians. Both at Parkland Hospital and UT Southwestern, this model is deployed. At Parkland Hospital, advanced practice providers-both certified nurse midwives and nurse practitioners-are a resource used to extend care across Dallas County. Among the 10 women's health care clinics and central high-risk clinic, there are more than 100 advanced practice providers delivering prenatal and postpartum care. The certified nurse midwife program established by Dr. Kenneth Leveno celebrated 30 years of service in 2017. Today, more than 30 certified nurse midwives with more than 500 combined years of experience integrate with physicians as such a team. In 2017, our team published a manuscript as one of the three "Editor's Choice" articles discussed for the July 2017 edition of *Obstetrics & Gynecology-the* official journal for the American College of Obstetricians and Gynecologists. This was a four- year prospective study of nearly 4,000 women evaluated in our triage unit and discharged to home after standardized assessment by our advanced practice providers under the supervision of physicians. We found that women discharged with false labor at term after a standardized assessment were not at increased risk for adverse perinatal outcomes or cesarean delivery. The results of this manuscript have far-reaching implications to providers and patients by providing some evidence-based information regarding the safety of clinical decision-making for discharge home with the diagnosis of false labor by extension of care with advanced practice providers.

Although the role of physician leadership is important, accountability of *all* health care providers-both physicians and non-physicians-should be our collective goal. Quality assurance and performance improvement programs should be highlighted with monitoring of deviations in practice or care by any healthcare team member. An example would be tracking timeliness of antihypertensive medication to women with severe range blood pressure (>160/110 mmHg). It is our hope that this is an ongoing process in quality improvement. Ultimately, it is our hope that more physician leadership and care extension with advanced practice providers coupled with accountability within the "chain of command" will lead to improved maternal health in the future.

Question la: Follow-up: Are there improvements in elements of the electronic health record or any other parts of the provider-to-provider communication system that could address this issue?

Response la: Yes, absolutely. There are elements of the electronic health record that are good examples of technology assisting delivery of care to our patients. For example, as part of our ongoing, quality improvement for maternal services at Parkland Hospital, we have implemented an "urgent request to the bedside" function with our nursing partners to electronically track and monitor timeliness to a patient's bedside for immediate care. This initiative identifies immediate, life-threatening conditions such as elevated blood pressure and hemorrhage, with an organized response by a nursing-physician team. All activations for "mother-baby" ward unit urgent responses to the bedside are reviewed within the Parkland Women and Infant Services (WISH) Adverse Event quality meeting held monthly as an organization. Each case is also reviewed by a team of nurses for opportunities of improvement.

Outside of Parkland, there is a network of hospitals that utilize the electronic medical record platform of EPIC that has a function titled, "Care Everywhere," that allows specific medical record features to be shared across organizations. This network is in more than 25 hospitals in Texas and is a feature utilized both at Parkland Hospital and UT Southwestern Medical Center. Utilizing this resource can provide relevant information from care in a prior hospitalization at another facility. To date, Parkland Hospital has shared over 25.2 million records with other organizations using the "Care Everywhere" function. Similarly, we've received over 10.5 million records from other organizations for patients we care for at Parkland. In all, over 650,000 unique patients have had records sent or received. This year alone, Parkland as an organization sent and received 1.4 million and 1.9 million records respectively. We have shared with literally every state in the country. To provide context to the value from this information exchange, year to date alone, we have avoided over 15,000 medication orders being entered inappropriately thanks to outside information received.

The Honorable Gus M. Bilirakis (R-FL)

Question l: As I've alluded to, maternal mortality is a bipartisan problem deserving bipartisan attention and response. Recently, my colleague on this Committee, Dr. Bucshon, introduced the bipartisan Excellence in Maternal Health Act to help reduce maternal mortality by improving health care provider education and training, and to develop and disseminate best practices to help ensure women get proper care, and to help reduce discrimination and bias? (a) To this end, collaboration is key. Is it important to include epidemiologists and statisticians at the table when formulating a program to help identify, develop, or disseminate best practices- why or why not?

Response 1: There can be no doubt that teamwork in healthcare is key, and this includes partnership amongst physicians, epidemiologists, and statisticians in developing and understanding the importance of relevant quality data. To advance the national effort in improving both maternal mortality and morbidity, it is critical that accurate, relevant clinical data are reported and are used by statisticians and epidemiologists to guide decisions for healthcare policy. Clinicians and statisticians must work together. Clinicians have a responsibility to identify clinically relevant quality metrics so that appropriate healthcare performance can be measured in a meaningful process. By not doing so, statisticians are left "connecting dots" without understanding the clinical context of what is in the "dot."

Incorrectly connecting dots can lead to unintended consequences. For example, one method of assessing "quality" of maternal care is measuring rates of severe maternal morbidity (SMM), or near-misses. These are unexpected outcomes that result in significant short- or long-term consequences to a woman's health, such as hysterectomy and transfusion. These SMM rates are also almost universally derived from hospital billing codes-simply because no other data sources are available. It is critical that clinical leaders and epidemiologists work together to understand the potential unintended consequences of tracking such "SMM" metrics, especially transfusion of blood. Blood transfusion is the single greatest contributor to the SMM rate both at Parkland Hospital and nationally. In 2014, blood transfusion accounted for more than 80% of the SMM rate in the United States. We caution, however, that this can become a perverse surrogate of quality. If a provider hesitates, or worse, withholds a transfusion of blood to a patient to avoid the "label" of SMM, then there is an unintended risk of mortality. Indeed, the reason obstetric hemorrhage is deadly is because of failure to promptly restore a woman's circulating blood volume. This can have far-reaching consequences in quality measurement across hospitals. For example, a hospital with a high rate of transfusion could be considered inferior to a hospital with a low rate of transfusion. Is it possible that this evaluation is upside down? The hospital with the higher transfusion rate may actually be higher in quality than the hospital with a low rate of transfusion as measured by mortality. We must be careful to not inadvertently worsen mortality while trying to avoid a surrogate of morbidity by careful selection of quality metrics. By aligning clinicians, epidemiologists, and statisticians, such missteps can potentially be avoided.

Our team at Parkland Hospital and UT Southwestern Medical Center have such a program with clinicians and biostatisticians working together in healthcare outcomes research. Dr. Don Mcintire, a biostatistician, has been integrated into our team for more than 20 years. This partnership has produced more than 200 peer-reviewed publications that are almost exclusively clinically-based. Dr. Mcintire and his team of trained research nurses are an integral part of promoting and improving healthcare quality by conducting healthcare outcomes research alongside physician partners. It is this partnership that fosters continuous quality improvement, and it should be encouraged among other healthcare systems.

Dr. Nelson - Conclusion

In closing, thank you again for the opportunity to testify at the September 10, 2019, hearing entitled, "Maternal Health: Legislation to Advance Prevention Efforts and Access to Care." I would also like to thank the members for their questions and interest in this important subject. This interest is producing meaningful results by encouraging national, regional, state, and local stakeholders to work together in multidisciplinary collaboratives and regionalization programs. The state, regional, and federal-sponsored programs, such as Maternal Mortality Review Committees and Maternal Levels of Care, are tangible examples of this orchestrated response among hospital administration and health care teams. Because of this interest and support, caregivers in obstetrics have been galvanized to study and lower maternal mortality rates in the United States. And although we do not yet have all of the answers, some of these efforts show promise for the future.

David B. Nelson, MD, FACOG
Chief of Obstetrics, Parkland Hospital
Dedman Family Scholar in Clinical Care
Assistant Professor, Maternal-Fetal Medicine
Department of Obstetrics & Gynecology
University of Texas Southwestern Medical Center
Dallas, Texas

ADDITIONAL QUESTIONS FOR THE RECORD, SUBCOMMITTEE ON HEALTH, HEARING ON "IMPROVING MATERNALHEALTH: LEGISLATION TO ADVANCE PREVENTION EFFORTS AND ACCESS TO CARE," SEPTEMBER 10, 2019, MS. USHA RANJI, ASSOCIATE DIRECTOR, WOMEN'S HEALTH POLICY, KAISER FAMILY FOUNDATION

The Honorable Nanette Diaz Barragan (D-CA)

Question 1: An important step to ensure that we are reducing the rate of maternal mortality is to guarantee that everyone has access to affordable quality health insurance. That is why crucial programs like Medicaid must be protected and strengthened. A report from the Georgetown university Center for Children and Families found that expanding access to Medicaid under the Affordable Care Act was associated with 1.6 fewer maternal deaths per 100,000 women compared with states that did not expand. Additionally, a study published in the American Journal of Public Health found the mortality rate among African-American infants declined by 14.5% from 2010 to 2015 in expansion states, which was more than twice the decline in states that didn't expand Medicaid.

1. Can you talk about the importance that access to Medicaid has on reducing maternal mortality, and the impact to women's health if Medicaid were cut?

Response 1: Medicaid, the nation's health coverage program for poor and low-income people, provides millions of low-income women across the nation with health and long-term care coverage. Women comprise the majority of the adult Medicaid population, and two-thirds (67%) of adult women on Medicaid are in their reproductive years (19 to 49). Medicaid covers a wide range of reproductive health care services, including family planning, and pregnancy-related care including prenatal services, childbirth, and postpartum care-all without cost-sharing.

Medicaid is the largest single payer of pregnancy-related services, financing 43% of all U.S. births in 2016. In five states and DC, Medicaid covers more than 60% of all births. By federal law, all states provide Medicaid coverage without cost sharing for pregnancy-related services to pregnant women with incomes up to 133% of the federal poverty level (FPL) and cover them up to 60 days postpartum. Many states set higher income thresholds, recognizing the importance of coverage during the perinatal period. Infants born to women covered by Medicaid are covered through at least the first year of life.

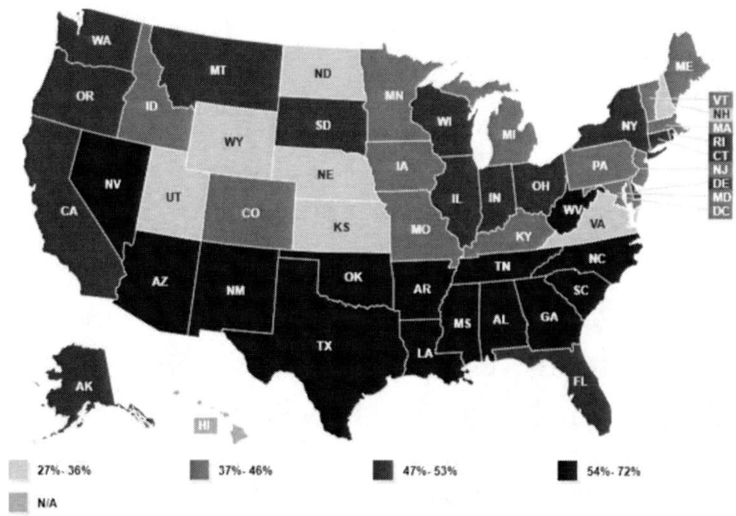

Note: In the 2016 Kaiser Family Foundation Medicaid Budget Survey, states were asked to report the share of all births in the state were financed by Medicaid in the most recent 12 month period for which data were available. States reported data from 2010-2016, which varied by calendar year, state fiscal year, and federal fiscal year.

Source: Kaiser Family Foundation, Implementing Coverage and Payment Initiatives: Results from a 50-State Medicaid Budget Survey for State Fiscal Years 2016 and 2017.

Figure 39. Medicaid is the Leading Financer of Maternity Care in Many States.

To date, 36 states and DC have adopted expanded eligibility for Medicaid under the ACA and offer low-income women the opportunity to continue their pregnancy related Medicaid coverage after the 60 days postpartum period. In the 14 states that have not adopted the ACA's Medicaid expansion, postpartum women need to requalify for Medicaid as parents to stay on the program. While the eligibility thresholds for pregnant women typically go higher than the minimum federal requirement of 138% FPL, Medicaid income eligibility levels for parents are much lower than for pregnant women in all of the states, as low as 17% FPL ($3,636 for a family of three) in Texas). As a result, many women in non-expansion states become uninsured after pregnancy-related coverage ends 60 days postpartum because, even though they are poor, their income is still too high to qualify for Medicaid as parents.

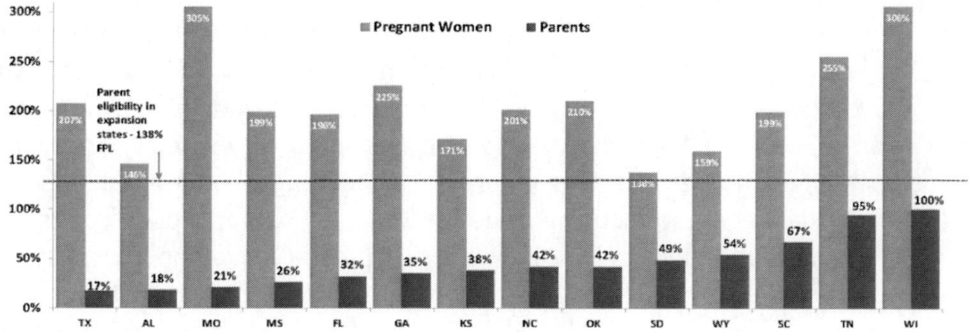

Note: For pregnant women, reflects highest eligibility limit for pregnant women under Medicaid, CHIP, or the unborn child option. For "Parents," eligibility limits calculated as a percent of the Federal Poverty Level (FPS) & are calculated based on a family of three for parents. In 2019, the FPL was $21.330 for a family of three. Thresholds include the standard five percentage point of the FPL disregard.

Source: Based on national survey conducted by Kaiser Family Foundation (KFF) with the Georgetown Universuty Center for Children and Families, 2019.

Figure 40. Medicaid Eligibility Thresholds for Pregnant Women Compared to Parents in Non-Expansion States, 2019.

Several research studies have demonstrated the important role of Medicaid for accessing sexual and reproductive health services as well as pregnancy-related care. Examples include:

- An analysis of the impact of pre-ACA state Medicaid expansions for low-income parents on insurance coverage before pregnancy that found an association between the expanded eligibility and an increase in health coverage among mothers before and during pregnancy, as well as earlier initiation of prenatal care.
- A synthesis of peer-reviewed literature that concluded that states' expansions for pregnancy eligibility in the 1980s contributed to "improvements in prenatal care use,"
- Having continuous insurance coverage facilitates a woman's access to care before, during, and after pregnancy. Access to care before and after pregnancy helps women obtain care for some of the conditions that might put them at risk for maternal mortality and morbidity, including heart disease, diabetes, and depression just to name a few. Research finds that insurance "churning" is common among low-income women around the time of pregnancy, with one-third of women who had recently given birth experiencing a change in insurance status or type during the perinatal period. However, this phenomenon was more pronounced in non- expansion states. In particular, more than one in five mothers in non-expansion states became uninsured during the postpartum period, three times the rate as expansion states.

- According to the Maternal and Infant Health Assessment (MIHA), one in five postpartum women in California experience symptoms of depression during or after pregnancy. California has approved a policy to extend Medicaid coverage for a year to any individual with a maternal mental health condition. For a new mother who needs medications, for example, to manage postpartum depression, this extension of coverage could fill an otherwise unaffordable gap, particularly since Medicaid would not impose cost sharing charges. Furthermore, in 2016 CMS approved coverage of postpartum depression screening for women during well child visits. Under this initiative, if the woman is enrolled in Medicaid, treatment services can be covered under Medicaid. If a woman is uninsured, for example in a non-expansion state, in order for Medicaid to cover the treatment under the child, the treatment must involve the child, such as family therapy.
- In a survey of women of reproductive age in Michigan covered by Medicaid expansion, the expansion was associated with improved access to family planning services, which may enable low-income women to plan and space pregnancies, obtain preconception and interconception care, and acquire postpartum contraception.

For women, the Medicaid program offers coverage of a wide range of primary, preventive, specialty, and long-term care services that are important to them across their lifespans. Given the critical lifeline that Medicaid provides for low-income women and their families, changes to the program financing and structure have significant implications for low-income women's access to coverage and care.

Question 2: An issue that must be addressed in the fight to reduce the rate of maternal mortality is eliminating doctor's implicit biases, as well as having doctors more effectively listening to patient's concerns. The National Partnership for Women and Families conducted a survey and issued a report entitled Listening to Latina Mothers in California. One finding that stood out to me was almost one-third of Latina m others reported that they did not feel that the deli very room staff encouraged them to make decisions about how they wanted their births to progress, while only 21 percent of white women said they felt this way.

2. How can we ensure that doctors more effectively listen to their patients, and take their patient's concerns to heart?

Response 2. As this topic is outside my area of expertise, I would refer you to the following resources on this topic:

- Black Mamas Matter Alliance (BMMA)
- National Birth Equity Collaborative
- Mclemore, M., "To Prevent Women from Dying in Childbirth First Stop Blaming Them," *Scientific American,* May 1, 2019.
- Council on Patient Safety in Women's Health Care. Reduction of Peripartum Racial/Ethnic Disparities (+AIM), October 2016.

Question 3: The California state Department of Public Health calculates that between 2006 and 2013, California lowered its maternal mortality rate by 55 percent To do this, they created a- pregnancy-related mortality review board to examine the causes of every death, and developed comprehensive "how to" manuals detailing the best practices to address specific medical complications. While other states have implemented similar programs, they haven't had the same success as California.

3. Based off California's success, what can be done to help other states be as effective in reducing their rates of maternal mortality?

Response 3: In contrast to the rest of the nation, the rates of maternal mortality in California declined by 55% between 2006 and 2013. The California Maternal Quality Care Collaborative ICMQCC\ has been a leader in efforts to improve maternal health quality in the state. In their recent article, the leaders of CMQCC identify four key steps in their work:

1. "engage as many disciplines and partner organizations as possible;
2. mobilize low-burden data to create a rapid-cycle data center to support the quality improvement efforts;
3. provide up-to-date guidance for implementation using safety bundles and tool kits;
4. make available coaching and peer learning to support implementation through multihospital quality collaboratives. "

For more information about the maternal health care quality efforts and trends in California, I would suggest you contact the staff at CMQCC.

I would add that in addition to the delivery system reforms, California is a Medicaid expansion state, providing continuous coverage to all qualifying individuals up to 138% of poverty. This means that most pregnant women on Medicaid in California have a pathway to coverage after pregnancy, either through Medicaid or with subsidies for private insurance by through the ACA Marketplace. In non-expansion states, many women are dropped from Medicaid after 60 days postpartum. In expansion states, the federal government pays 90% of the expansion costs.

In: A Look at Maternal Health and Reproductive Rights ISBN: 978-1-53619-760-0
Editor: Lisa R. Flores

Chapter 2

EXAMINING STATE EFFORTS TO UNDERMINE ACCESS TO REPRODUCTIVE HEALTH CARE*

Committee on Oversight and Reform

Thursday, November 14, 2019
House of Representatives
Committee on Oversight and Reform
Washington, D.C.

The committee met, pursuant to notice, at 2:19 p.m., in room 2154, Rayburn Office Building, Hon. Carolyn Maloney, presiding.

Present: Representatives Maloney, Norton, Clay, Lynch, Connolly, Krishnamoorthi, Raskin, Rouda, Wasserman Schultz, Sarbanes, Speier, Kelly, DeSaulnier, Lawrence, Khanna, Gomez, Pressley, Tlaib, Jordan, Foxx, Massie, Hice, Grothman, Cloud, Roy, Miller, Green, Armstrong, Steube, Keller, and Norman.

Also present: Representatives Chu, Schakowsky, Schrier, and Lee.

Chairwoman Maloney. The committee will now come to order.

Good morning to everyone. The purpose of this hearing is to examine how state policies, like those in Missouri, are impacting residents' access to comprehensive reproductive healthcare services, including abortion.

Without objection, the chair is authorized to declare a recess of the committee at any time. For audience purposes, we welcome you and respect your interest in being here. In turn, we request and we ask you to respect the proceedings as we go forward in today's hearings. With that, I will now recognize myself to give an opening statement. I would like to begin by acknowledging that this is the first full committee hearing we have held since our friend, our colleague, and our beloved chairman,

* This is an edited, reformatted and augmented version of Hearing before the Committee on Oversight and Reform, House of Representatives, One Hundred Sixteenth Congress, First Session, Serial No. 116–71, dated November 14, 2019.

Elijah Cummings, passed away. Chairman Cummings spent his entire life fighting for justice and equality for everyone, and he was a fierce champion for women's access to healthcare.

Across the country extreme forces in some state governments are taking draconian steps to violate women's rights by restricting access to reproductive health services, including abortion. These state actions include prerequisite undue burdens, restrictions, and outrageously invasive procedures for patients seeking abortions. Let me be clear about what these restrictions are. They are a denial of basic healthcare services that women have a right to receive no matter where they live.

I want to thank my very good friend, Congressman Clay, for his leadership in requesting today's hearing. Missouri has taken some of the most extreme actions to limit access to reproductive healthcare. Missouri is one of six states with only one remaining abortion provider, and as we will hear today, it is at risk of having no providers at all. Missouri's one remaining clinic is Planned Parenthood, and we thank that clinic's director, Dr. McNicholas, for testifying here today and for her brave service to the women in her community every single day.

Earlier this year, Dr. Randall Williams, the director of the Missouri State Health Department, ordered Planned Parenthood to perform medically unnecessary pelvic examinations on every single woman seeking an abortion. This was an invasive state-sponsored abuse of women seeking care. After significant public backlash, the State suspended this cruel practice. But Dr. Williams also recently was forced to admit that he directed state employees to collect information about patients' menstrual cycles to advance his ideological crusade. That is what they were spending taxpayers' dollars on.

I cannot begin to describe my disgust at these violations of privacy and breaches of trust by government officials. Sadly Missouri's actions are not taking place in isolation. Other states have pushed for similar restrictions. I believe these states have been emboldened by the Trump Administration's systemic attacks on reproductive healthcare and general disrespect for women.

In 2012, our former chairman, Darrell Issa, held a hearing in this room in this committee with an all-male panel of religious leaders who were trying to take away contraceptive coverage for women. They did not invite one single woman to testify on that panel. Then they refused our request to have Sandra Fluke, who was a Georgetown law school student at the time, testify about the importance of health insurance coverage of contraceptives. They said she was, and I quote, "not qualified." It was at that hearing that I asked in protest, where are the women. It is time to let women speak, and it is time for everyone to listen. It is time for elected representatives here in Congress and in state houses across the country to protect the right to privacy and a woman's right to abortion services rather than attack it, undermine it, and try to eliminate it.

I want to thank Jennifer Box for sharing her family's story with us. No one should ever have to make the heartbreaking decision that you and your husband had to make, but it is your decision and it does not belong to anyone else. I also want to thank Marcela Howell from In Our Own Voice, which is part of the National Black

Women's Reproductive Justice Agenda, and Fatima Goss Graves from the Women's National Law Center, for all their work and for being here today, and for helping the committee and me on this subject.

I now recognize the Ranking Member Jordan for his opening statement, and I yield back.

Mr. JORDAN. Thank you, Mr. Chair. I want to thank our witnesses for being here today. In the Declaration of Independence, signed 243 years ago, our Founding Fathers enshrined the principle that life, liberty, and the pursuit of happiness are unalienable for everyone. I think it is always interesting to note the order the founders placed the rights they chose to mention. Can you really pursue happiness, can you chase down your goals and dreams if you first don't have freedom, if you first don't have liberty? Do you ever enjoy true liberty, true freedom if government won't protect your most fundamental right, your right to live, your right to life? Life is precious. It is a sacred gift from God.

During an earlier time here in Congress, whatever disagreements that we had, colleagues who didn't share those beliefs, there was a common understanding about this fundamental principle, that life, in fact, is precious. Over the past few years, it seems our two sides have moved away from this basic understanding. Today my colleagues on the other side of the aisle will charge me and Republicans as being against women. Democrats will say if you are not for them and this position and their position on this issue, then you are against all women. We want all people, including women and babies, to have access to world-class healthcare. Statements to the contrary are simply false and are meant to divide our country.

Today, this Congress is in the midst of an unprecedented impeachment inquiry against President Trump. I am proud that President Trump is one of the most pro-life presidents to ever lead our Nation. President Trump has taken bold steps to stop Federal funding of abortions and enable better legal protections for healthcare workers who are opposed to providing, assisting, or participating in these procedures. The hearing today is an attack on that pro-life record.

Today's culture, standing for life, is not easy. I am always guided by one of my favorite Scripture verses, II Timothy 4:7, "Fight the good fight, finish the course, keep the faith," and that is what we have to do, keep the faith in those basic principles outlined in that document that started our Nation over 200 years ago. We came to this Congress to fight for the right of all Americans to have life, liberty, and pursue happiness. I yield back.

Chairwoman MALONEY. I will now yield one minute to the member from the great state of Missouri, Lacy Clay, who requested this hearing.

Mr. CLAY. Thank you, Madam Chairwoman. I along with my constituents appreciate your calling this hearing today on an urgent issue that threatens the health and personal freedom of millions of American women. The assault against a woman's right to make their own healthcare decisions is an insult to the basic values of individual freedom and limited government. Nowhere in the Nation is that assault more urgent than in my home state of Missouri, specifically in the city of St. Louis, which I am so proud to represent.

Planned Parenthood of St. Louis is the last remaining women's healthcare clinic in the entire state of Missouri that also provides abortion services. I visited the clinic staff and physicians this past June as the battle was elevating, and I wanted to lend my support and voice to their efforts. As a husband, father, and brother, I support and trust the private personal health choices of women. I am truly amazed at the Missouri Department of Health would, along with efforts to shut down the clinic, intimidate patients and threaten providers, and would allegedly and bizarrely track women's menstrual periods on spreadsheets to determine if they had had an abortion. No woman should be subjected to this violation of their personhood. This is America, it is her body, it is her healthcare, and it is her decision.

I stand with Planned Parenthood because they are truly on the front lines of defending women's healthcare across America. Madam Chairwoman, I would also like to introduce into the record a personal statement by Ms. M'Evie Mead, the director of policy and organizing of Planned Parent Parenthood advocates in Missouri.

Chairwoman MALONEY. Without objection, so ordered.

Mr. CLAY. Thank you. I yield back.

Chairwoman MALONEY. I will now yield time to the member from the great state of North Carolina, Dr. Foxx.

Ms. FOXX. Thank you, Chairwoman Maloney. I welcome you to your first hearing as acting chairwoman and look forward to continuing working together in your new role. We have had a productive working relationship over the years, and I commit to continuing in that spirit.

I want to say that my sympathy goes out to any woman who feels she must seek an abortion. It must be a horrible situation to be in, but I will admit that I am perplexed by the scope of the hearing. After all, my colleagues on the other side are quick to assert that Roe v. Wade is "the law of the land. However, Planned Parenthood V Casey clearly allows states to implement abortion restrictions, even ones that apply during the first trimester of pregnancy. States are grappling with issues of how to defend and preserve life and support high standards for women's healthcare. As states continue to explore ways to do so in recent years, we are now at a reflection point.

After the Governor of Virginia's horrific comments earlier this year, there has been a national outcry over the apathy shown by the pro-abortion movement toward babies that have been born after an abortion. This is an issue that is very close to my heart and the hearts of millions of Americans. I am going to quote the Governor: "If a mother is in labor, I can tell you exactly what would happen. The infant would be delivered. The infant would be kept comfortable. The infant would be resuscitated if that is what the mother and the family desired, and a discussion would ensue between the physicians and the mother. Governor Northam unfortunately does not stand alone in this appalling stance. He echoes Planned Parenthood's lobbyists, who during testimony on Florida's Born Alive Bill, expressed support for leaving an abortion survivor on the table to die, if that is what the patient and abortionist decided.

In New York, the Reproductive Health Act signed into law by Governor Andrew Cuomo removes protections for children born alive during abortion attempts, leaving them at the mercy of the abortionist who just minutes earlier was trying to kill them. Illinois has also enacted a law that repeals the Illinois Partial Birth Abortion ban Act, and removes licensing requirements for abortion facilities. Still other states, notably, Massachusetts and Virginia, having proposed legislation equally as alarming. Only two-thirds of the states have any laws to protect infants who survived abortion and that positively enshrine their right to life into law. That is simply unacceptable.

Madam Chairwoman, respectfully, in light of these events, I hardly find that anyone is losing access to anything, anyone save the defenseless, the unborn, and now even the born alive. They are the ones having their rights deprived, and the American people find this intolerable. I find it to be an abomination. The pendulum in the states is not one that swinging against women, not in the slightest. Some of my colleagues used to espouse the idea that abortion should be safe, legal, and rare. They espouse it no longer. Instead, on-demand access to abortion up to and, tragically, even after birth is the new mantra. And the fact that extremists are working to keep this ever-expanding restriction on the right to life buttressed against the lives of babies born outside the womb, this should be a wake-up call to us all.

I call on Speaker Pelosi to end her blockade against the bipartisan Born Alive Survivors Protection Act. This bill would protect babies born alive in the remaining one-third of state jurisdictions that fail to do so. Life is sacred, and the regard with which we hold it is what defines who we are as a society. We live in a society that mistakes choice for liberty and denies the dignity of unborn life. But the beauty of living in a free country is that we can use our liberty for love. We must put love into action every day, affirming the value of life at all stages, no matter the difficulties it presents. Striving to love daily is not easy, yet it is the greatest exercise of our freedom, and there is no life unworthy of that love. I yield back, Madam Chairwoman. Thank you.

Chairwoman MALONEY. I will now briefly yield to Congressman Clay to introduce his constituent, Dr. McNicholas.

Mr. CLAY. Thank you, Madam Chair, and I am happy to introduce to the committee one of my distinguished constituents, a highly skilled physician, who has dedicated her life to providing exceptional healthcare for all women, the chief medical officer of Planned Parenthood of the St. Louis Region in Southwest Missouri, Dr. Colleen McNicholas. Dr. McNicholas has also served as a distinguished assistant professor of obstetrics and gynecology at Washington University of Medicine in St. Louis, and Dr. McNicholas is also a champion for closing healthcare disparities, like high maternal and infant mortality rates, that affect minority and low-income patients, mostly because of a lack of access to basic medical care.

Dr. McNicholas performs her duties with skill and compassion. She is a compassionate healer who fiercely defends her patients' rights and their privacy as well. Dr. McNicholas is a warrior for access to quality healthcare for women, not just in St. Louis, but across Missouri and across the Nation as well. Welcome, Doctor, and I yield back.

Chairwoman MALONEY. Thank you, Congressman. We are also joined by Jennifer Box from St. Louis, Missouri, and she was holding that beautiful baby girl. Also we are joined with Fatima Goss Graves, president and chief executive officer of the National Women's Law Center, and Allie Stuckey, from Carrollton, Texas, and Marcela Howell, founder and president, chief executive officer, In Our Own Voice: National Black Women's Reproductive Justice Agenda.

If you would all please rise and raise your right hand, I will begin to swear you in, and raise your right hand.

Do you swear to affirm that the testimony you are about to give is the truth, the whole truth, and nothing but the truth, so help you God?

[A chorus of ayes.]

Chairwoman MALONEY. Let the record show that the witnesses answered in the affirmative. Thank you, and please be seated.

The microphones are sensitive, so please speak directly into them. Without objection, your written statement will be made part of the record. With that, Ms. Box, you are now recognized for your opening statement.

STATEMENT OF JENNIFER BOX, ST. LOUIS, MISSOURI

Ms. BOX. Good afternoon, Acting Chairwoman Maloney, Ranking Member Jordan, and members of this committee. My name is Jennifer Box. I am a mother of three living children, and, as you saw, I am here today with my three-month-old, Astrid, and my husband, Jake. I am a small business owner, a wife, and a Missourian.

I am here today to tell you the story of our daughter, Libby. I am also here to share with you as someone who was in need of an abortion, how difficult my home state of Missouri makes it for pregnant people to access abortion. Libby's story is heartbreakingly linked with the political landscape in Missouri, something I never imagined I would have to navigate when the learning the most devastating news of our lives.

It was almost in the same breath that I learned my pregnancy had a fatal fetal diagnosis that I learned my home state of Missouri would insert itself in the middle of my grief. I searched for answers everywhere, and yet we found no solace in them. Our daughter, if not stillborn, would be born into a life of immediate and repeated invasive medical intervention. She would essentially have been born onto life support. With broken hearts, we knew that the greatest act of love that we could undertake as her parents would be to suffer ourselves instead, to end the pregnancy, grant Libby peace, and spare her tiny, broken body a short life full of pain.

We had made our decision and were still grappling with the reality of it, but there was little time to spare. Missourians like me who seek abortion are confronted with a litany of onerous restrictions, including mandatory waiting periods, private and public insurance bans, informed consent laws, and more. This means that I moved at the direction of the government. For example, my doctor's Catholic hospital, where I delivered my two older children, refused me care. We had to pay thousands of dollars out of pocket because of the state's insurance bans against abortion coverage. And perhaps most surprising, our procedure was rushed due to the state's consent and mandatory delay laws.

Despite how difficult it was to access the medical care I needed, my actual abortion procedure was the most compassionate care I have ever received from a physician. Jake and I left that day knowing that we had made the most loving and merciful choice for our daughter.

I thought after the procedure was over my family could begin to heal privately. I never imagined watching the State of the Union and hearing the President refer to women like me, women who have had abortions later in pregnancy, as murderers. I never fathomed my Governor would weaponize the health department in an attempt to end safe, legal abortion in Missouri. I did not anticipate my state legislature enacting an eight-week abortion ban that would have made it impossible for me to make the best decision for our family.

And let me be clear. My story does not give anyone the right to make judgments about good reasons and bad reasons for abortion. A fetal diagnosis was my reason, but nobody should have to explain themselves or compare their stories to justify a deeply personal decision. I tell my story knowing I am a woman of privilege with means and resources to access the care I needed despite a complicated landscape of laws. Every day women and people of color who fear racist and discriminatory policies carry the heaviest burdens when navigating abortion access.

Politicians like Governor Parson are hellbent on finishing off what little remains of the reproductive healthcare in my State. Members of Congress, I urge you to remember who you represent. I am the one in four women who will have an abortion in her lifetime. You have the power to change a broken system working against us, and I ask that you work in our best interest. I am not asking you to condone my choice. I am simply begging lawmakers like you, who have the power to create change, to allow families to make that choice for themselves.

I speak for Libby. It is an honor to share her name with this committee and the country today. Libby Rose Box. I have a rose tattoo above my heart so that she is with me every day. I am her mother, and she is my daughter and will always be my daughter. I made decisions from day one as her mother, and I made the most important decision of Libby's life, when together with my husband we decided to terminate the pregnancy. It was a sacred, painful, personal decision. That is our story unique to our family, and one that never should have included any politicians. Thank you for your time.

Chairwoman MALONEY. And thank you for sharing your story. I will now call upon Dr. Colleen McNicholas.

STATEMENT OF COLLEEN MCNICHOLAS, MD, OB/GYN, CHIEF MEDICAL OFFICER, PLANNED PARENTHOOD OF THE ST. LOUIS REGION AND SOUTHWEST MISSOURI

Dr. MCNICHOLAS. Thank you, Acting Chairwoman Maloney, Ranking Member Jordan, and members of the committee. Special thanks to Representative Clay for that very kind introduction.

My name is Dr. Colleen McNicholas, and I am a practicing OB/GYN in the state of Missouri. And as you heard, I am the chief medical officer of Planned Parenthood of the St. Louis Region in Southwest Missouri. For more than a decade, I have been honored with the trust of patients seeking a broad spectrum of reproductive healthcare services, including abortion.

As you may know, there is only one health center left in Missouri that provides abortion to meet the needs of more than 1.1 million women of reproductive age in my state, Planned Parenthood's Reproductive Health Services in St. Louis. I am here today because if Governor Parson and Health Director Williams get their way, Missouri could soon become the first state since Roe v. Wade without a single health center that provides abortion care.

I want to tell you how we got here and the dangers that we face when state officials abuse their power and disregard patients' lives to pursue a political agenda. Despite the reality that abortion is safe, Missouri politicians have layered restriction upon restriction, ranging from long waiting periods to insurance coverage bans, in a deliberate attempt to end abortion access. Over the last 30 years, Missouri has gone from nearly 30 clinics to just one clinic today.

Earlier this year, Governor Parson signed one of the most restrictive abortion bans in the country, banning abortion as early as eight weeks, and all together if Roe were overruled. Fortunately, that ban for now is blocked in the courts. Unable to get the job done through legislation, though, Parson's administration weaponized the licensure process to deny our abortion facility license. Health officials admitted under oath that they singled out Planned Parenthood for extra inspections, additional scrutiny, including at the behest of anti-abortion protestors and legislators.

They came to our clinic five times in the first five months of this year, all while they conceded that hospitals and surgery centers providing much riskier procedures went years without a single inspection. During this year's inspection process, the department also admitted to keeping a spreadsheet of my patients' menstrual cycles, a brazen abuse of power and misuse of data motivated by an agenda to find something, anything, that they could use to justify further scrutiny. As shocking as that sounds, more egregious was Director Williams' reinterpretation of a 1988 regulation which forced over 100 patients to undergo multiple invasive pelvic exams. My colleagues and I could not in good conscience force patients to take their clothes off unnecessarily and endure and extra statemandated vaginal exam. Due to public outcry, the department relented, but that only confirms that there was no real medical reason for that exam.

Missourians want to believe that state officials charged with protecting public health have their best interests in mind. They want to trust that when they go to the doctor, their private medical information will not be mined by the department of health as part of a political fishing expedition. Governor Parson and Director Williams have repeatedly violated the trust of our community and compromised my patients' safety, all to push a political agenda.

And it is not just Missouri. Anti-abortion politicians in other states, including Louisiana, refuse to license abortion facilities simply because they do not agree with the healthcare that is provided there. This year alone, 12 states have enacted 25 different abortion bans, and that is on top of the nearly 500 abortion restrictions enacted in the states since 2011. This obsession with abortion has not only proven detrimental to our patients, but it has lasting effects on the health of an entire community. While Missouri goes to incredible lengths to ban abortion, maternal mortality is rising, and black women are dying in pregnancy at three times the rate of white women. Despite this and many other serious public health crises anti-abortion politicians continue to divert precious resources to the overregulation and targeting of abortion providers.

In Missouri, I am happy to say that despite the unrelenting attacks on reproductive healthcare, our doors remain open for now. Planned Parenthood will continue the work of ensuring that every patient who needs and wants an abortion is able to access that care with dignity and respect, and consistent with their values in spite of this impossible landscape. In my exam room, abortion is not political. It is simply healthcare, and it is time we listened to the majority of Americans and put an end to this rampant abuse of power, and do what is necessary to keep abortion safe, legal, and accessible. Thank you.

Chairwoman MALONEY. Thank you. Thank you for your work and for your testimony today. I am now going to recognize Fatima Goss Graves.

STATEMENT OF FATIMA GOSS GRAVES, PRESIDENT AND CHIEF EXECUTIVE OFFICER, NATIONAL WOMEN'S LAW CENTER

Ms. GOSS GRAVES. Thank you, Acting Chairwoman Maloney, and Ranking Member Jordan, and members of the committee. Thank you for the invitation to testify today, and especially on this first hearing following Congressman Cummings' passing. He was a champion for justice and on these issues.

My name is Fatima Goss Graves. I am president and CEO at the National Women's Law Center. At the Law Center, we know that access to reproductive healthcare, including abortion, is vital to gender justice. Access to abortion is a key part of a person's liberty and equality and economic security, and everyone, no matter where they live, no matter their financial means should have access to abortion when they need it.

As the Supreme Court said in Planned Parenthood v. Casey, the ability of women to participate equally in the economic and social life of this Nation has been facilitated by their ability to control their reproductive lives. We also know that legislators passing restrictions on abortion want to control the lives and futures of women. And it is not lost on me that we are facing the biggest threat to the right to abortion on the eve of the 100th anniversary of the Nineteenth Amendment when some women first gained the right to vote. The fight to secure the vote was symbolic of a broader societal change regarding women's ability and right to be politically equal and make politically independent decisions. Now, too, there is a broader movement in this country that will transform the relationship between gender and power. And it is against this backdrop that we must view Missouri's regulatory and legislative efforts to shut down the state's last abortion clinic.

Missouri is not the only or even the first state to seek to end abortion in this country, of course, but what is unique in this moment are the types of abortion bills that are being introduced and passed, before this year, bans on abortion that represented direct challenge to Roe. For example, banning abortion two weeks after a missed period before most people would even know that they are pregnant, were typically seen as too radical, even by many antiabortion advocates.

What is also unique to this moment is state legislators' willingness to express up front why they are pushing these extreme measures. Their goal is to propel a case that presents the Supreme Court an opportunity to overturn or to grossly undermine Roe v. Wade. These legislators believe that between President Trump, Vice President Pence, and the newly constituted Supreme Court, that their goal will be realized. During his first campaign, President Trump even promised some form of punishment for women who have abortions, and that he would automatically overturn Roe v. Wade. In the three years that Trump has been in power, he has reshaped our Federal judiciary in shocking terms to fulfill that promise.

It is disturbing then that earlier this year, the Fifth Circuit upheld a Louisiana law that is identical to a Texas law struck down by the Supreme Court in Whole Woman's Health v. Hellerstedt in 2016. The Supreme Court has just agreed to review this rogue decision this term in June Medical Services v. Gee. This should be an easy decision. Nothing relevant has changed in the last three years except for the composition of the Supreme Court, but the law at issue in June also does nothing to make abortion, an already extremely safe procedure, safer. Instead, such laws are intended to close clinics, and they have done just that.

The resulting shortage of abortion providers has led to longer waiting times for appointments, increased travel to clinics which often result in increased costs, long distance travel, hotel stays in different cities, additional childcare expenses, more time off work when people don't have it, and ultimately delays in getting the care that they are seeking. These costs compound the other restrictions that are already in place, including restrictions on insurance coverage of abortion, all intended to make abortion unaffordable and, therefore, inaccessible. What these politicians are doing is not representative of the will of the people. The public doesn't want the right to abortion overturned. In fact, in the wake of these extreme abortion bans, the public sentiment showed its strength as people flooded the streets this past summer to protest these laws in the middle of the week.

As president of an organization that fights for gender justice in our schools, in work, in healthcare, and improving income security for women in their families, I have a bird's eye view of how all of these fights are connected. The same misogyny that is driving these abortion bans drives much of the opposition that we are seeing in other gender justice battles. That is why at this moment of reckoning on the constitutional right to abortion, we need Congress to lead. We think they can start with passing laws, such as the Each Women Act and the Women's Health Protection Act. Thank you.

Chairwoman MALONEY. Thank you so much. Allie Stuckey.

STATEMENT OF ALLIE STUCKEY, CARROLLTON, TEXAS

Ms. STUCKEY. I would like to thank Chairwoman Maloney, and Ranking Member Jordan, and the rest of the committee for the opportunity to appear before the committee today. My name is Allie Stuckey. I am an author, a podcast host, a commentator, a wife, and a mom. I have spent the last few years studying the pro-abortion movement, observing the growing radicalism of the abortion agenda, and speaking out about the injustice occurring on the state and Federal [level] against preborn children and their mothers.

I am here today as a mom fighting for a future for her kids in which rights are not dependent on whether a person is wanted, but upon their humanity. I am here as a woman who believes that female empowerment, equality, and freedom are not defined by her ability to terminate the life of her child. I am here as an American, afraid for the fate of a country that no longer considers the right to life a prerequisite to liberty and the pursuit of happiness. I am here as a human being horrified by the violence, the oppression, and marginalization of a defenseless people group based solely on where they reside, in the womb.

It's surreal to be here, and not because I'm testifying before Congress, but because of the subject at hand. It is incomprehensible to me that we are having a debate over whether or not it is acceptable to kill a baby before they are born. And while we discussed Democrats' concerns about abortion restrictions today, I want to remind the committee of the true victims of radical legislation, and that is preborn babies.

There was a time perhaps when we could claim ignorance as our justification for allowing and approving of abortion. Only a few decades ago, we knew relatively little about preborn babies in early stages of development. It seemed appropriate to some to deem abortion a privacy issue or an issue of bodily autonomy. Even then the motto was "safe, legal, and rare." Pro-abortion advocates have abandoned these three qualifications in favor of on-demand through all nine months for any reason.

Barbaric laws, like those of New York, Illinois, and a bill in Virginia, aim to codify what Roe and its companion cases allow, the virtually unrestricted access to abortion until the point of birth. As its defendants' position on abortion has radicalized, science and technology have advanced. We now know that a baby's heart begins to beat as early as six weeks. The child can feel pain as early as 20 weeks, only halfway through the pregnancy. Babies born as early as 21 weeks' gestation have survived outside of the womb. By 24 weeks, still only the second trimester, a fetus has a significant probability of surviving if born premature. Babies at this age have also received lifesaving procedures to treat diseases like spina bifida.

Any woman who has been pregnant or has seen her child on an ultrasound knows the undeniable humanity of their preborn babies. Even as someone who is pro-life, I was shocked to see my daughter in the womb at just 11-and-a-half weeks kicking, punching, flipping around. Eleven-and-a-half weeks is still the first trimester. Embryology tells us that at the moment of conception onward, a baby is a living human being with a distinct DNA, and yet the abortion advocates have doubled down on their dehumanizing rhetoric and legislative efforts. Remarkably many members of the so-called party of science insist upon referring to preborn children as no more than clumps of cells.

In speaking of abortion, its defenders ignore the existence of the child entirely. Terms like "reproductive freedom" or "bodily autonomy," "women's empowerment" are used as euphemisms to obscure the reality that the life inside the mom's body is a human, a baby, her baby. If abortion were truly a winning issue for women, if it were, as an article in New York Magazine recently argued, a moral good, this kind of deception wouldn't be necessary. But abortion advocates know that using accurate terminology to describe abortion is ineffective PR, and, therefore, it doesn't make for a profitable business model.

Late-term abortions are typically performed, of course, by emptying the uterus of amniotic fluid, then dismembering the baby with forceps. There are other cases of more grotesque methods utilized, like with Kermit Gosnell. Witnesses before Congress have testified to the neglect of babies who survived abortions, many of whom were reportedly left to die alone. Virginia Governor, Ralph Northam, declared earlier this year that a baby who survives an abortion would be delivered, kept comfortable, and resuscitated if that is what the mother and the family desired.

While tragic, pro-lifers shouldn't be surprised by pro-choice radicalism. This is the end of the logic of the pro-abortion case. There is no logical argument for abortion that doesn't also apply to people who are born. America is included on a list of only seven countries, including China and North Korea, to allow abortion after 20 weeks' gestation. The same legislators who are pro-abortion were happy to vote "yes" on the bill criminalizing animal cruelty on the Federal level. And while I'm am thankful for this, I only wish the same basic compassion could be extended to the most vulnerable members of our own species. Thank you.

Chairwoman MALONEY. Thank you very much. And Marcela Howell.

STATEMENT OF MARCELA HOWELL, FOUNDER AND PRESIDENT, CHIEF EXECUTIVE OFFICER, IN OUR OWN VOICE: NATIONAL BLACK WOMEN'S REPRODUCTIVE JUSTICE AGENDA

Ms. HOWELL. Acting Chairwoman Maloney, Ranking Member Jordan, and honorable members of the committee, thank you for the opportunity to testify at today's hearing. I would like to take a moment first to mourn the passing of Chairman Cummings, a fearless champion of human and civil rights. We promise to pick up his mantle and continue his fight for universal justice.

I am Marcela Howell, founder and president of In Our Own Voice: National Black Women's Reproductive Justice Agenda, a national state partnership with eight black women's reproductive justice organizations: Black Women for Wellness, Black Women's Health Imperative, New Voices for Reproductive Justice, SisterLove, Sister Reach, SPARK Reproductive Justice NOW!, the Afiya Center, and Women With a Vision.

Reproductive justice is the human right to control our bodies, our sexuality, our gender, our work, and our reproduction. That right can only be achieved when all people have the complete economic, social, political power and resources to make healthy decisions about our bodies, our families, and our communities in all areas of our lives. This includes the right to choose if, when, and how to start a family.

When it comes to abortion, we focus specifically on access rather than rights, asserting that the legal right to abortion is meaningless for pregnant people when they cannot access such care due to the cost, the distance to the nearest provider, or other obstacles. Across the country, we are faced with the ever-complicated wave of abortion restrictions that continue to compound already existing barriers making access to quality abortion care a privilege for the few rather than a human right for all.

After the 1973 landmark Roe v. Wade decision, the Supreme Court victory was immediately undermined and invalidated for people with low incomes with the passage of the Hyde Amendment. As the Guttmacher Institute notes, "Because of social and economic inequality linked to systemic racism and discrimination, women of color are disproportionately likely to be insured through Medicaid, therefore subject to the Hyde Amendment's cruel ban on insurance coverage of abortion." The decision of when and how to have a family or when to start or grow a family is a decision that should be made by a pregnant person and those they trust, not politicians.

Over the last decade, abortion access in the U.S. has become increasingly fraught with restrictive laws. Such abortion restrictions include everything from parental consent laws for individuals under 18, often coercive mandated counseling, mandated waiting periods, and unnecessary and burdensome regulations on providers and clinics. This web of restrictions and bans has ultimately created an unjust landscape. As the country grapples with the maternal mortality crisis, one that disproportionately impacts black women, research has found that the states with the higher numbers of abortion restrictions are the exact same states that have poor maternal health outcomes. That is not a coincidence.

Reproductive justice is economic justice. One reason people choose to have abortions is because of the significant expense of having and raising another child given that many are already parents. We cannot afford to endure another abortion ban because we are already battling discrimination in healthcare, wages too low to put food on the table, debilitating childcare costs, attacks on immigrants, and threats to our voting rights. These issues cannot be separated or siloed. Together, they are an attack on our ability to live with full agency over our lives and to raise our children with dignity.

I thank the committee for its dedication to addressing these issues through a lens of justice and equity, and centering the valued, lived experiences of marginalized communities, including black, Latinx, Asian-American/Pacific Islanders, and Native and indigenous women, transgender and gender non-binary people, LGBT people, people with low income, people in rural communities, those with disabilities, youth, and immigrants. I explicitly name us all because all of our struggles are tied together, and many of us live at the margins of multiple oppressed identities.

I urge the committee to address these abortion restrictions with urgency as we collectively work toward bodily autonomy and a world where full reproductive justice can be actualized. Thank you.

Chairwoman MALONEY. Thank you. I want to thank all of the panelists for your important testimony.

Without objection, the following members are authorized to participate in today's hearing: Congresswoman Chu, Congresswoman Schakowsky, Congresswoman Schrier, and Congresswoman Lee.

I will now call on Lacy Clay to begin the questioning. He is the originator of this hearing.

Mr. CLAY. Madam Chairwoman, let me thank you again for convening this hearing to call attention to the intrusive restrictions that are threatening the health and well-being of thousands of women in my congressional district and home State. In Missouri, we are down to one last abortion clinic. State health officials are doing everything in their power to try to shut that clinic down. They are trying to regulate Missouri's last clinic out of existence by imposing rules and regulations that are medically unnecessary, overtly intrusive, or virtually impossible for any healthcare provider to comply with.

And as you heard Dr. McNicholas explain, the health department began enforcing a medically unnecessary requirement that women submit to an additional pelvic exam three days before being allowed to have an abortion. Dr. McNicholas, as a physician, is there any medical reason for such a requirement?

Dr. MCNICHOLAS. Thank you for the question, Representative Clay. So as I previously stated, and I think you noted as well, forcing women to undergo medically unnecessary pelvic exams shows clear disregard for the potential traumatic impact that that has. We are talking about a country where every 73 seconds an American is victimized with sexual assault, and that rate is 12 times higher for women with intellectual disabilities. Within days of having to comply with that mandate, we saw a patient, a minor accompanied by her mom, who was a victim of sexual assault, who had never had a pelvic exam before, who didn't even know what her parts were.

And as a reminder for those of you who have never had a pelvic exam in this room, that means putting your fingers inside someone's vagina. Forcing somebody, this minor, never having had a pelvic exam, to have that invasive procedure when there was absolutely no medically relevant reason to do so, was traumatic for her, for her mother, and for the physician who was required to do it.

Mr. CLAY. How did that make you and your staff feel?

Dr. MCNICHOLAS. So I can tell you that in the times when we had to comply with this regulation, I am not sure who cried more, the physicians, the staff, the patients. We had patients apologizing to us that we were forced to do this to them. Our patients are accustomed to jumping through hoop after hoop to get an abortion, so when told they had to do this, too, they were resigned to the fact that that was just part of the deal. But it was traumatic for everyone.

Mr. CLAY. And if that wasn't outrageous enough, just weeks ago we learned that the state staff were ordered to keep spreadsheets tracking the menstrual cycles of women who visited St. Louis' Planned Parenthood Clinic. Doctor, do you find the practice of tracking the dates of patients' periods problematic?

Dr. MCNICHOLAS. I find it bizarre and a complete violation of the trust that the community puts in the public health department, and the trust that our patients put in us. It was clearly part of an orchestrated attack on Planned Parenthood, and really demonstrates an abuse of power in misuse of data.

Mr. CLAY. And what do you make of the fact that a trained physician has imposed these medically unnecessary and intrusive requirements on providers and patients?

Dr. MCNICHOLAS. So it is shocking that our department of health is headed by a physician, Dr. Randall Williams, and more shocking is that he is an OB/GYN. He knows better. But instead of relying on the medical ethics that he was taught and the many patient experiences that he has had over the course of his career, he instead decided that his job was to act at the behest of a politician to end abortion as part of a political agenda, and forgetting what it is like to treat patients.

Mr. CLAY. What would it mean for patients in Missouri if your clinic closes?

Dr. MCNICHOLAS. You know, the consequence of that, there are so many consequences to that. Certainly people will be forced to carry pregnancies that they can't and shouldn't and don't want to, continuing the cycle of poverty for some. Many will be forced to travel long distances, expending resources they already don't have to access that care. And people will have really lost the trust that they have in the state of Missouri who would then have abdicated its responsibility to providing very basic healthcare.

Mr. CLAY. I thank you for your responses. I thank the entire panel for being here today. And, Madam Chair, I yield back.

Chairwoman MALONEY. I will now recognize Clay Roy. Representative Roy?

Mr. ROY. I will take the name "Clay." It is all right.

Chairwoman MALONEY. Okay.

Mr. ROY. Thank you. Thank you, Madam Chairwoman. In 2015, I got a call from a young woman who is one of my dearest friends. She is like a little sister to me. She said that the baby that was in her belly, her third, might be missing part of his brain, the part that connects the left and right hemispheres. She was terrified and couldn't ask questions fast enough. She had a monthly checkup with her OB/GYN the following week. Her husband had to work, but she took her two boys with her. They liked going to hear the baby's heartbeat, and the checkups were usually routine and quick.

She went into the appointment expecting her doctor would reassure her and, in her answer, review the file. Then the doctor looked our friend straight in the eye and asked her if she wanted to terminate the pregnancy. She called us right after that appointment, understandably angry and terrified. Terminate? What? She explained the doctor had asked the question in the same tone as she might have used when ordering coffee at Starbucks. She didn't blink an eye. She asked it in front of her two little boys. She asked without her husband there. She offered no explanation or comfort. It was cold.

The doctor told her she had to decide quickly because she was approaching 22 weeks, which is as long as you can legally wait to have an abortion in Virginia. Our friend's response was such a source of pride for us. She told us she almost laughed, and then politely responded that termination was not an option. She walked out of that doctor's office and never returned.

So how did it all turn out? Her ultrasound was completely normal at 24 weeks. They just couldn't get a good read at her 20-week appointment. Her baby was born in May 2015 and is completely healthy. It was a boy, by the way. None of us, but particularly his loving and courageous mother, can imagine life without him. He is my godson.

In the winter of 1996, a couple went in for a checkup. They were excited. They had recently been informed they had twins. The doctor came in and performed more tests. Time passed by and the doctor returned. The doctor seemed concerned as they believed the twins had cystic fibrosis. If they were born, they would only survive for a few hours, they were told, if that. "I recommend termination," said the doctor. The couple said the first thing that came into their mind, no, and walked out. They chose life. Those twins would grow up to become excellent men. I know this because Jonah works for me right here. He's one of my staffers.

Ms. Stuckey, Planned Parenthood is not about healthcare. It is about abortion, no?

Ms. STUCKEY. Yes.

Mr. ROY. Planned Parenthood that took in $1.67 billion in total revenues, a 14 percent increase over the year before. Private donations totaled $630 million. Does that sound right to you?

Ms. STUCKEY. Yes.

Mr. ROY. Government funding amount to $563 million of that amount. Does that sound right to you?

Ms. STUCKEY. Yes.

Mr. ROY. Planned Parenthood received nearly $60 million dollars annually under Title X under the Protect Life Rule, which ensures compliance with statutory prohibition against using Title X funds for programs where abortion is a method of family planning. In August 2019, Planned Parenthood confirmed they would withdraw from Title 10 funding rather than comply with the new rule. Does that sound right to you?

Ms. STUCKEY. Yes.

Mr. ROY. Do we need Planned Parenthood for healthcare for women?

Ms. STUCKEY. Planned Parenthood is not in the business of healthcare. They are in the business of abortion as they demonstrated by refusing Title X care. They could have financially and physically separated their abortion services from the rest of their healthcare services, but they refused to do that. They have decided that abortion is central to their mission, which is exactly why they fired CEO Leana Wen, who, in her words, was ousted because she didn't prioritize abortion high enough.

Mr. ROY. That is right, and if I might direct you to the chart behind me, in Texas we have 301 rural health clinics in Texas, 434 federally qualified health centers, to total 735 federally funded community health clinics. There are 327 pregnancy centers, 130 of which are medical pregnancy centers. And according to the Planned Parenthood website, there are 40 Planned Parenthood centers in Texas. Does that number sound right to you?

Ms. STUCKEY. Yes.

Mr. ROY. Does Texas, at least in the state which I represent, provide healthcare solutions for women throughout the state of Texas.

Ms. STUCKEY. Yes, they do. I am from Texas as well.

Mr. ROY. Yes, ma'am. Texas's Program, Healthy Texas Women, was established in 2016, has been helping women in Texas with services and with more providers than Planned Parenthood. Does that sound right to you?

Ms. STUCKEY. Yes.

Mr. ROY. In Fiscal Year 2018, Healthy Texas Women served 172,000 clients. According to the Planned Parenthood website of Greater Texas, in 2018 Planned Parenthood served only 83,000 patients compared to that larger number, and it has only been in existence since 2016. Does that sound right to you?

Ms. STUCKEY. Yes.

Mr. ROY. My point is simply this. The state of Texas I can speak to. I can't speak to the other 49 states. We take women's health very seriously, and we should. We should entities and we should allow the market to thrive, and, frankly, if we could get some of the regulations out of the way of a healthy healthcare system, we could have more options. But could you please, as my time is running out, please share your view of the ways in which we can provide healthcare and better ways than allowing an organization like Planned Parenthood, which takes unborn babies, puts them in plastic bags, and throws them in garbage bins, to be the center of healthcare provision for women? Thank you.

Ms. STUCKEY. Abortion is not healthcare. I think that's all I have time for.

Chairwoman MALONEY. The chair now recognizes Congress-woman Norton.

Ms. NORTON. I thank you very much, Madam Chair. Dr. McNicholas, just to follow up here. What kind of health services do you provide?

Dr. MCNICHOLAS. I appreciate that question, Ms. Norton. So Planned Parenthood provides a broad spectrum of reproductive healthcare services, including well people care, cancer screenings, the full spectrum of birth control options, transgender care, primary care. Some Planned Parenthoods also provide prenatal care, and the list goes on.

Ms. NORTON. So it look like you provide the kind of across-the-board care that a young woman may need. You go in this one stop fits all.

Dr. MCNICHOLAS. The goal is to meet our patients' needs both in the clinical services that they need and require and that the community needs, and also to make sure that it is accessible for them.

Ms. NORTON. And abortion would be only one of those services.

Dr. MCNICHOLAS. That is correct.

Ms. NORTON. I have a question. Perhaps I should start with Ms. Graves or perhaps also Dr. McNicholas. I represent 700,000 residents. They pay the highest Federal taxes–this is a little-known fact–highest Federal taxes per capita in the United States. We are trying to make the District of Columbia the 51st state, but when look at where there are intrusions into healthcare, you will find that they are all Federal bans that include Federal employees, Federal prisoners who are included in this list, low-income residents of the District of Columbia.

Our jurisdiction wants to provide on their own, pay for abortion services for low-income women the way almost 20 states already do. We are not demanding that the Federal Government does this. My question is, why we are finding that restrictions on coverage are related to economic mobility for women on coverage for abortion and others such as services? And apparently there is a correlation here for not only for women generally, but especially for women of color. So why do restrictions on abortion relate to economic mobility? Why are they correlated in that way?

Ms. GOSS GRAVES. Well, I very much appreciate you raising that issue also as a resident of the District that lacks the range of voting rights that you described. And oftentimes there has been a deep focus on the levels of restrictions that are in places like Missouri. But even in the District, because of restrictions on insurance, for low-income women, in particular, what that means is that abortion is inaccessible and unavailable, and having to scrap together the money to be able to afford it is not possible.

And what it also means is that for the most vulnerable of folks, the right to abortion does not feel very meaningful. And that connection between the ability to have economic security for yourself and for your family is deeply tied to your ability to access the healthcare you need. This is a travesty that is deeply felt by people who live in the District, in part because, you not only have the restrictions on like Medicaid. You also see them show up in Federal health insurance, and so many people who live here are also working for the Federal Government.

Ms. NORTON. So you can see that there are many reasons why the District of Columbia wants to become the 51st state. I just want to say to my Republican colleagues, you know, whose mantra is we want government out of our business, my friends on the other side of the aisle vote against the government doing things which the American people want government to do. All the District of Columbia is asking is that you get out of their business so that we can deal with our business alone.

Thank you very much, and I yield back.

Chairwoman MALONEY. The chair recognizes—

Mr. CONNOLLY. Might I just yield to her 20 seconds? Ms. Norton, would you yield?

Ms. NORTON. I will be glad to yield.

Mr. CONNOLLY. I thank my friend. I just wanted to give Dr. McNichols an opportunity. We just heard a stunning statement that Planned Parenthood is not in the health care business, doesn't provide health care. I want to give you the opportunity to respond to that. Thank you.

Dr. MCNICHOLAS. I appreciate the question. Abortion is health care, and I think the best way to demonstrate that is to share a story about a patient who, when unable to access her abortion, died, because her comorbidities and the complications she had prior to pregnancy worsened during that.

A patient from out of state visited my clinic for a consultation after understanding that her current medical condition would worsen with pregnancy. She returned to her out-of-state home, having to wait the mandated amount of time between those visits before she can receive that care. When she didn't return and we called to followup we were later told that she passed away from complications of her pre-pregnancy medical condition.

This is the very definition of why abortion is health care and is needed and is necessary, when people need it, where they live.

Chairwoman MALONEY. Thank you very much. Dr. Foxx.

Ms. FOXX. Thank you very much, Chairwoman.

Dr. McNicholas, earlier this year, Governor Northam of Virginia said, "If a mother is in labor I can tell you exactly what would happen. The infant would be delivered, the infant would be kept comfortable, the infant would be resuscitated, if that is what the mother and the family desired, and then a discussion would ensue between the physicians and the mother."

Do you support Governor Northam's comments?

Dr. MCNICHOLAS. So I can't speak for Governor Northam, but what I can say is that there is no way to oversimplify the– sort of the medical conditions in which people present in the second trimester, that I think that he was referring to.

Ms. FOXX. So as a physician, then, what would be the harm in legislation such as the Born Alive Abortion Survivors Act, to make sure that a child born alive would not be put to death?

Dr. MCNICHOLAS. So there are several harms. The first is which, using that language and perpetuating the notion that that is actually a real thing is harmful in and of itself, and it only serves two purposes. The first is to shame people, like

Jennie, who need life-saving care in the second and third trimesters of pregnancy. It also creates an environment in which abortion providers like myself and my colleagues are targeted and harassed. So first and foremost, it is dangerous for those reasons.

The second reason is because medicine is complicated. There really is no way for me to boil down more than a decade of education and practice to give you a single reason why doing such things is harmful to patients.

Ms. FOXX. The answer should have been either yes or no.

Earlier this year, thousands of fetal remains were found in the home of deceased abortionist, Ulrich Klopfer. Who do you believe–do you believe that all fetal remains should be disposed of in a manner that treats them with dignity and respect?

Dr. MCNICHOLAS. Just like I believe that patients are capable of making a decision to continue their pregnancy or not, to expand their family or not, I believe that patients are capable of deciding what should happen to the remains of their pregnancy.

Ms. FOXX. So is it okay for those fetal remains to be sold for profit by Planned Parenthood?

Dr. MCNICHOLAS. Planned Parenthood has never sold fetal tissue, and current doesn't, and never has.

Ms. FOXX. Does Planned Parenthood v. Casey give states the authority to regulate abortion in accordance with the opinions of their respective constituencies?

Dr. MCNICHOLAS. I believe that the most recent decision, and we have some policy experts on the panel who can speak more to this, but the more recent decision in Whole Women's Health set a precedent that restrictions must be based and grounded in science, and that is all we are asking for is that abortion is treated to the current standards of medical evidence and science.

Ms. FOXX. Ms. Stuckey, thank you very much for being here. Are there more federally qualified health centers than abortion clinics in the United States?

Ms. STUCKEY. Thank you for the question. Yes, the ratio is about 26 to one of health care centers that are federally funded, to Planned Parenthoods.

Ms. FOXX. And which offers more comprehensive health services to women?

Ms. STUCKEY. Of course, the health care centers that are not Planned Parenthood.

Ms. FOXX. So if we wanted to support access to comprehensive health care services for women, would we be better off supporting abortion clinics or federally qualified health care centers?

Ms. STUCKEY. The federally qualified health care centers.

Ms. FOXX. Thank you. In 2005, a Planned Parenthood-funded study found a majority of women seeking an abortion did so because having a baby would interfere with education and work, cost too much, or they did not want to be a single mother or having relationship problems. What are your thoughts on the findings of this study?

Ms. STUCKEY. It shows that– it belies this notion that abortion is only used in very extreme cases. The extreme, rare cases are typically used to cast pro-lifers into a negative, extremist, radical, misogynous light, which is just not accurate. The majority of abortions, according to Planned Parenthood's own research, are done on the basis of convenience, and I just don't see a logical or moral justification for killing an unborn child on the basis of simply not being wanted.

Ms. FOXX. Thank you. Madam Chair, earlier Dr. McNicholas said that Dr. Williams was a physician and had taken an ethics oath and show know better than to do what he had done. I just want to quote from the classic Hippocratic Oath: "I will use those regimes which will benefit my patients according to my greatest ability and judgment, and I will do no harm or injustice to them. I will not give a lethal drug to anyone if I am asked, nor will I advise such a plan, and similarly, I will not give a woman a pessary to cause an abortion."

Dr. McNicholas, did you swear a Hippocratic Oath when you were licensed?

Dr. MCNICHOLAS. I did, and I continue to live that every single day.

Ms. FOXX. Amazing.

Madam Chair, Mr. Roy asked me if I would enter into the record this article.

Chairwoman MALONEY. Without objection.

Ms. FOXX. Thank you, Madam Chair. I yield back.

Chairwoman MALONEY. The chair now recognizes Representative Lynch.

Mr. LYNCH. Thank you, Madam Chair. I want to thank you for holding this hearing, and also to my friend and colleague, the gentleman from Missouri, Mr. Clay, thank you for your leadership as well.

I want to thank all the witnesses here today, especially Ms. Box–Mrs. Box, for your willingness and your courage to come before this committee to share our own experience, and all of you for sharing your perspectives.

As I noted in my op-ed in the Boston Globe back in May, when this onslaught of state legislation arose, in Missouri, Alabama, Ohio, and Georgia, the legislatures have recently adopted draconian measures on abortion. Alabama has banned abortion at any stage of pregnancy, apparently even in the case of rape or incest, while several other states have banned abortions as early as six weeks, which, as some of our witnesses have noted, is often before many women would even know they are pregnant. In Georgia, a woman terminating a pregnancy after six weeks could be charged with homicide.

These laws are far more punitive than those in place before the Roe v. Wade decision. They are so intrusive and so restrictive that the basic core constitutional right to privacy and protection from government intrusion into health care decisions would be effectively and totally eliminated. Meanwhile, other states are actively considering similar restrictive measures.

This all occurs against a backdrop in which Republicans in Congress have repeatedly attempted to eliminate women's access to contraceptive services offered by groups such as Planned Parenthood, ironically, even though those contraceptive services actually prevent unwanted pregnancies, and thereby reduce the number of unwanted pregnancies and abortions. Ironically, and seeking to shutter many of these clinics, they would also be cutting off expectant mothers, especially in those low-income areas, who rely on their services for the prenatal and postnatal care they need to ensure that they have safe and healthy pregnancies.

It is to be noted that to be pro-life includes supporting the health of pregnant women. It includes feeding and educating and housing children. Simply opposing abortion does not make you pro-life.

The Supreme Court's decision on reproductive rights, as controversial as they may be in our country, have sought to acknowledge and balance the constitutional interests that are at stake on this issue. And while critics are bound, even without the onslaught of restrictive state legislation, the number of abortions that are performed in the United States each year has dropped dramatically, and that is largely due to the impact of effective and widely available contraception, family planning, and education.

Women are and should be in charge of their reproductive health, and their efforts to reduce unwanted pregnancies are actually working, all of which leads many to believe that the timing and the similarities of this multistate campaign reveal a purely political strategy to energize and motivate the religious right, and that is truly shameful.

While I am personally informed by my faith, my actions as a legislator must be in support of, in defense of the Constitution. That is the oath that I took and I stand by it. And as I said back in May, if these recent developments, closing all clinics, obstructing contraceptive services, denying women every option in their health care decisions, if this defines the new pro-life movement then you can count me out.

I have one question for either Counselor Graves or Ms. Howell, and thank you for your kind words regarding Mr. Cummings. So there are millions of women each year– and Ms. McNicholas, you might have some – Dr. McNicholas, you might have some input on this as well – if we have millions of women who come to Planned Parenthood and other contraceptive services providers, and yet the government steps in to deny funding– and this came to the floor. I spoke against it. This actually came to the floor when the Republicans were in control of the House, and they proposed to zero out– zero out– any Federal funding for Planned Parenthood to carry on its contraceptive services. What would the impact on the abortion rate be, the rate of unwanted pregnancies and the abortion rate, if that measure had been implemented?

Dr. MCNICHOLAS. So I think you raised a very important point, which is one of the strategies– one of the best strategies we have to reduce unintended pregnancy is– it is actually multilayered. It is, first, improving the sexual education that we provide to our young children, helping them know how their body works and being very positive about understanding how sex works and how you get pregnant.

Second, it is providing them access to the available contraceptive method of their choice when they need it, and without barrier, including going to a clinic in their neighborhood, making sure that it is affordable for them, and making sure that they can change that method as often as they need to, when their history or their preference changes.

Mr. LYNCH. Counselor Graves, on this, do you want to add to that?

Ms. HOWELL. Many people actually go to Planned Parenthood for a number of different health care services. They go not only for birth control but also to have tests for diabetes, for mammogram screenings. A lot of the people that we represent, and that we work with, go to Planned Parenthood clinics as their primary provider. And so to remove services that they think are vital to them, because people are opposed to the fact that some Planned Parenthoods also do abortions, means that you are cutting off health care for people who most desperately need it.

Mr. LYNCH. Thank you.

Ms. GOSS GRAVES. The only thing I would add, it is a good opportunity for me to correct something Ms. Stuckey said about Planned Parenthood. We should be really clear about what happened with this gag rule that the Administration put out.

Planned Parenthood wanted to do right by its patients. It was not going to lie to them. It was not going to misinform them. And the idea that we are now in a situation where providers are being forced to make that sort of decision about whether or not they can continue to serve the lowest income population in communities is really, really terrible, and patients are going to suffer for it.

Mr. LYNCH. Thank you very much. Madam Chair, I yield back.

Mr. HICE. Madam Chair, I have a unanimous consent request. I have a unanimous consent request.

Okay. Thank you, Madam Chair. Being from Georgia I just want to clarify that the law is not according to what was just identified by my colleague, and I would like to ask unanimous consent to be added into the record an article by David French that goes into the details of the law that the Georgia Heartbeat Bill would not imprison women who have an abortion.

Chairwoman MALONEY. Without objection.

Chairwoman MALONEY. I now recognize Mr. Massie.

Mr. MASSIE. Thank you, Madam Chair.

Dr. McNicholas, what is the medical consensus for age of viability of a fetus?

Dr. MCNICHOLAS. I appreciate the question. So viability is a complicated medical construct. There is no particular gestational age. There are some pregnancies in which a fetus will never be viable. There are a number of different factors that we think about when we are considering if a pregnancy is or is not viable.

Mr. MASSIE. So is there a legal consensus on the age of viability?

Dr. MCNICHOLAS. Not to my understanding, but I am a physician, not a lawyer.

Mr. MASSIE. In your 10 years as a doctor, how many abortions have you performed?

Dr. MCNICHOLAS. So I provide a variety of different services, and as you—

Mr. MASSIE. I am not asking about the other services.

Dr. MCNICHOLAS. Right.

Mr. MASSIE. How many abortions have you performed?

Dr. MCNICHOLAS. So I can't tell you how many hysterectomies I have done and I can't tell you how many abortions I have done. I have had a long career taking care of people for a variety of things.

Mr. MASSIE. So you manage a facility. Can you tell me– or you are the medical overseer– can you tell me how many abortions the facility in Missouri performs each week?

Dr. MCNICHOLAS. I can tell you– I believe it is probably available, so I can give you a rough estimate of how many abortions we perform per year, which is, I think roughly around 3,000.

Mr. MASSIE. How do you dispose of 3,000 fetuses every year?

Dr. MCNICHOLAS. So Missouri has a state law that requires that we send all of the remains of pregnancy to pathology.

Mr. MASSIE. What is the latest-term abortion that you have performed, like gestation period, in weeks?

Dr. MCNICHOLAS. So my practice includes the provision of abortion up until the point of viability, and again, we already had a discussion about viability not being——

Mr. MASSIE. So just give me the number in weeks them.

Dr. MCNICHOLAS. I don't know.

Mr. MASSIE. You don't remember the number of weeks?

Dr. MCNICHOLAS. That is correct. So I—

Mr. MASSIE. What about size of the unborn baby? Do you know the largest baby that you have aborted?

Dr. MCNICHOLAS. I am not sure how I would even quantify that.

Mr. MASSIE. If I use the word fetus could you– do you know? You have no idea the age or gestational period of the fetuses that you are aborting.

Dr. MCNICHOLAS. So again, as I said, my practice includes abortion care through the point of viability, and as we previously discussed, that could be—

Mr. MASSIE. Let me put it this way.

Dr. MCNICHOLAS [continuing]. at any point, yes.

Mr. MASSIE. Is there any point of gestation beyond which you personally would not abort a fetus?

Dr. MCNICHOLAS. You know, medicine is not black and white. I recognize, in my 10 years of practice, informs this opinion, that pregnancy can be really complicated, and given that there are pregnancies for which a fetus may never be viable, I think it is really important that we allow physicians and patients to have every medical resources to make decisions that are appropriate for them and their health.

Mr. MASSIE. In the absence of a law preventing it, would you abort a viable fetus?

Dr. MCNICHOLAS. Again, every patient is different and I can't make any—

Mr. MASSIE. I am just asking about a viable fetus. If the law didn't prevent it, would you consider it a limitation, morally, for you to abort a viable fetus?

Dr. MCNICHOLAS. So I think you are forgetting that there a number of reasons that go into a patient's—

Mr. MASSIE. If the reason—

Dr. MCNICHOLAS [continuing]. choice.

Mr. MASSIE. At your clinic, does it matter what the reason is for the abortion?

Dr. MCNICHOLAS. At my clinic, I trust that women have a valid reason. Every reason that they have is valid.

Mr. MASSIE. Okay. So given that you think that every reason is valid, would you abort a viable fetus, if there was not a law preventing it?

Dr. MCNICHOLAS. Again, given that the reality for people choosing abortion is that there are many reasons, there isn't a single thing that defines somebody's choice.

Mr. MASSIE. You seem to have a—

Dr. MCNICHOLAS. It is a reflection of their—

Mr. MASSIE [continuing]. hard time– you seem to have a hard time saying this. This tells me you have a heart, or at least you know that people watching this have a heart, and they would be concerned if you would just admit, but you won't admit here, that you would abort a viable fetus for any reason if the law did not prevent it.

Dr. MCNICHOLAS. Mr. Massie, abortion is moral. It is important. It is health care. And I support people being the experts in their own lives and making decisions for themselves.

Mr. MASSIE. It gives me some hope that you here understand that people do not support you when you abort– when you say– or if you would say that you would abort a viable fetus for any reason. But given what you told us in your opening statement, and knowing what you have said, we know that you would. But it does give me hope that you still know, in your heart, that is wrong.

Mrs. Stuckey—

Dr. MCNICHOLAS. I am not sure– can I respond to that really quickly?

Mr. MASSIE. If you would answer my question you could, but you won't, so I am going to use my remaining time asking Mrs. Stuckey, should any reason be a good reason for having an abortion?

Ms. STUCKEY. Absolutely not. It is a child. It is a life inside the womb from the moment of conception onward. And I am very troubled by how flippantly she said that there are 3,000 abortions performed every year, of defenseless human beings, and the remark that abortion is moral—

Mr. CLAY.

[Presiding.] The time has expired.

Ms. STUCKEY. You cannot have that kind of logic—your lifestyle.

Mr. CLAY. No. The time has expired. I recognize—

Mr. HICE. You gave the others over two minutes, Mr. Chairman. Mr. Chairman, we need to be fair on both sides of the aisle, please.

Mr. CLAY. You want to finish your answer?

Mr. MASSIE. Please. I would like for her—

Mr. CLAY. No, no. Finish your answer. Go ahead.

Ms. STUCKEY. I don't quite understand the illogic of saying that killing a child inside the womb for any reason whatsoever is moral, it is health care. In what other situation, besides when a child is defenseless in the womb, do we call killing someone health care, do we call killing someone moral? Can anyone on the pro-abortion side tell me a situation, outside of a defenseless child inside the womb, in which it is morally justifiable to kill someone simply because they are not wanted?

That is the answer that I would like. That is the question that I have. I, unfortunately, don't think anyone is able to answer it for me.

Mr. CLAY. I recognize the gentlewoman from Illinois, Ms. Kelly, for five minutes.

Ms. KELLY. Thank you, Mr. Chair, and thank you for this hearing.

My Republican colleagues have suggested that earlier restrictions on abortion have become necessary because advances in medicine are moving the point of viability earlier and earlier. Dr. McNicholas, I am interested in hearing your thoughts on this point.

Dr. MCNICHOLAS. Thank you for the question. So I think, as I previously alluded to, viability isn't an easy thing to assess. It requires—

Ms. KELLY. It is different with every pregnancy.

Dr. MCNICHOLAS. That is exactly right. It requires knowledge of multiple things about any individual's pregnancy.

Ms. KELLY. Thank you for clarifying. First of all I want to thank the witnesses for being here. Thank you for sharing your story with us. And I want to let you know that I was a proud board member of Planned Parenthood in Peoria, and I am very proud that my state of Illinois is an oasis in the sand, very proud that we are a shining light in the dark.

And, Mrs. Stuckey, you said you want to see the same basic compassion. You made that comment. Well, I wanted to see the same basic compassion for maternal mortality. I had to water down the bill I had because the compassionate Republicans, not one would sign onto the bill to extend Medicaid.

We have not been able to get a gun violence prevention bill passed because we don't have the same basic compassion once the unborn fetus becomes a baby, and they grow up. We don't seem to have compassion in that area. We don't have the same compassion when it comes to feeding our young people. We don't seem to care about that. We are looking at cutting that, so 500,000 people don't have the food they have.

So where is the compassion once you are born? That is the question I have?

Ms. STUCKEY. Well, Ms. Kelly, thank you so much for bringing up these points, because I agree that we should have compassion from the womb to the tomb. That is what I believe. I don't necessarily—

Ms. KELLY. It is not fair.

Ms. STUCKEY [continuing]. I don't necessarily agree with all of your legislative solutions to that. I do believe the private sector does a much better job. But your premise is that these things are mutually exclusive, that we either have to be on your side of the debate, and for violently murdering children inside the womb—

Ms. KELLY. No, you never heard me—

Ms. STUCKEY [continuing]. or we are not—

Ms. KELLY [continuing]. no, I am just saying—

Ms. STUCKEY. They are not mutually exclusive.

Ms. KELLY [continuing]. you are saying we are violently murdering, but there is a lot of kids being murdered every day—

Ms. STUCKEY. And why can't we care about—

Ms. KELLY [continuing]. and we don't do anything about that. I am reclaiming my time. Reclaiming my time.

In the wake of many draconian measures, my own state of Illinois recently signed into a law a bill to protect abortion access for our residents. The Illinois Reproductive Health Act ensures coverage for abortion care and updates clinic regulations to lift that burden from abortion providers.

Ms. Goss Graves, how does eliminating coverage bans improve access to abortion care for women who are working to make ends meet?

Ms. GOSS GRAVES. It will mean that the right to abortion, which has been legal for almost 50 years, will actually be a right that is accessible for women, for women no matter their income. Whether or not that right is accessible to you should not be depending on your financial means. That is not what the court said.

Ms. KELLY. Because the other thing we never talk about is, you know, wealthier women who tend not to be women of color, they have been having abortions for a long time, whether they are in red states or blue states, or however they vote—

Ms. GOSS GRAVES. That is right.

Ms. KELLY [continuing]. or whatever their political interests are. And how will rolling back targeted regulations of abortion providers improve access?

Ms. GOSS GRAVES. Here is what we know. These targeted regulations of abortion providers are designed really to shut down clinics. They are designed to shame patients. They are designed to confuse people and disrupt the doctor-patient relationship. All of that makes abortion less accessible. And all of that– I mean, listening— I have to say, the rhetoric that is surround it, on top of the sorts of regulations and restrictions, have made all of this so difficult for people who are just trying to live their lives and get the health care that they need.

Ms. KELLY. And I know from a lot of college students that they are not going to Planned Parenthood to get an abortion. They are going for health. That is their place of choice to get health care, not for abortions.

Dr. MCNICHOLAS. Yes. Planned Parenthood is very proud to be able to provide services to people who are financially insecure, and to do that in a way that serves their needs and respects their dignity.

Ms. KELLY. Thank you, and I yield back my time.

Mr. CLAY. The gentleman from Georgia, Mr. Hice, is recognized for five minutes.

Mr. HICE. Thank you, Mr. Chairman. It seems to me that a lot of this debate and argument centers around whether or not the baby is a person or a fetus, and I recognize that many on the other side of the aisle refuse to recognize the baby as a baby, refuse to recognize it is a person, it is humanity.

Ms. Stuckey, there have been a lot of medical advances, certainly, over the last several decades. Can you tell us about some specific scientific evidence supporting the personhood, the humanity of the baby, and the viability?

Ms. STUCKEY. Well, embryology tells us– thank you for your question, first of all– embryology tells us that the child, from the moment of conception, has a separate DNA, and so when we hear these euphemisms thrown around, like my body, my choice, immediately obscuring the life of the child, it shows me that the proabortion argument doesn't deal with fact. It deals with feeling, which is exactly why we have had such a hard time getting any kind of clear answer from any of the panelists of what abortion actually is. What does it do? Because, talking about tearing a child apart, limb by limb, with forceps just isn't a very good P.R. strategy for Planned Parenthood or the abortion industry.

All I am trying to do is to remind us, when we are having this conversion, that there are two people. There are two people. And I don't believe we have to pit a mother against her child in order for a woman to be successful.

We talked about, you know, legislative solutions and showing compassion for children after they are born. I absolutely believe in that. Every pro-life pregnancy center that I have ever been a part of, that I have ever donated to, they don't just counsel women. They also offer parenting classes. They are also offering help from abusive situations. They are offering programs for these young women to be able to get affordable baby clothes and baby products and things like that.

Every pro-life organization I know cares about children, in the womb, after they are born, and the mother, who is pregnant with these children. That is what I am trying to argue, that let's not ignore the scientific reality that a baby is a baby, and, therefore, in my opinion, is deserving of the right to life.

Mr. HICE. In a way this is even going beyond abortion in the womb. As we all were horrified, many of us, Virginia Governor Ralph Northam, and his description of however it could possibly be described as a post-birth abortion, one of the most horrifying things I have ever heard in my life, where the baby would just sit there on the table and we would decide what to do with it. How do you respond to this?

Ms. STUCKEY. Yes. That is a great point that you bring up. Unfortunately, this has been a reality in other places across the country. We like to act like this is not a thing. The CDC itself says that over a span of 11 years, at least 143 babies were born alive and then not resuscitated, or born alive and not attended to and cared for. Only six states actually require this kind of reporting, so the number of 143 is probably a lot higher than that.

So what we see, that this is not just a degradation of children inside the womb. It is a degradation of babies, in general. It is a degradation of life based on whether or not this child is wanted by the mother. And again, I ask, in what other context, in what other stage of life do we decide that someone gets to die simply because they are not wanted? And not provoke a slippery-slope fallacy, but truly, what we have seen from Governor Northam's statements and from other statements that we have heard, is that it truly is a slope. There is a logical and a moral slope to this, and it seems like the pro-abortion side is sliding down very quickly.

Mr. HICE. Well, and to that point– and I think it is, likewise, an excellent point you brought forth a while ago, Planned Parenthood's own study, that the majority of women have abortions not because of their own personal health but because of convenience sake, whether it be a job or whatever it may be.

How does those findings from Planned Parenthood itself undermine the narrative, particularly about late-term abortions, that it has something to do with the health of the mother?

Ms. STUCKEY. Yes, and we can have conversations about the health of the mother in those very rare circumstances. But as you mentioned, and that Planned Parenthood has noted the vast majority of cases are for any reason whatsoever, including just not wanting a child, it not being convenient, wanting to finish school. And if the pro-abortion side were honest, they are completely fine with that. They are completely open to the normalization– there are organizations now that exist to normalize abortion, to destigmatize abortion. That means that they believe abortion to be not only normal but good.

Actually, we heard the doctor say that she believes that abortion is good. If you believe that abortion is morally good, of course you don't think it should be limited to the life of the mother or any of those very rare circumstances. It is all nine months, on demand, without apology. That is the new motto of the pro-abortion side.

Mr. HICE. And the fact is the baby is a person, and for that reason how could it be moral to kill it?

Ms. STUCKEY. I don't know what else it is if it is not a person. Mr. HICE. Thank you. I yield back.

Mr. CLAY. The gentleman yields back. I recognize the gentlewoman from Michigan, Mrs. Lawrence, for five minutes.

Mrs. LAWRENCE. Thank you, Mr. Chairman, and I am glad to be here for this hearing. This hearing should be substantive discussion on how to expand access to care for women. I am disappointed that my Republican colleagues are using this hearing to make such blatantly false claims, the young lady who speaks in generalization. And for the record, while one side calls themselves pro-life, there is not a person I know that says they are pro-abortion. They are pro-choice.

So abortions are not infanticide. That is not how abortion works, and this type of deceptive rhetoric is yet another attempt to distract from efforts to make abortion out of the reach for women, to shut down clinics.

And just constantly I have had this debate a number of times on this panel. The mistruths that are spoken about, ripping full-sized babies out of wombs and killing them, that is not true. Selling of parts is not true. And it just seems like it is enjoyed to say, because it paints this horrific picture, and we should say the truth, statistics.

Mrs. Box, I am so sorry to hear about the pain your family had to suffer, and thank you for bringing your beautiful baby in the room. Have you considered whether this law that is being proposed or passed in Missouri would have prevented you from having an abortion if it had existed two years ago?

Ms. BOX. Thank you. It absolutely would have prevented me from having an abortion. At eight weeks, which is when the ban that my state legislature passed, it is impossible to know of the chromosomal abnormalities, as far as my understanding. I am not the doctor here today. We did the early genetic testing because I am of advanced maternal age– another one of my not-favorite terms—

Mrs. LAWRENCE. Yes.

Ms. BOX [continuing]. and so believe that we found out before most women and families would find out, because we found out earlier. Most people would not find out until the 20-week anatomy scan. And I can say that after Libby I was obviously able to successfully get pregnant again, as evidenced by beautiful daughter, who is now being quiet, thankfully. So I was pregnant during the time that the state legislature was enacting this ban and that Governor Parsons signed this into law.

And at our 20-week ultrasound for Astrid they couldn't get a couple of views of the heart. Everything looked good. Physicians weren't concerned. But what should have been a happy day, to know that we were having a successful pregnancy– because a pregnancy after a fetal diagnosis is a very stressful pregnancy– ended with me being in the car, my husband and I walking out of the appointment, and me being in the car sobbing hysterically, because they wouldn't see me again until I was 24 weeks along, and in Missouri– because they weren't worried, right? That was my next regularly scheduled appointment. And in Missouri, that would have been too late. And what I kept saying to Jake, to my husband, is, "What if they find something devastating now? I can't protect my daughter."

And I understand that Mrs. Stuckey and I don't agree on things, but I would like to ask you to remember that you are calling me and my husband murderers, and you believe in compassion and love, and I would ask for compassion and respect, ma'am, when you speak about these decisions, because Americans make these decisions that are difficult and personal, and we deserve to be treated with respect, whether or not you condone our choice. I don't need your approval, Mrs. Stuckey, but I would ask for your respect.

Mrs. LAWRENCE. I appreciate what you are saying. In the few minutes I have left I just want to bring another issue to the table. We, in this country, have the highest maternal mortality rate of any civilized country in the world, and for women to be dying to give birth in America is unacceptable. And with the same energy that we are making health decisions and decisions about our bodies, and we should, as women in America, have the same choices that men have, without the government telling them what to do.

I often use the comparison because now there is discussion about birth control. I would love to have a debate about Viagra and whether the government should regulate or restrict Viagra for me. That has never been on the table.

And so women, we are targeted, and for us to have the same passion of a discussion about saving women who want to have their babies, and this medical industry is failing us, we need to have the same passion.

I yield back my time.

Mr. CLAY. The gentlewoman's time has expired. I want to say to Ms. Box, we are sorry that you and your family had to experience what you did.

And now I recognize the gentleman, Mr. Grothman, for five minutes.

Mr. GROTHMAN. Correct. A couple of quick questions for Dr. McNicholas. If someone came to you who is eight months pregnant with a healthy baby girl and said they wanted to have an abortion because they didn't want another girl, would you perform that abortion?

Dr. MCNICHOLAS. So that sensationalized hypothetical isn't real and I have never had that happen before.

Mr. GROTHMAN. Well, you said you performed an abortion– you know, it is up to– I am just giving you an example. Well, let's say, okay, someone came in with an eight-month pregnancy and just wanted to have an abortion because they didn't feel they had time to care for a baby. Would you do the abortion then?

Dr. MCNICHOLAS. So I first want to reject the notion that people make decisions about continuing their pregnancy out of convenience. I have never, in 10 years of taking care of pregnant people, had somebody request an abortion because it just wasn't convenient.

Mr. GROTHMAN. Okay. Do you report– people presumably come to Planned Parenthood for contraceptive care as well. If a 14-year-old or 13-year-old came to you, would you give them the contraceptives?

Dr. MCNICHOLAS. So we talk to all of our patients about the availability of all of their contraceptive methods.

Mr. GROTHMAN. Right—

Dr. MCNICHOLAS. And particularly for young people we would have an in-depth discussion about—

Mr. GROTHMAN. Okay.

Dr. MCNICHOLAS [continuing]. healthy behaviors, prevention of sexually transmitted infection, the importance of making informed decisions.

Mr. GROTHMAN. What I will say is, if a 13-year-old is sexually active, by definition that is a serious sexual assault. Do you make any efforts to report the person who is engaging in illegal activity with the young lady?

Dr. MCNICHOLAS. So we at Planned Parenthood follow all the rules and laws, and so we would—if, by law, we were required to do it, we would do it.

Mr. GROTHMAN. Would make any efforts—

Dr. MCNICHOLAS. If we are required to do it—

Mr. GROTHMAN [continuing]. any efforts to—

Dr. MCNICHOLAS [continuing]. we would do it.

Mr. GROTHMAN. If you weren't required to do it, you wouldn't do it.

Dr. MCNICHOLAS. You know, talking to young people about their sexual health can be a—

Mr. GROTHMAN. I will ask you another question. If someone comes in, is a 13-year-old girl, and wants to have an abortion, would you– which means, inevitably, or almost certainly something illegal was done, a serious sexual assault—would you probe into that anymore, or would you just do the abortion and not worry?

Dr. MCNICHOLAS. So one of the most impactful times I have with patients is discussing particularly around issues of sexual assault. We provide our patients with the space to discuss what happened, if they want to discuss that, recognizing that it can be incredibly traumatic to discuss that experience in any single health situation. And so I would respect whatever is comfortable for her.

Mr. GROTHMAN. I will give you another question. If someone comes in and doesn't have the money for an abortion, says they are broke but "I want an abortion," maybe seven or eight weeks pregnant, do you perform the abortion, or do you say that "we don't do the abortion"?

Dr. MCNICHOLAS. We make every effort to take care of patients' every needs, regardless of their financial insecurities.

Mr. GROTHMAN. So as I understand it, talking to people in your industry, you will find a way to do an abortion, whether the government is paying for it or nobody is paying for it. Somehow you will find the money to do that abortion. Correct?

Dr. MCNICHOLAS. So to set the record straight, the government does not pay for abortions. People are navigating the complexity of paying for basic health care because the government has abdicated its responsibility to pay for that.

Mr. GROTHMAN. So you don't turn people down. That is what I want to know.

Dr. MCNICHOLAS. We do not turn people away.

Mr. GROTHMAN. Correct.

I have toured some abortion clinics, and one thing that struck me about the abortion clinics, at least– and this was like 20 years now since I toured them—is they never used the word "abortion" and they never used the word "fetus." They always used the words "procedure" and "tissue." Do you still follow that policy, in which we try to avoid using the words "fetus" and "abortion" and use the words "procedure" and "tissue"?

Dr. MCNICHOLAS. Twenty years is a long time. I invite you back to our clinic to see what happens there. And I absolutely use the words "fetus" and "abortion." And, actually, I take the direction from my patients, who absolutely understand the potential life that is in their uterus. Most patients who have abortions are parents. They are well– aware of the fact that what would happen if they didn't have an abortion is that they would have a baby.

Mr. GROTHMAN. We– I am running out of time here. We did pass a 24-hour waiting period bill in Wisconsin. Do you have a similar bill in Missouri?

Dr. MCNICHOLAS. We have one of the most restrictive waiting period bans in Missouri.

Mr. GROTHMAN. Okay.

Dr. MCNICHOLAS. It is 72 hours, and requires the same physician.

Mr. GROTHMAN. Okay. The question I have for you, it came out as part of a lawsuit, in Madison, Wisconsin. Because of the waiting period bill, about 10 percent of the women who came in the first time around, I believe, and gave an amount of money, did not come back the second time, which would indicate they were very much on the fence, and given some more time to think about it they decided not to have the abortion.

Percentage-wise, of all the women who come in to see you the first time, what percent don't come back the second time, in Missouri?

Dr. MCNICHOLAS. I think you made an assumption about what that 10 percent means. My informed assessment of that would be that those 10 percent of women really struggled to figure out a way to get back, because they didn't have the financial means, the secure transportation needs, the ability to navigate additional time off of work or find somebody to watch their children while they were trying to access that care.

Mr. GROTHMAN. So you are not going to answer my question.

Mr. CLAY. The gentleman's time has expired.

Mr. GROTHMAN. Thank you for being so—

Mr. CLAY. I recognize the gentleman from California, Mr. Khanna, for five minutes.

Mr. KHANNA. Thank you, Representative Clay. Thank you for your leadership in convening this hearing.

I would like to discuss state and Federal restrictions to abortion access and the disproportionate impact that they have on LGBTQ patients.

Dr. McNicholas, a few questions for you. First, could you briefly describe the need for abortion care among the LGBTQ+ community?

Dr. MCNICHOLAS. Absolutely. Thank you for your question. I think the first, most basic thing that most people forget is that your sexual orientation does not define who you are having sex with, and so people in all of those communities may experience pregnancy.

Similarly– and I have had the honor of taking care of many trans and non-binary folks in my career– so long as you have a uterus you have the capability of getting pregnant, and if you think that accessing abortion care is stigmatizing when you present as a woman, imagine what it is when you are presenting as your authentic male self.

Mr. KHANNA. I appreciate you mentioning that there are transgender men and non-binary individuals who rely on reproductive health services and abortion services.

In 2015, when the National Center for Trans Equality surveyed transgender Americans, 23 percent of respondents did not see a doctor when they needed to because of, quote, "fear of being mistreated as a transgender person."

As a doctor, can you describe some of the challenges gender-diverse patients face in accessing health care, and abortion care, specifically?

Dr. MCNICHOLAS. So in my practice I have, again, had the great honor of taking care of many specifically trans men seeking hysterectomies in their transformation process, and one of the things I hear from them, unequivocally, each one of them, is that there have been tremendous delays in accessing very basic care, one, because they are afraid that they won't be treated with dignity and respect, and the second is because that is their lived experience. They have been turned down by many patients– excuse me, physicians– and have been intentionally degraded with, for example, use of intentional misgendering of the patient in front of them.

Mr. KHANNA. And can you also describe some of the specific challenges that gay, lesbian, and bisexual patients may face in abortion care, specifically?

Dr. MCNICHOLAS. Sure. So I think it is important to remember that gay and lesbian folks also want to build families. They are parents. I, myself, have a wife and a child, so I fit into that group as well. It is important that they are able to access that care in a place where they feel respected and dignified, and Planned Parenthood is happy to be one of those places.

Mr. KHANNA. Thank you so much for speaking to those issues. Turning to you, Ms. Howell, transgender people are four times more likely than the general population to live below the poverty line, and close to one in four lesbian bisexual women in the United States live in poverty. Yet current laws prevent Federal Medicaid dollars from being used to cover abortion services.

How do these funding restrictions overlap with identity to make abortion even less accessible for the LGBTQ communities?

Ms. HOWELL. The discrimination that people go toward, because they are either trans or gender nonbinary or LGBTQ, it really does hit them harder because, as was already mentioned, they are afraid to go and get services, and when they go to get services they find that some of the current regulations allow people to discriminate against them, and that they then find that they don't have any access to getting good reproductive health services, much less regular health care services.

Our organization does believe that all people have the right to get reproductive health services, regardless of whether they identify as LGBTQ, whether they are trans, whether they are low income. All of these factors should be taken into account to allow them to get the kind of services that they deserve. And so laws or regulations that allow—that have been done by this government that allow other people to discriminate against them puts them at higher risk, and those are the kind of laws and regulations that we fight against.

Mr. KHANNA. Well, thank you, Ms. Howell. Thank you, Dr. McNicholas, for your advocacy for some of the most vulnerable populations, and I believe we need to really consider their access to health care as we craft these laws.

I yield back my time.

Chairwoman MALONEY.[Presiding.] Thank you. Representative Cloud.

Mr. CLOUD. Thank you all for being here. I appreciate you all coming to take part in a discussion that is, no doubt, very emotionally charged with very deeply held beliefs of conscious on both sides of the issue.

For me, the most difficult decisions we have to make as law-makers are those in which individual rights are in conflict with each other. And so for me, on this issue, where I come down, is to the whole life living in pursuit of happiness, where which rights supersede. And I do believe that while having compassion for anyone who has to go through a difficult situation that the right to life is more– supersedes the right to liberty and the pursuit of happiness.

So in that context I approach this conversation.

Dr. McNicholas, could you describe what happens in the process of an abortion, to the baby?

Dr. MCNICHOLAS. So I appreciate your question and I want to first note that abortion was around before there was any concept of life, liberty—

Mr. CLOUD. Answer the question.

Dr. MCNICHOLAS [continuing]. and the pursuit of happiness.

Mr. CLOUD. I have only five minutes.

Dr. MCNICHOLAS. The abortion procedure really depends on the clinical situation. When I speak to patients about their options for terminating a pregnancy I start with where are we in pregnancy.

Mr. CLOUD. I only have five minutes. Could you speak to the process please?

Dr. MCNICHOLAS. So I realize it is difficult, but in medicine things aren't short. There are 100 shades of gray. So it is impossible for me to take what is often a 50-minute conversation with a patient and answer it in 30 seconds for you.

As I approach patients, I talk to them about what their options are for pregnancy termination, and that really depends on a variety of things, including what stage of pregnancy they are in, what are their other medical comorbidities or health problems that they have, whether any particular instances in previous pregnancies, for example—

Mr. CLOUD. Okay. I am going to have to—

Ms. Stuckey, could you describe what happens in the process of an abortion?

Ms. STUCKEY. Well, apparently I am the only one willing to talk about specifics, and this is free online. Anyone can go look. Even Planned Parenthood's website describes pretty clearly what, for example, a D&C abortion is, which is taking out of the amniotic fluid, drying that up from the uterus, which is what, of course, the fetus, the baby, needs to survive, and then dismembering the baby, limb by limb, with forceps. And Ms. Lawrence spoke to that being deceitful or hyperbolic. It is not at all. Please, go look online and you can see what an abortion actually is.

But again we see that it is not me that is speaking in generalities. It is the pro-abortion side that is speaking in generalities, because they know the grotesque nature of what an abortion procedure is. You don't have to be an abortion provider to know what an abortion is. That is exactly why I am here, to talk about the absolute brutality of the killing of life inside the womb.

And I also want to address Ms. Box, who I have the utmost compassion for. One, I actually did not say the term "murderers," to my recollection, and I don't think me being passionate about this subject we do disagree on means that I disrespect you. I think that we can agree, or disagree, even passionately, without taking that as a personal slight, and I certainly didn't mean it that way. I just care about life inside the womb and protecting babies unborn.

Mr. CLOUD. Okay. I have very little time left now, but, Ms. Graves, you mentioned that nothing has changed since Roe v. Wade except for the makeup of the Supreme Court. The reality is—

Ms. GOSS GRAVES. I actually said– I just want to correct you, because I was talking about the whole women's health decision, which was three years ago—

Mr. CLOUD. Okay.

Ms. GOSS GRAVES.—and the case that is going to be before the court this term, the June Medical Services—

Mr. CLOUD. But a lot has changed. We– science has developed a whole lot. Back in the 1970's, it was rare for an ultrasound– for a woman to have an ultrasound. Isn't that correct? Now we know a whole lot. We know that a baby can be viable at 20 weeks. We know that a baby feels pain.

I ask unanimous consent to submit this peer-reviewed scientific article on fetal pain that a baby feels during abortion.

There is a lot that has happened since this is– and certainly I think the scientific advances merit us relooking at this.

Ms. GOSS GRAVES. The Supreme Court did, three years ago, in the Whole Women's Health decision, it considered—

Mr. CLOUD. Dr. McNicholas, you mentioned a number of health inspections at your abortion clinic when you just took over. Were you aware of the history of health violations at your clinic before you took over?

Dr. MCNICHOLAS. So our clinic has been subject to repeated inspections every year, which we have passed, with a single inspection every single year, up until this year when clearly it became–it was no longer about ensuring the safety of patients and it became about a quest to end abortion access.

Mr. CLOUD. Okay. Well, I ask unanimous consent to submit to the record. This is only seven states, the violations at abortion clinics from a—

Chairwoman MALONEY. No objection. We accept this entry. Thank you.

Chairwoman MALONEY. And your time has expired.

Mr. CLOUD. Unfortunately, my time is up.

Chairwoman MALONEY. Okay. I now recognize Congresswoman Pressley, for her questioning. She has been a tireless advocate for these issues on this committee, so thank you for your leadership.

Ms. PRESSLEY. Thank you, Acting Chair Maloney, for holding the line on this full committee hearing since the transition of Chairman Cummings. Thank you, Ms. Box, for modeling that which he spoke of often, which is turning your pain into purpose. We thank all of you for being here.

Elijah Cummings often reminded us that we are to be in efficient and effective pursuit of the truth, and so we are still trying to arrive at that, it seems, today.

This conversation cannot be more timely, as we bear witness to and experience this Administration's calculated and systemic attacks on our constitutional rights and freedoms. The right to determine our own economic future and the audacity to determine our own fate, and the freedom to determine when, if at all, to have a child.

Even in states like the Commonwealth of Massachusetts, which I represent, individuals, particularly low-income and young people, LGBTQ and black and brown folks, continue to face barriers in accessing comprehensive reproductive health care. And let me be clear, health care is abortion care.

But in these times, we have seen many states emboldened by this Administration pass additional restrictions that further hinder individuals' access to abortion, endangering lives and criminalizing individuals for decisions that should be kept between themselves and their doctor.

It is important to discuss these draconian state restrictions, but as chair of the Abortion Rights and Access Task Force of this firstever pro-choice majority in this history of Congress, I would be remiss if I didn't also shed light on the impact that Federal coverage bans are posing on our most vulnerable communities.

Current law restricts Medicaid funds from covering abortion care for women in communities across the United States. To be clear, the Hyde Amendment functioned as the original abortion ban for low-income individuals.

According to the Guttmacher Institute, restrictions on Medicaid coverage for abortion services force one in four low-income women to carry unwanted pregnancies to term.

Ms. Goss Graves, how do coverage bans like the Hyde Amendment force low-income individuals further into poverty?

Ms. GOSS GRAVES. So just at, for some women, is the hardest time in their life, you know, around being pregnant, they are now in a situation where they, because they are on Medicaid or because they are on a Federal health plan or other Federal restrictions, they no longer have, or are in a situation where their health care can be covered by insurance, like the rest of their health care. So all of a sudden you are having to scrap together money, on top of a range of other barriers. Those barriers may look like having to travel long distances. Those barriers may look like having to pay for child care because of multi-day waiting periods. So it is not only the restrictions on coverage. You also have these other costs.

And for the right to abortion, which has been legal for 50 years almost, and reaffirmed again and again and again by the Supreme Court, most recently just three years ago, that right is not just for those who are affluent. That right is not just for those who happen to live in a state where the state is trying to make up for the very serious gaps in Federal coverage. That right is a fundamental right. It is a right that is tied to your ability to have dignity in this country, it is a right that is tied to your ability to have freedom in this country, and it is fundamental to your economic security.

Ms. PRESSLEY. Thank you. I would be remiss if I did not acknowledge, sitting next to me, a champion in the efforts for decades now to repeal Hyde. I want to acknowledge my other sisters in service from our Pro-Choice Caucus were waived on today, Representatives Chu and Schakowsky, respectfully. Thank you for being here.

Each year, 700 women in the U.S. are likely to die during childbirth. These numbers are even worse for black and Native American women. Ms. Howell, could you speak to your report recently issued connecting the impacts of abortion bans on the maternal health crisis?

And I would be remiss– I just wanted to acknowledge, since there was this conversation about compassion for the innocence– earlier today I rolled out the People's Justice Guarantee, which calls for the abolishing of the death penalty, and, in fact, 1 in 25 are wrongfully convicted and innocent. So I look forward to my colleagues on the other side of the aisle signing on to my legislation.

Ms. Howell?

Ms. HOWELL. The report that you refer to looks at the correlation between maternal mortality and states that have placed these bans against abortion. And what we know is that trying to– if you decide that you need to terminate a pregnancy and you are denied that care, it puts additional stress on you.

We also know that women who are denied abortion care tend to delay prenatal care. So, again, there is an additional stress as well.

And I might add, I want to give you some of the states that have some of the worst abortion bans and also some of the worst maternal mortality outcomes.

Alabama, Georgia, Ohio, Missouri, unfortunately, and a lot of the Southern states– South Carolina, Texas. Those are the states that primarily have these outrageous abortion bans that prevent people from actually accessing abortion care, but they also have—

Chairwoman MALONEY. The gentlelady's time has expired.

Ms. HOWELL [continuing]. the highest mortality—

Chairwoman MALONEY. Could you please wind down?

Ms. HOWELL. They also have some of the highest mortality rates for maternal mortality. So we have to look at both of those things together in terms of what it means to access good reproductive healthcare for people.

Ms. PRESSLEY. Thank you, Ms. Howell.

Ms. HOWELL. Thank you.

Ms. PRESSLEY. Thank you, Madam Chair.

Chairwoman MALONEY. Thank you. The chair recognizes Representative Miller.

Mrs. MILLER. Thank you, Madam Chairman and Ranking Member Green, and thank you all for being here today.

As a mother, I have had the privilege to feel life quicken in my womb. As a grandmother, I know the joy of grandchildren. I have gotten to experience endless joy having grandchildren because it is just unconditional love.

I have had family members and friends who have yearned to be parents but were unable to have children of their own. I have had friends and family who have been adopted, and they are very grateful. I have friends and family who have adopted children, and they are very grateful. They have brought such blessings to their family.

However, I have become increasingly concerned as of late about the actions taken by my colleagues across the aisle. Washington Democrats refuse to protect babies even after they are born alive after an abortion attempt, and it is so heartbreaking. Our most vulnerable and youngest citizens deserve our utmost protection.

Ms. Stuckey, speaking of medical innovation, I think we can all agree that women having access to all healthcare is important. That being said, not every Planned Parenthood provides comprehensive women's healthcare. Can you elaborate on the positive steps that the Trump administration has done to not only protect life, but to ensure that women have better access to healthcare through federally Qualified Health Centers?

Ms. STUCKEY. Yes, thank you for that question.

First, I do want to address an issue that I think that we can all say– all agree on, that the maternal mortality rate in this country, in a developed country, is way too high. And it is, I think the number is 3.3 times higher for African-American women than it is for white women, and I fully believe that we need to address that. And I would encourage the Trump administration to address that.

I don't understand why the exclusive solution that we discuss when we talk about the maternal mortality rate is abortion. Why is that the only solution that we discuss? Can we not come together and talk about how can we best care for a woman and her child? Why do we have to sacrifice the child for the health of the mother when it is not medically necessary?

President Trump has been the most pro-life, most– if you want to call it anti-abortion, I am fine with that, too– anti-abortion administration since Ronald Reagan, maybe even more so than Ronald Reagan, with the Mexico City policy. And of course, we know enacting the final rule for Title X that says you have to physically and finally separate your abortion services from the rest of your contraceptive care in order to receive Title X funding.

I heard earlier a comment about this gag rule. Well, it is actually not a gag rule that the Trump administration enacted. It is you cannot encourage someone to get an abortion, but you can counsel them neutrally. So that is not actually a gag rule. It is not a limit on free speech.

President Trump has ensured that these policies can go forth and, of course, given states the freedom to protect life inside the womb. And for that, I am very thankful.

Mrs. MILLER. You might be familiar with efforts by House Republicans to protect babies who are born alive after an abortion attempt. Many argue that the Born Alive Act is unnecessary because doing so violates existing criminal law.

Do you believe Federal law should be clarified to ensure babies born alive after a failed abortion should receive critical medical care?

Ms. STUCKEY. Yes. It needs to be clarified. So this new law the Democrats have tried so hard to blockade simply criminalizes the neglect of an abortion provider to attend to the medical needs of a child who survives an abortion, further recognizes this child's personhood, and says this is the medical treatment that is required for a child outside the womb. We are not even talking inside the womb anymore.

And unfortunately, Democrats cannot even get onboard with that. There are not any undue burdens, undue regulations. This is not preventing abortion providers from even giving abortions. It is simply saying if a child survives an abortion, attend to that child.

It should be really simple. If you really are pro-choice and you are really not pro-abortion, as I have heard many times during this hearing, that should be a no-brainer.

Mrs. MILLER. I understand a baby can survive as early as 23 weeks old. Can you elaborate on how age of viability has changed in the recent years, and what has made that possible?

Ms. STUCKEY. Well, as technology and medicine advances, thankfully, hospitals are able to give incredible perinatal care, so that a child as young as 21 weeks actually has been known to survive outside of the womb. I mean, that is pretty early in the second trimester. That is only halfway through the pregnancy.

At 24 weeks, that is generally accepted as the age of viability. What that means is that that child has a really good chance, if she were to be born prematurely, to live outside the womb, to grow. She would spend some time in NICU, but she would grow up, you know, if everything went well and she was healthy, into a normal functioning child. You wouldn't even be able to look back and tell that the child was premature.

So when we are talking about these children as if they are not children, as if they are not babies, we are talking about mere location. I mean, on the one hand, we talk about them as if they are just these parasites to be discarded as these remains of pregnancy, I think is what I heard the doctor say earlier.

And then a second later, when they are outside of the womb, they are all of a sudden babies. Although, unfortunately, as you pointed out and other congresspeople have pointed out, even then, even then they don't seem to be respected by the pro-abortion side.

Mrs. MILLER. Thank you. I yield back.

Chairwoman MALONEY. Thank you.

I understand that the witness, Ms. Stuckey, has a flight she has to catch. So I will dismiss her, noting that there may be other additional questions that I request that she answer them in writing.

And thank you for your testimony, and I hope you don't miss your flight.

Ms. STUCKEY. Thank you.

Chairwoman MALONEY. So the next speaker will be Debbie Wasserman Schultz from Florida. Congresswoman Schultz?

Ms. WASSERMAN SCHULTZ. Thank you, Madam Chair.

Madam Chair, I have a question of you, and in fairness, I would like Ms. Stuckey to hear my question because I wouldn't want there to be any assumption that I was saying it as she was no longer in the room.

I just want to clarify that Ms. Stuckey is here expressing her own opinion exclusively and has no scientific or particular expertise in this subject matter whatsoever. Is that accurate?

No, I want to ask you, from what your knowledge of her experience is in the description of the witness's experience.

Chairwoman MALONEY. That is my understanding.

Ms. WASSERMAN SCHULTZ. Thank you. I just wanted to clarify that particular fact.

Chairwoman MALONEY. But I think the witness should answer, in all fairness, as she is here.

Ms. STUCKEY. I think it says something that when I, the one without the scientific or medical background, am the only one to give you specifics on what is—

Ms. WASSERMAN SCHULTZ. Reclaiming my– reclaiming my time.

My question—

Ms. STUCKEY [continuing]. what an abortion procedure actually is. Ask the doctor for yourself.

Ms. WASSERMAN SCHULTZ. Reclaiming my time, Ms. Stuckey, my question was not of you, and you have essentially acknowledged that you are here expressing your own opinion, which we appreciate.

So the other thing I wanted to point out was that no one here today has said that abortion is the only solution to address the maternal mortality rate. How about access to– better access to prenatal care? How about the passage of the Affordable Care Act and making sure that it remains the law of the land so that women are no longer considered preexisting conditions just because of our existence as women and the potential for us to be dropped or denied coverage because of our propensity to get pregnant and have babies, which happened all the time before the Affordable Care Act was the law of the land.

I could go on with many other provisions that we advocate to make sure that we can reduce the maternal mortality rate. Certainly, abortion is not the only thing we suggest and, in fact, is not a solution that we ever suggest to reduce the maternal mortality rate. It is a ridiculous suggestion.

What isn't a ridiculous suggestion is that the decision to become a parent is one of the most important and most personal life decisions that we make. Watching the rapid expansion of state laws that limit a woman's autonomy to make this personal choice for herself is deeply troubling.

This fight for reproductive freedom is one that we are all too familiar with in Florida. I have seen Republicans in my home state in the legislature introduce bills that ban abortion after six weeks, ban abortions that are based on certain medical diagnoses, and right now are fast-tracking a proposed Draconian parental consent law.

We need to be unequivocal about calling these laws out for what they are, sinister attempts to interfere with a woman's right to make her own personal health choices and decisions and obvious steps in a larger political plan to ban all abortions. As we have heard, Missouri has enacted so many restrictions on providing abortion care that only one clinic is left standing.

Because my time is limited, I want to ask Dr. McNicholas, the excuse that a patient can just drive to another state to receive medical care, is that an acceptable rationale for any other type of medical service? And is it accurate to say that requiring medically unnecessary patient delays, whether that is to gather travel funds or make lodging and caregiving arrangements, would lead to women having later abortions, which were more expensive and can pose a higher health risk?

Dr. MCNICHOLAS. Thank you for the question and acknowledging the sort of many intersecting realities that people are navigating when they are trying to access basic care. And in Missouri, for many of them, that means driving hundreds of miles multiple times.

I am reminded, actually, of a patient I took care of recently in the second trimester, who actually was able to get to the clinic the first time very early at six weeks of pregnancy. She went home and scheduled her clinic procedural date for about a week and a half later but, unfortunately, was in a car accident on the way to that appointment.

Because Missouri's law not only requires a waiting period, but requires it to be with the same physician who will ultimately perform your procedure, she was then– her two-visit abortion became a four-visit appointment visit, and she was pushed from seven weeks to 15 weeks. This is exactly what happens when there is no context and no medical or scientific grounding in abortion restrictions. Patients are pushed to later and later in pregnancy, which is quite ironic for a cohort of folks who want to limit abortion later in pregnancy.

Ms. WASSERMAN SCHULTZ. Thank you.

Ms. Box, I want to end with you, and I am so sorry for your loss. But I know you are overjoyed in your daughter that you brought with you.

You received test results that revealed your daughter Libby had a chromosomal anomaly when you were around 13 weeks pregnant. But if H.B. 126, the Missouri law that would ban abortion after about eight weeks, had been the law in the state of Missouri at that time, would you have considered leaving the state to have an abortion? How difficult would have it have been for you and your family if you had needed to travel out of state to obtain your abortion care?

Ms. BOX. So the answer is, yes, I would have looked at how I could have protected my daughter, regardless of what regulations the state tried to interfere with. The truth is, even though abortion, the ban had not come into effect yet, the eight-week ban, we did look at leaving Missouri and going to Representative Kelly's state of Illinois because the restrictions there are fewer. There is an opportunity for—

Chairwoman MALONEY. The gentlewoman's time has expired. If you could please wrap up real quick?

Ms. BOX. Yes. So, yes, we would have done whatever we could to protect our daughter, regardless of governmental intrusion.

Ms. WASSERMAN SCHULTZ. Thank you for sharing your personal story, and I yield back the balance of my time.

Chairwoman MALONEY. I now recognize Representative Green.

Mr. GREEN. Thank you, Madam Chairwoman.

My first question is for Dr. McNicholas. Am I pronouncing that correctly? Yes. If the DNA from a fetus and a mother were found at, say, a crime scene, say it is two blood samples. We take fetal blood. We take mother's blood. We put them at the crime scene. The investigators know nothing. They find two samples. Would the investigators see these as two separate people?

Dr. MCNICHOLAS. I have no idea.

Mr. GREEN. Of course, they would. The answer is yes. You know, as a physician, it is two different DNAs, and they would see two DNAs, and so they would say it is two people.

My next question, question for you as well. Recently, in California, a mother was charged for killing her unborn baby by excessive methamphetamine usage. If the mother had just gotten an abortion and killed the baby that way, she wouldn't have been charged. Do you see the hypocrisy in this?

Dr. MCNICHOLAS. I think it is tragic that we are criminalizing people who need basic healthcare and treatment for their drug addiction problem. That is what I think is a problem in this country.

Mr. GREEN. Absolutely. Someone who uses methamphetamine should get help. There is no doubt about it. And she was charged with a crime for the death that she caused of her baby with methamphetamine use. The child was stillborn.

I just– I find that hypocritical that if she had just gone a week prior to Planned Parenthood and gotten an abortion, she wouldn't be charged.

You know, I am going to transition a little bit here. I want people to make their own choices. I am for freedom. But when one person's freedom impinges on the freedom of another, and for example, if someone in this room yelled "fire," that would be against the law because, potentially, a stampede could occur, and people would be hurt.

Abortion is a decision where one person makes it, and it leads to the death of another person. So that is something to take into consideration.

My next question I was going to actually ask of Ms. Stuckey, but she is gone. I will just read the question and let the audience and others consider it.

A few years ago, a freezer unit protecting previously fertilized human eggs, meaning a sperm and ovum where they had combined to form a fertilized egg, was broken. And thousands of these fertilized eggs were lost. I just want to ask people in the room whether or not they would agree with the headline in the newspaper the following day that said it was a human tragedy that these lives were lost. Just consider that.

My next question again is back to you, Dr. McNicholas. In regards to ABO and Rh incompatibility, why do I, as an ER physician, have to treat the mothers with RhoGAM to prevent her antibodies from attacking the blood supply of the baby?

Dr. MCNICHOLAS. Oh, so two minutes for this?

Mr. GREEN. No, you got 30 seconds.

Dr. MCNICHOLAS. Oh.

Mr. GREEN. Or I can do it because I do it all– I treat these patients all the time. Go ahead.

Dr. MCNICHOLAS. Sure. So in the instance in which the fetus has a different type than mom, there are occasions where mom can create her own defense mechanism to that situation, which would in a subsequent pregnancy attack a subsequent pregnancy and have some serious conditions for the fetus.

Mr. GREEN. That was pretty good, and I mean, you did it in about 30 seconds. But she is absolutely correct. Basically, the mother's immune system sees that second child as foreign and attacks it because it has got a different blood type than the mother.

Let us see, I also want to share a few quick observations, in the little bit of time that I have left, as an ER physician. I know that there are a lot of statements about the safety of abortion. I just want to tell you that I have treated many, many patients in the emergency department where the abortion hasn't gone as intended, where products of conception, the medical term– or baby parts– are left inside the mother, and sepsis results.

Those patients come to us, and we take care of them in the emergency department. We save their life from that infection.

I also want to say that I have taken care of many, over the years as an emergency medicine physician, patients who have come in bleeding from an abortion. And the unfortunate thing is that the obstetrician who has to take care of that patient didn't do the abortion. So he doesn't know the patient's history, and they are rushing them into surgery to stop the bleeding and save the patient's life. That does happen.

And it happens more frequently than many people would want you to know, but it is a reality. And I just want to say that is why I support abortion providers having credentials at a hospital where they can treat the complications of the surgical procedure of an abortion that they– that results when they do that.

Chairwoman MALONEY. The gentleman's time has expired.

Mr. GREEN. Oh, am I out? Okay, thank you, Madam Chairwoman. Thank you.

Chairwoman MALONEY. Thank you. I would now like to recognize Congressman Raskin.

Mr. RASKIN. Madam Chair, thank you. And thank you for calling this important hearing.

Big Brother seems to have come to Missouri, the Leviathan state has arrived in Missouri, and all of our colleagues who like to strike a libertarian note when it comes to people possessing AR– 15s and military-style assault weapons, the kinds that are wreaking havoc across the land, suddenly become the champions of Leviathan, Big Brother, Gilead, and the all-powerful state. Politicians making healthcare choices for our people.

Ms. Goss Graves, let me start with you. You are the president of the National Women's Law Center. Presumably, you know something about the history of sterilization in our country, where certainly tens of thousands of women at least were sterilized. If Government has the power to prevent a woman from having an abortion against her will, won't Government also have the power to sterilize women against their will, which was so much a part of our history?

Ms. GOSS GRAVES. You know, I think it is important to put the right to abortion, which is so core and fundamental, in the context of a range of rights. The right to abortion is in the context of the right to make reproductive healthcare decisions broadly, including contraception, including around sterilization and not having forced sterilization. But it is also among the set of rights around the right to be intimate, the right to marry.

All of those things follow a long line of decisions that emanate from the Fourteenth Amendment's guarantee around liberty and around your ability to sort of live with dignity.

Mr. RASKIN. Thank you.

Dr. McNicholas, officials in Missouri, including Dr. Randall Williams, the Director of the Department of Health and Senior Services, and Governor Parsons, have asserted that the restrictions adopted in Missouri are necessary for the health and safety of people seeking abortions. In your opinion, is the requirement that a physician have admitting privileges at a local hospital necessary for the health or safety of a woman seeking an abortion?

Dr. MCNICHOLAS. So the short answer is no, and the longer answer is it is not my opinion. It is what science and fact and ACOG and the most recent publication out of the National Academies of Science has told us.

Mr. RASKIN. Well, what about this 72-hour waiting period between a woman seeking an abortion and being able to get one? And then also I understand they adopted a provision for two pelvic exams during that time. Is that necessary for the health and safety of women in Missouri?

Dr. MCNICHOLAS. None of those are required to maintain health and safety.

Mr. RASKIN. But how do you know that?

Dr. MCNICHOLAS. Science. There is plenty of published literature supported by the American College of OB/GYN, again supported by the National Academies publication that has demonstration that not only are they not medically relevant or necessary, but they actually cause harm.

Mr. RASKIN. Well, what about from the standpoint of the patient? Ms. Box, let me come to you. Did you feel that any of the procedural hurdles and hoops that were set up in Missouri and you were forced to jump through were necessary for your health and safety?

Ms. BOX. No. I found them insulting. They presumed that my husband and I didn't have the ability to make a decision for ourselves. The waiting period that Dr. McNicholas was talking about and the mandatory same physician rule meant that my abortion, which happened at around 15 weeks, had I not been able to do the available date that the physician had, I actually would have been outside of when is the legal timeframe in Missouri.

And I was well short of it. I would have had to reconsent, been given another booklet of medically inaccurate information, which my husband and I refer to as the "book of shame," and that– all of that presumes that– and I think what I find most insulting as a patient is that I didn't have the ability to think for myself, that I needed my state government to put that time in for me.

Mr. RASKIN. I thank you for that really important insight. You talk about this "book of shame." I think you started your testimony by saying that one quarter of American women will have an abortion over the course of their lifetime, most of them also mothers, as you are. You have how many kids? Two kids?

Ms. BOX. I have three living children.

Mr. RASKIN. You have three living children. Okay. Well, they want to throw the "book of shame" at tens of millions of American women. How does that feel to you as a citizen in Missouri? That you get hit by the "book of shame"?

Ms. BOX. I mean, it is devastating. I mean, in our particular case, we were in the middle of a very grief-stricken process, and we were in a crisis. And to have confusing and misleading information when you are trying to make a medical decision is horrifying that we would ever allow patients to get mischaracterization and misinformation and hope they can make the best decision for themselves.

Mr. RASKIN. Okay. And finally, I wanted to ask this question while all the witnesses were there. I was thinking we could make history by getting the pro-choice witnesses and the anti-choice witnesses to agree on a pro-life program, which is a universal criminal and mental background check on all gun purchases.

At least for the witnesses who are still here, would you reach across the aisle to the pro-life witnesses to say you would stand for that?

[Response.]

Chairwoman MALONEY. The gentleman's time has expired.

Mr. RASKIN. I would let the record reflect I think they all nodded their heads, Madam Chair.

Chairwoman MALONEY. Congressman Connolly?

Mr. CONNOLLY. Thank you, Madam Chairman. And thank you for holding this hearing.

And thank you, Mr. Clay, for being our inspiration in highlighting what is happening in your state.

I think we need to be honest here. Everything designed to make your very difficult decision, personal decision—not a state decision, Ms. Box—was designed to take away your choice. What Mr. Green described was insidious logic. Because there might have been complications from some abortions, all abortions should be eliminated.

Even though the overwhelming majority of legal abortions, because of Roe v. Wade, they are done under medically supervised conditions and are safe and allow women and families to have choices. The changes in Title X are designed, again, to take away or limit choices. The attack on Planned Parenthood insidious, designed to take away choices and being willing to deny women healthcare as the price you have to pay for their ideological stance.

And Ms. Stuckey's misguided moral absolutism for all the rest of us. And of course, the sacrifice of science, as you point out, Dr. McNicholas, that has to be in there, too, because science is an inconvenient source of information and truth, again denied you and your family, Ms. Box, at a critical moment in the decision you had to make. Go ahead.

I thought you wanted to comment.

All right. Dr. McNicholas, how many women patients does Planned Parenthood see every year?

Dr. MCNICHOLAS. The Planned Parenthood of the St. Louis region, so—

Mr. CONNOLLY. No, no. Nationwide?

Dr. MCNICHOLAS. Oh, I don't know.

Mr. CONNOLLY. All right. St. Louis?

Dr. MCNICHOLAS. Our Missouri– our Missouri affiliates see more than about 50,000 women a year.

Mr. CONNOLLY. How many?

Dr. MCNICHOLAS. Fifty thousand.

Mr. CONNOLLY. Would you guess that is a lot more than Dr. Green sees in a year?

Dr. MCNICHOLAS. It is. And I would actually like to highlight, to Dr. Green's point about safety, that I have yet to see an oral surgeon be brought in front of Congress to talk about the risks of wisdom teeth, but having an abortion is safer than having your wisdom teeth removed.

So I think mischaracterizing abortion as anything other than safe is inappropriate. It is healthcare. So, yes, unfortunate outcomes will happen for some people, but by and large, it is safer than colonoscopy, wisdom teeth, and I will also mention it is far safer than carrying a pregnancy to term.

Mr. CONNOLLY. And it is safe because Roe v. Wade made one law for the whole United States, including Missouri. Is that correct?

Dr. MCNICHOLAS. We have lots of examples internationally to show that legalization of abortion is one of the most important public health and lifesaving interventions for women.

Mr. CONNOLLY. And would it be fair to say that absent Roe v. Wade, it is not that abortion will disappear, it is that people will be forced once again to go into the shadows to secure those services, to make those decisions, or go to states that do protect it legally? Is that a fair statement?

Dr. MCNICHOLAS. So as I mentioned before, abortion was around before the Constitution, and it will not go anywhere if we remove those barriers.

Mr. CONNOLLY. So our choices make it safe. Hopefully, it is rare because contraception is available. Family planning is available, but it has to be an option. As Ms. Box's personal experience tells us, it is a health decision, a hard one, a heartbreaking one for many people.

But to deny them access to it because you have decided on the morality of it or you have made up science to justify your own personal belief is to impose your will on the majority of Americans, including women who are affected by this choice.

Title X, Dr. McNicholas, Planned Parenthood decided to pull out of Title X, even though it does not provide funding for abortions. Is that correct?

Dr. MCNICHOLAS. That is correct.

Mr. CONNOLLY. Why did Planned Parenthood decide to leave Title X?

Dr. MCNICHOLAS. I think, as was previously mentioned by Ms. Goss Graves, there is a really fundamental issue for Planned Parenthood, which is that the new rule would force us to lie to patients and intentionally exclude information that could be important and lifesaving for them.

Mr. CONNOLLY. And real quickly, because Title X provides other healthcare for women, they are now going to be denied that coverage because of Planned Parenthood's being forced out of the program. Is that correct?

Dr. MCNICHOLAS. We are going to try our very best to meet all of the needs of our patients, including those who were previously receiving Title X, but I think the point is well taken that with reduction of Planned Parenthood seeing Title X patients, there will be a tremendous gap in services for patients, particularly who are low-income or people of color.

Mr. CONNOLLY. My time has expired, but I thank you all for being here and for the courage of sharing, especially you, Ms. Box.

Chairwoman MALONEY. I would now like to recognize Congresswoman Tlaib.

Ms. TLAIB. Sorry. I didn't know I was next.

Thank you so much. It really is incredibly important that you all are here to talk about this particular issue. Especially as a woman serving in the U.S. Congress, I just want to personally thank you for defending my right to choose.

One of the things I want to discuss is the impact of politically motivated restrictions of abortion that we have been talking about, access to maternal health. But even more, even around infant mortality.

When I served six years in the Michigan state legislature, I was always taken aback by so much time and effort and debate and conversation around the right to choose versus infant mortality, you know, maternal health. All of those things that I think are interconnected with some of the, you know, reasoning behind folks that want to support life, right?

And there is an issue that is particularly concerning to me is that parts of my home district have among the highest maternal mortality rates in the country. In 2014, a woman giving birth in Detroit was three times more likely to die in childbirth than the rest of the country. Infant mortality in Detroit is double the national rate in the country, and it just goes on and on.

Dr. McNicholas, you know, Missouri was one of the highest rates—has the highest rates of maternal mortality in the country, and that continues to rise, especially among women of color. In fact, black women in Missouri are three times more likely to die from pregnancy complications than other women. Is that correct?

Dr. MCNICHOLAS. That is correct.

Ms. TLAIB. Which state official again is responsible for addressing maternal mortality in Missouri?

Dr. MCNICHOLAS. That would be the Director of our Department of Public Health, Dr. Randall Williams.

Ms. TLAIB. So Dr. Williams is, in fact, the same official that has spent state dollars on enforcing unnecessary pelvic exams on women and tracking their menstrual cycles of Planned Parenthood patients. Correct?

Dr. MCNICHOLAS. Yes.

Ms. TLAIB. How do you think that he should be spending time? I mean, what do you think he should be doing right now? And again, around the same ideals, right, that they are supporting this, they won't support the women that are having children.

Dr. MCNICHOLAS. Yes, you raise a great point. Under Dr. Williams, Missouri went from 42nd in the country to 44th in the country in maternal mortality. And while he is spending his time visiting– his time and resources on visiting Planned Parenthood multiple times, he could be focusing on things like addressing maternal mortality, addressing the systemic and institutional racism that is engrained in that rate of three times higher for black women.

He could be working on improving access, particularly for our rural women. You know, Missouri is one of the states who, because we haven't expanded Medicaid—hey, that is another thing he could do– we have rural hospitals closing at alarming rates. So if you want to continue your pregnancy, your chance of having a healthy pregnancy is sabotaged by the fact that there is no hospital that you can go to to get care during that pregnancy.

There are a number of things that he could be doing to address maternal mortality.

Ms. TLAIB. I know, and the hypocrisy is so unjust and absurd. Ms. Howell, your organization did a phenomenal study, finding that black women face greater barriers to access to reproductive healthcare, including abortion care. What are some of the factors that you think account for the discrepancy in health outcomes?

Ms. HOWELL. Some of the factors are that black women disproportionately get their health insurance from Medicaid, which already then bans their access to abortion care and to get coverage. So what happens is that when they find they are pregnant and they decide they want to terminate a pregnancy, they have to go through a number of steps. They have got to figure out how to afford it, how they can take off work, how they can get childcare, how far they have to travel.

One of the things that we did is we asked black women in a poll what are all the factors you take into account when you are deciding whether or not to have a child? And it wasn't just about having money. It was also about having a neighborhood where neighborhood services were happening. It was about being able to get quality food sources. It was about clean water. There were a number of factors.

And if you are a woman of low income and you get your healthcare from Medicaid, you also have all these other factors that come into it. And that is why when we were talking about no one knowing all the reasons why someone might decide to terminate a pregnancy, our organization trusts black women to make those personal decisions that are best for themselves and their families. And the other side clearly does not trust us to make those decisions.

Ms. TLAIB. No, they want to control us.

Thank you so much, and I yield the rest of my time.

Chairwoman MALONEY. I thank my friend from Michigan for her powerful voice for her state, and I now call upon one of Congress' most outstanding leaders, my good friend and colleague Barbara Lee, for her– and I want to publicly thank her for her tireless and for being such a powerful advocate for progress, gender justice, and equality.

Thank you for sitting here all day long. She is not even a member of the committee. So I really appreciate your being here, and I appreciate your voice.

Ms. LEE. Well, thank you, Chairwoman Maloney, for holding this hearing and for your tremendous work and leadership and also for allowing me to sit through this very, very important hearing.

I also want to thank my colleagues from the Pro-Choice Caucus, especially our chairs of our task forces, Congresswoman Ayanna Pressley and Congresswoman Judy Chu, who have been such clearthinking and passionate leaders on so many issues since they have been here in the House of Representatives.

First, let me just– and throughout their lives, quite frankly. Let me start by just stating a couple of statistics.

Banning access to safe, legal abortion is not what the majority of this country wants. According to recent polling published in September, 77 percent of Americans support access to abortion. And we know and we see how many of these restrictions disproportionately, which we have talked about, impact women of color and lowincome women.

Access to the full range of reproductive healthcare should be accessible to all and not based on one's race, income, or zip code.

Now fighting for equitable access to abortion is deeply personal for me, and I do, and it is hard to talk about this, but I think today, you know, I will mention it again. I remember very clearly the days of back alley abortions before Roe v. Wade. I was a teenager, only 16 years old, and had to go to Mexico for a gut-wrenching back alley abortion.

Again, before Roe v. Wade, abortions were not safe nor legal in my own country. So I refuse to stand by and see even one more woman's life put in danger because of lack of access to safe and legal abortion.

Now many of my Republican colleagues here today and the minority witness, they want to portray women who have had abortions as evil or as murderers. But I am here today with several of my sisters, several who have personally had an abortion. And when you say these comments, they also say them to me, they say them to you, and we are not going to stand for it.

Many– and I serve on the Appropriations Committee, and let me tell you what I see. Many of our Republican colleagues, they opposed teen pregnancy prevention programs. They oppose comprehensive sex education. They oppose family planning. They oppose contraception. They oppose abortions.

Again, as an appropriator, I see these budgets zeroing out funding for healthcare programs that would prevent pregnancies, prevent pregnancies. Also I see budget cuts every day to childcare, SNAP benefits, nutrition, early childhood education, everything that would help raise families and children in a way that they deserve to be raised.

So I want to just ask you your feedback, maybe Ms. Howell, could you just– we know that these programs are disproportionately impacting women of color, and how do you see this whole movement now, what we are seeing? I still call it a war on women's health because when you look at the comprehensive nature of these cuts and the policies and the restrictions, what else is it? What are we to do as women in this country?

Ms. HOWELL. I think that one of the things that we have—we have seen over the last couple of years is women taking back their rights, and it is not just women. It is people. It is LGBTQ people. It is trans people. Basically, standing up and saying we won't allow this to happen anymore.

And we saw it in the 2018 election. We saw it where women of color, for instance, came out and voted to change the House of Representatives. Voted very strongly. And one of those issues that they voted on was Hyde, eliminating Hyde and having the EACH Woman Act.

So they were very clear about what they were looking for and the right to make decisions for themselves without political interference. And I think that that is critical.

Ms. LEE. Thank you.

Ms. Graves, would you like to comment? We have just a few more seconds. I want to thank Ms. Box for your being here today and your stories and for being so brave in terms of giving the real deal about what women go through as a result of trying to exercise their constitutional right.

So thank you. Ms. Graves?

Ms. GOSS GRAVES. I just want to add that it is true that people are outraged and are rising up against the bans that are sweeping this country, but this is a dangerous time. It is dangerous to ban abortion. It is dangerous to have states where people think they can't get care, even though abortion is legal in every state of this country.

And it is dangerous, the rhetoric that we heard in this room today and that we hear outside of this room that demonizes patients, that demonizes women, and that goes sort of to the core of who we are as a country. This is– today has reminded me how dangerous these times are.

Ms. LEE. Thank you.

Thank you, Madam Chair, very much.

Chairwoman MALONEY. I want to thank my friend Barbara Lee for sharing really one of the most personal and heartbreaking events of her life. She is sharing it not only at this hearing, but with the whole world, and Barbara Lee, your courage has made us all stronger.

Thank you. And your leadership.

I now call on an incredible woman, a newly elected woman to our Congress, Congresswoman Kim Schrier. She is from the great state of Washington. She is a physician and a powerful advocate for science and women across this country.

Thank you for being here. She is not a member of this committee, but she wanted to be here and to speak out, and I thank you for being here all day, supporting our efforts.

Thank you. Dr. Schrier?

Ms. SCHRIER. Thank you, Madam Chair. I laughed because I thought you were going to talk about Ayanna Pressley, who is a member of our freshman class.

[Laughter.]

Chairwoman MALONEY. I already talked about her.

Ms. SCHRIER. I came here today to talk about these unnecessary restrictions on a woman's access to full reproductive care, access to abortion. And we have heard about a million ways that local governments and state governments are trying to restrict a woman's access to a safe and legal medical procedure.

And every one of these unnecessary ultrasounds, bogus scripts, hallway signs, admitting privileges at local hospitals, second pelvic exams, even first pelvic exams, admitting privileges I mentioned, and even waiting periods, all of those are unnecessary. They make it harder for women. They especially make it harder for women who are poor, who would have to take additional time off work, who would have to travel great distances.

These do not stop abortions. If you want—that is your goal, you should be doubling down on funding for Planned Parenthood for pregnancy prevention. These do not stop abortions. They make them later. They delay them, or they make them less safe. They are totally inappropriate.

Now I came to talk about that, and I want to reinforce that this is a safe and legal procedure. It is something that 1 out of 4 women have before she is 45 years old. This is more common than a tonsillectomy. This is common. Chances are excellent, pretty much 100 percent, that everybody in this room knows somebody who has an abortion. That is how common it is.

So I came to discuss those things, but then I heard all kinds of rhetoric, all kinds of rhetoric. And as a doctor, and thank you all for being here, I really feel like I need to push back on a lot of Ms. Stuckey's comments. Pseudoscience, total baloney, and I don't feel like I can let those things just stand.

I mean, it is everything from not understanding a difference between an embryo and a baby, which, by the way, if she believes they are the same, that is a personal philosophical and religious decision. That is not a medical distinction, and that is not something that Congress should be involved in. It is not something that she should have any say over any other woman's decision.

But there are other things that she talked about, like 20 weeks in pain. Totally unproven, bogus. She talked about the gag rule not being a gag rule. It is. When a physician cannot mention that one option for her patient is abortion, that is a gag rule. And by the way, it is a dangerous gag rule because if a woman is diagnosed with pregnancy and cervical cancer at the exact same visit, an abortion would save her life. Let us be clear.

The other one she mentioned was she painted a very happy picture of a 23-week micro preemie. I am a pediatrician. I spend a lot of time in NICUs. Let me tell you what the real picture is. The real picture is that you have got about a 50/50 shot at survival. And you have got, if you do survive, a very high likelihood of having consequences later down the line.

Now that doesn't mean that I didn't resuscitate those babies and take care of them and take care of them in the NICU, but it does mean that she is not giving you the full correct picture of the situation.

But the most egregious one is this discussion that somehow you could pull a baby out 3 days before delivery and call that an abortion. We call that an induced delivery. That is a baby who is pulled out and handed to their mother or taken to the NICU, where a doctor like me would take care of them if they are in trouble or in distress.

If you want to have a conversation about pregnancies and abortions later in pregnancy, let us have a really honest discussion about it. About 1 percent of abortions happen after 20 weeks, and none of these are because a woman just decided one morning I don't want to be pregnant anymore. That does not happen.

These are all for a reason. Some devastating turn, something devastating has taken a turn in a pregnancy. Something has happened, either with the health of the mother or the health of the pregnancy, and it is so important that Congress not get into that discussion.

This is a decision between a woman and her God and her doctor and her life, and only she knows how to make this decision, and there is absolutely no place for me or anybody in Congress to get into that discussion. What we owe that woman is a little grace and a little trust to make the best decision about her body.

I will end there. Thank you. And I am sorry that you had to put up with such harassment today. Thank you for your services.

Chairwoman MALONEY. Thank you. I now recognize Mr. Keller.

Mr. KELLER. Thank you, Madam Chair.

What I want to start out with is I heard some testimony during today's hearing about the viability of a pregnancy being difficult to determine because they are all based on a different diagnosis, different situation. And I will get to that later in my comments.

I just want to start out with knowing that, and I know that it was just mentioned that some babies have a 50/50 shot at survival. You know, Dr. Schrier mentioned that. I just want to say this. Every life has opportunity and hope. And sometimes doctors, despite their best efforts, do not calculate the appropriate outcome for their diagnosis.

I have had personal experience with this. When my son Freddy was three years old, he had an injury resulted in a– led to a devastating head injury. He had an accident. The doctors, despite their best efforts, thought Freddy was not going to live.

He was put on life support. As we waited and prayed, the doctor's prognosis was that the mortality rate of children in his condition was not 50 percent, was not 98 percent, but we were told was 100 percent. He was not going to live.

They even tried to convince us to disconnect life support and end his treatment since they did not believe he was going to live. He was on a vent for 28 days. We chose life. We chose hope. And Freddy started to recovery.

Even then, the doctors said he would have permanent brain damage and would not have a meaningful or full life. I am happy to say that today Freddy has fully recovered. Freddy's outcome was different.

He graduated from college and now works for the hospital that saved his life. It was a different outcome than what the doctors told us it would be. His accident is now a memory, but also an opportunity to learn about the value of human life.

As this pertains to today's hearing, in this country, we have countless situations where people determine the value of an unborn human life. Abortions are sometimes planned and executed based upon diagnoses that have uncertain outcomes.

Sometimes as a result, babies are born. They are alive, and they are killed as part of a planned abortion procedure. This should not only shock the conscience, but should make the American people sick.

I am not asking for an answer to the next question I am going to ask. I am just going to leave it up to the people that are watching. But where does it stop when we have people determining the value of human life?

I yield back.

Ms. FOXX. Mr. Keller, would you yield to me?

Mr. KELLER. I yield to Dr. Foxx.

Ms. FOXX. Thank you, Mr. Keller.

Mr. Keller, thank you for that moving story about Freddy. I think you illustrated something very important to us. Doctors can make predictions, but they are not God, and they don't know what is going to happen.

We have heard a lot of things here today, but I could not let this hearing close without saying that there are many things we have heard that should make us shudder, but I believe that what Mr. Keller said leads us into what I want to say next.

But comparing killing a baby to removing wisdom teeth is absolutely beyond the pale. And when we have people, as Mr. Keller asked the question, where is this decision to kill innocent life going to take us in this country?

To say it is terminating a pregnancy, and as Ms. Stuckey said, never, ever facing up to what you are really doing, is scary to me. And I want to say that Ms. Lee said that Republicans characterize women who have had an abortion as evil. I have never heard a Republican say that.

We grieve– and I said that at the beginning. We grieve for the women who find themselves making that decision. I cannot imagine that it is ever easy. I hope it is never easy for any woman to decide to kill her unborn child. I hope and pray that is not easy, and I would never characterize a woman who is faced with that decision and makes that decision as evil.

Thank you, Madam Chair.

Chairwoman MALONEY. I thank the gentlewoman. She yields back.

And I yield myself five minutes.

And this hearing is very important to me and very meaningful because usually when I am attending a hearing on women's healthcare and women's needs, I am talking to an all-male panel and usually have to ask "Where are the women?" especially on hearings that affect their well-being and their healthcare. It is personally thrilling and inspiring to me to see a panel made entirely of women's voices, and America should listen to women's voices.

I want to thank all of the panelists, but I particularly want to thank Mrs. Box. I believe that your voice is the most important of all the important voices that we have heard today. Because to me, you represent every person who has been shamed and judged for making a deeply personal decision about their own body and their own healthcare and for them wanting to access the very best healthcare that they need to take care of themselves and their families.

I just want to ask you, Mrs. Box, and I know it is difficult to testify before Congress on anything, but especially something that has been so personal, how did it feel to hear officials in your state and across the country say hateful, hateful rhetoric about the decision that you were making, your own personal decision? How did it feel?

Ms. BOX. It is insulting, and I appreciate Representative Foxx's sympathy for me, but I would like to say that while my particular reason for abortion of fetal diagnosis was sad for our family, most women, including myself– not all, but most– experience relief after having an abortion.

And I said in my– I think when I answered a question that our abortion, it was the first day that we began to heal from the grief of our diagnosis. I have cried a lot of tears about Libby, but they have all been in grieving my daughter and never once in regret for my decision to make a medical choice for her as her parent.

And you know, I also wanted to say– I am sorry, sir. I can't see your name. But I am really glad that your son had a positive outcome, and I believe in supporting parents in making the best decisions for their family and their children, and that is what my husband and I did for Libby.

Chairwoman MALONEY. Thank you. Thank you for sharing your experience.

Dr. McNicholas, you cared for hundreds of patients in Mrs. Box's situation. What impacts have you seen on the patients you care for in Missouri, as these restrictive laws are enacted and forced upon them?

Dr. MCNICHOLAS. So I think, first and foremost, the outright confusion that people have about what is happening in terms of their access to abortion, and reproductive care more broadly, is really important to lift up.

As abortion bans are passed, whether they are enacted or not, patients automatically think that means they can't access abortion. So we have done a tremendous amount of work in patient reassurance, in making sure that the country knows that abortion is still legal in every single state in this country.

Chairwoman MALONEY. What are you most worried about for your patients?

Dr. MCNICHOLAS. I worry that they have the realization, the full realization that the people who are charged with protecting their health have completely abdicated their responsibility based on an ideologic viewpoint.

I 100 percent people who don't believe in abortion choosing not to have one. But I also think it is the right of every other individual to make that choice based on their values.

Chairwoman MALONEY. I thank you really for the—

Mr. CLAY. Madam Chair?

Chairwoman MALONEY.– courage that all of you have in your work and what you have done for other women and for our country.

I want to share that I have within my district two Planned Parenthood centers, and if you go to them at the end of the day, when women are getting off of work, women are lined up through the halls of the building, outside to the sidewalk, down the street into the next block, waiting to get basic healthcare services. And Planned Parenthood centers provide primary and preventive healthcare to many who otherwise would have nowhere else to turn for care.

And I want to point out that 54 percent of Planned Parenthood centers are in areas where there is healthcare shortages, and we have heard testimony from medical experts that if Planned Parenthood is defunded, there is no other health facility that can address these needs and help these women. I cannot tell you how many women come to my office and tell me that at certain times in their life, the only place they could get healthcare was Planned Parenthood. And I want to put that on the record that I think it is a scandal that anyone would ever try to defund a service that is providing so much help to people that need it.

This has been an important hearing to me, and I intend to continue working on this area and helping women receive the respect and the healthcare they deserve. I would now like to call on my good friend Jackie Speier and give her five minutes and thank her for her relentless leadership in support of women's issues and women.

Ms. SPEIER. Thank you, Madam Chair.

And thank you to a remarkable panel of very persuasive and committed women to the service of other women.

Ms. Box, when you testified earlier, I was sitting here, and I started to cry because I share the same experience that you have had. I lost a child, a fetus, when I was 17 weeks, and I told my story on the House floor in part because I sat there and listened to such false information coming from my colleagues on the other side of the aisle that it outraged me so much that I said you have no idea what you are talking about. You have not lived through this kind of experience.

And to hear you talk about Libby Rose and keep her on your chest is just very powerful because it underscores what we all go through when we lose a fetus at late term. It is never by choice. And I find it so offensive that we continue to have Members here in Congress think that they can somehow take hold of our bodies and tell us what we can do.

So thank you. Thank you for your presence here, for your new infant's presence here. Having the gurgling of your child was just music to all of our ears.

And thank you to all of you as well.

I am going to share one story, though, that relates to Missouri. My daughter went to the University of Missouri and graduated there. She had a girlfriend who became pregnant, who then drove an hour and a half to St. Louis to be seen and then was told that she had to wait three days. And so then she had to drive an hour and a half back. And then, of course, she couldn't get the abortion in three days because there was such a long waiting list.

Now this friend of my daughter's then finally called her mother, who lived in another state, who was not pro-choice. And her mother came and picked her up and took her to another state to get the abortion.

We cannot force women to have to jump through hoops and travel long distances to get the healthcare that they deserve and that is legal under the law in this country. And to see what Missouri has done with their laws and how difficult they have made it is so repugnant to me and should be repugnant to every woman in this country.

Now, Ms. Box, let me ask you the question that I think about a lot. When you were required to wait your 72 hours and received this counseling, what was the counseling that you received?

Ms. BOX. Well, first, I want to say that I thank you for sharing your story with me, and I am sorry for your loss. I know how painful that is.

I am not the legal expert, but you don't really have is it counseling?

Ms. SPEIER. You didn't recognize it as counseling.

Ms. BOX. Oh, the book? Oh. Okay. I am sorry. Yes, you are right.

I didn't understand that was considered counseling.

Ms. SPEIER. What was it?

Ms. BOX. It is a booklet that has– so the consent process, I guess, is that– I apologize. So they had to go over this information, and they provided me with a booklet that is written by the state that has medically inaccurate information in an attempt to help me make an informed decision, which just doesn't make sense to me.

But what I will say is that how it works in Missouri currently is that you have to consent with the provider who will perform the abortion. So my consent and my counseling, the book, like I said earlier, I called "book of shame." But my conversation with the provider, with the doctor who works at Planned Parenthood, was the most compassionate care I have ever received.

She took something that was the worst experience of my husband and my life and showed us love and no judgment and counseled us in all of the options available to us, and gave us medically accurate, science-based information so that we could make a decision as parents that was informed and full of love.

Ms. SPEIER. Thank you. Thank you again, all of you, and I yield back.

Chairwoman MALONEY. Thank you. Thank you so much.

I would like to enter into the record a series of letters the committee has received in recent days from organizations, including the American College of Obstetricians and Gynecologists, Reproaction, the Guttmacher Institute, and the American Civil Liberties Union. These letters express grave concern over the impact that state restrictions on abortion access are having on the health, economic well-being of women in America and their families.

I ask unanimous consent that these letters be entered into the official hearing record, and I so order.

Chairwoman MALONEY. I would like now to thank our incredible witnesses for testifying and for their life's work.

And without objection, all Members will have five legislative days within which to submit additional written questions for the witnesses to the chair, which will be forwarded to the witnesses for their response.

I ask our witnesses to please respond as promptly as possible, and this hearing is now—

But before I conclude this hearing, I would like to thank the powerful women of this committee, especially Ms. Speier, Ms. Pressley, Ms. Kelly, Ms. Ocasio-Cortez, for their leadership on this issue and for encouraging the committee to examine it.

I would also like to thank Congresswoman Judy Chu, Congresswoman Jan Schakowsky, Congresswoman Barbara Lee, and Congresswoman Kim Schrier, for joining us this afternoon and for their tireless work to preserve access to abortion and reproductive healthcare for women across this Nation.

And I would also like to thank Lacy Clay, who has worked with me on this hearing and for his leadership on this issue.

This hearing is adjourned, but we are going to continue on this issue.

Thank you.

[Whereupon, at 5:24 p.m., the committee was adjourned.]

In: A Look at Maternal Health and Reproductive Rights ISBN: 978-1-53619-760-0
Editor: Lisa R. Flores

Chapter 3

THREATS TO REPRODUCTIVE RIGHTS IN AMERICA*

Committee on the Judiciary

Tuesday, June 4, 2019
House of Representatives
Subcommittee on the Constitution, Civil Rights,
And Civil Liberties
Committee on the Judiciary
Washington, DC.

The subcommittee met, pursuant to call, at 10:09 a.m., in Room 2141, Rayburn Office Building, Hon. Steve Cohen [chairman of the subcommittee] presiding.

Present: Representatives Cohen, Nadler, Raskin, Scanlon, Dean, Garcia, Escobar, Jackson Lee, Johnson of Louisiana, Collins, Gohmert, Cline, and Armstrong. Also Present: Representatives Chu, Roby, and Lesko. Staff present: Lisette Morton, Director of Policy, Planning, and Member Services; Madeline Strasser, Chief Clerk; Moh Sharma, Member Services and Outreach Advisor; Susan Jensen, Parliamentarian/Senior Counsel; James Park, Chief Counsel, Constitution Subcommittee; Sophie Brill, Counsel, Constitution Subcommittee; Will Emmons, Professional Staff Member, Constitution Subcommittee; Paul Taylor, Minority Counsel; and Andrea Woodward, Minority Professional Staff Member.

Mr. COHEN. Good morning, everyone. The Committee on the Judiciary Subcommittee on the Constitution, Civil Rights, and Civil Liberties, will come to order. Without objection, the chair is authorized to declare recesses of the subcommittee at any time. I welcome everyone to today's hearing on threats to reproductive rights in America. I will now recognize myself for my opening statement.

---

* This is an edited, reformatted and augmented version of Hearing before the Subcommittee on the Constitution, Civil Rights, and Civil Liberties, of the Committee on the Judiciary, House of Representatives, One Hundred Sixteenth Congress, First Session, Publication No. Serial No. 116–23, dated June 4, 2019.

More than 45 years ago, the United States Supreme Court recognized that women must have the right to control their own bodies, including by having the right to decide when to have children and when to terminate a pregnancy. Now, it was not an unlimited right, but it was a right. More than 25 years ago, the Supreme Court affirmed that right after years of sustained opposition.

Now in this year, the year of 2019, the rights of women across the Nation are under attack like never before. It started with a flurry of laws meant to scare and shame women and to regulate abortion providers out of existence. These laws require clinics to offer or perform ultrasounds on women and even to provide medically inaccurate counseling, counseling dictated by the legislature, not by doctors. They demean women by imposing "waiting periods," and some, such as my home State of Tennessee, compound the obstacles and red tape by requiring women to travel to a clinic to receive the State's mandated lecture, written by our general assembly, about her body in person, then undergo a waiting period, and then travel back to the appointment.

Other laws, also enacted under the guise of protecting women, have attempted to shut clinics down by requiring doctors to obtain admitting privileges at nearby hospitals and requiring the clinics to outfit themselves like surgical facilities. Ironically, because abortion is such a low-risk procedure, doctors are often unable to meet the requirements for admitting privileges because few or none of their patients ever require a hospital visit.

In Alabama, as Dr. Yashica Robinson will note, the State passed legislation that require her clinic to relocate to a new facility so that it could meet burdensome new physical requirements. Then when the relocation was complete, the State passed a law to try to chase the clinic away again by prohibiting it from operating next to a nearby school. It was only through the intervention of a Federal judge that the clinic was allowed to stay open.

A few years ago, there was some hope that the Supreme Court's ruling in Whole Women's Health v. Hellerstedt would put a stop to laws like these. In that case, the Court struck down a Texas law that required doctors providing abortions to obtain admitting privileges at hospitals, and required providers to have the physical capacity of a full surgical facility. The Supreme Court, with Justice Kennedy joining the majority opinion, held that these requirements had no medical benefit for women and would serve only to close down clinics, leading to particularly harsh results for poor women and women in rural communities.

But Justice Kennedy has now been replaced by Justice Kavanaugh, and it now seems that the gloves are off. Many States have dropped the pretense all together that they are somehow trying to protect women. This year alone, Georgia, Kentucky, Mississippi, and Ohio have enacted laws banning abortion once a fetal heartbeat is detected, which occurs approximately 6 months into a pregnancy, before many women even know they are pregnant.

Alabama has enacted a law banning abortion outright with exceptions only in cases where the life of the mother is in danger. There are no exceptions for rape or incest or for women's health. Missouri has enacted a law banning abortions after 8 weeks, and Arkansas and Utah have enacted laws banning abortions after 18 weeks, all periods in which Roe v. Wade protects a woman's right. Many other States have enacted the so-called trigger laws that would immediately ban abortion if the Supreme Court overturns its decision in Roe v. Wade. These States appear to be betting that the Court is about to take that step.

We cannot afford to go back. I would not presume to know what it is like for a woman to live in a world where she has to participate in a crime in order to end a pregnancy that she does not want, or cannot afford to have, or cannot put her body through, or was the result of rape or incest. Americans, Democrats and Republicans, are in strong, strong support of allowing abortion when it is the result of rape or incest or to protect the life of a woman. And in most of these States' new laws, those exceptions are not written into the law, making it a very, very minor, unpopular, and undemocratic approach.

I do remember what it was like for the women I knew growing up. I remember when a friend of my family needed to get an abortion when it was illegal in the United States, pre-Roe v. Wade. She was relatively lucky. She was wealthy, so she was able to fly across the country to California and go to Tijuana. And it made me realize—I was only 14 or 15 years old—what a poor person would be and the circumstance they would be in. They would be out of luck because they couldn't afford that first-class air ticket or the coach class air tickets. But air tickets were expensive in the 60s, and to go across country and to go to Mexico was an expensive ordeal, which people of means could afford to do. People not of means could not.

This had a disparate impact upon poor women, women of color, women of rural communities who couldn't take the time off or had the money to make that trip. If States are allowed to outlaw access to abortion again, these laws would doubtless have that disparate impact on these groups of women, just as it was when it was illegal before Roe v. Wade.

Women are fighting back. Our witnesses today include two legal experts who are raising awareness of these issues, one of whom is fighting day after day to keep these clinics open. We will also hear from two physicians who provide reproductive healthcare to patients, including abortion care when necessary. And we have two women with the courage to share their own stories about receiving abortions, because they have recognized how important it is to destigmatize this subject and stop shaming women for their choices and medical histories. I thank our witnesses for being here today, and I look forward to hearing from each of the women on the panel about this critical and timely subject.

It is now my pleasure to recognize the ranking member of the subcommittee, the gentleman from Louisiana, Mr. Johnson, for his opening statement.

Mr. JOHNSON of Louisiana. Thank you, Mr. Chairman. This is a serious issue, and there may be no more divisive issue in our country than the decades-long battle over the sanctity of human life. Indeed, many Americans regard this as the defining issue of our times.

In Congress, our Pro-Life Caucus and Republican Conference members work hard every day to advance measures to protect more children in the womb because they are the most vulnerable and threatened lives in our society. We do this work because we share the same deep and abiding conviction that so many of the founders of this extraordinary Nation did about the sanctity of human life. It is that seminal conviction, of course, that is recorded in the very birth certificate of our Nation, the Declaration of Independence, and has come to be known as our Nation's creed. You know the language well: "We hold these truths to be self-evident, that all men are created equal, that they are endowed by their Creator with certain unalienable rights, that among these are life, liberty, and the pursuit of happiness."

We believe, as the founders articulated, that every single human life is sacred because that value is given to us not by the State, but by our Creator in Whose image all of us are made. Because of this, every single human life has inestimable dignity and value, and our value is not related in any way to the color of our skin, our zip code, our socioeconomic status, our level of talent or education, or what we can contribute to society. Our value is inherent because it is given to us by our Creator.

During the first 2 centuries of our republic, most Americans accepted and revered the biblical truths that every human being is fearfully and wonderfully made, and personally known by our Creator, God, even before they were formed in their mother's womb. The rejection of that essential truth has now led to the murder of more than 60 million innocent pre-born children since 1973's Roe v. Wade. What an unspeakable tragedy this is.

In addition to the deeply-held conviction about the lives of the unborn, millions of conscientious Americans also support pro-life legislation and reasonable restrictions on the abortion practice because it is pro-women to do so. The abortion industry itself presents very real dangers for millions who are in difficult circumstances. I bring firsthand knowledge of those dangers to this hearing today. Prior to my election to Congress, I spent a good portion of my 20-year legal career in the courts defending commonsense, pro-life legislation when those laws are challenged, and litigation to protect vulnerable women who were irreparably harmed by the notorious practices of the abortion industry. In fact, I was co-counsel in the trial of one of the cases that the chairman's hearing memo today laments was upheld by the Fifth Circuit in 2018.

Over the course of my career, we uncovered and made public shocking evidence, including the documented use of rusted surgical instruments, filthy and dangerous conditions in the clinics, unlicensed doctors engaging in physical and emotional abuse of patients, falsifying health records, and so much more. I have spent many hours with and conducted extraordinary depositions of abortion providers, some of whom boasted about personally performing tens of thousands of abortions each. Their callous disregard for the barbarism of their practice and the countless precious lives they terminated merely for cash was always stunning to me. To so many of these abortion providers, women are merely objects and a source of revenue, and State health and safety regulations put in place to protect those vulnerable women are mere nuisances to be blatantly ignored. There is no one in this room that can tell me otherwise because I have seen and heard and documented all this in court records myself.

Today we also have indisputable scientific evidence and advanced medical technology, like 4–D ultrasounds, that clearly affirm the humanity of every unborn child. We know that when a human sperm meets and fertilizes a human egg at the moment of conception, there becomes an unborn living, genetically distinct, and biologically self-directed human being. That is an uncontroversial statement among embryologists and those who practice modern medicine generally. In other words, there is no such thing as a potential human being. There are only human beings from the moment of conception.

But today we see lawyers and politicians and activists straining logic and language past the breaking point for political reasons. They do their very best to avoid phrases like "unborn child," and try to defend and deny the gruesome reality of abortion, which expert witnesses have previous described before this very subcommittee as a typical procedure in which a living human being is literally and brutally ripped to pieces limb by limb. When I served in the Louisiana legislature, I authored and passed a ban on the barbaric dismemberment abortion procedure in my State. Of course, the abortion lobby immediately challenged it in Court.

Over the past several months, we have all witnessed liberals in high political office move aggressively to further expand abortion rights, even after the point when an unborn child can clearly live outside the womb on its own. The United States, by the way, you should know, is one of only seven Nations, including North Korea and China, that allow elective abortions after 20 weeks, a practice that kills thousands of innocent babies every year. New York's Reproductive Health Act allows all abortions up to 24 weeks and expanded access for later abortions. There is proposed legislation in Virginia, as we all now know, that the bill sponsor said would allow an abortion even during labor, and Virginia Governor Ralph Northam infamously endorsed allowing physicians and mothers to let children die in some circumstances.

When Senate Republicans in this Congress pressed for a vote on the Born Alive Abortion Survivors Protection Act, Federal legislation that the House has passed in previous years that would simply require doctors to provide medical care to babies born alive after failed abortion procedures, incredibly 45 Senate Democrats voted to block its further consideration and passage in the Senate. I stood in the back of the Senate chamber that night with dozens of our Republican colleagues, and we could not believe what we were watching.

Mr. Chairman, this hearing is entitled "Threats to Reproductive Rights in America," but rights must be accompanied by responsibilities. In this case, that responsibility includes our duty to protect unborn human beings. As the Declaration acknowledges, this is the first and most fundamental obligation of any civilized people.

My own mother had just turned 17 when she and my father decided to choose life and allow me into the world, and I am so grateful that they did. Countless millions of young women have made that same blessed choice, and their children are equally thankful. For women in vulnerable situations who have made the opposite decision and lived to regret it, I just want to say personally that you, too, are valued and loved, and that the Creator, Who gave us our inalienable rights, is so gracious that He offers hope, forgiveness, and redemption to every single one of us.

I look forward to hearing from all of our witnesses here today, and we thank you for your time. Mr. Chairman, I would ask unanimous consent that the full committee members, Mrs. Roby and Mrs. Lesko, be allowed to sit on our subcommittee today.

Mr. COHEN. Without objection, that will be done.

Mr. JOHNSON of Louisiana. Thank you. I yield back.

Mr. COHEN. I want to thank the ranking member for his statement. His positions are different from mine, but they are heartfelt and they are sincere. And another member who has heartfelt and sincere opinions at least is Mr. Judy Chu of California. She is here, and I want to recognize her for her attendance and her support.

And now I want to recognize the chairman of the full committee, one of the leading voices for many, many years for women's rights and choice and the Constitution, the chairman of the full committee, the gentleman from New York, Mr. Nadler, for his opening statement.

Chairman NADLER. Thank you, Chairman Cohen, for convening this hearing to address the ongoing assault against women's reproductive rights that we are witnessing across the Nation. This country has reached a crisis point for women's constitutional rights to control their own bodies and their own reproductive choices. States have passed unconstitutional bill after unconstitutional bill, imposing new extreme restrictions on abortion, setting the most direct challenge to Roe v. Wade we have seen in decades.

In the month of May alone, Alabama outlawed abortion outright, making no exceptions even in cases of rape or incest. Georgia and Louisiana effectively outlawed abortion at just 6 weeks into a pregnancy, and Missouri outlawed abortion just 8 weeks into a pregnancy. These laws would in many instances ban abortions before women even know they are pregnant. Meanwhile, the new conservative majority in the Supreme Court upheld portions of an extreme anti-abortion law from Indiana, and the last abortion clinic in Missouri came to the brink of being forced to close its doors after the State refused to reissue its license. Had the Court not intervened, Missouri would have been the first State, but surely not the last, without a single abortion clinic.

Let me add a word here about some of the rhetoric we have heard already today. The rhetoric from the ranking member of the subcommittee is heartfelt and sincere. It is also arrogant in that it seeks to impose his and certain other people's moral commitments on people who don't share those moral opinions. The power of the State should not be used by one segment of society to impose its moral or religious beliefs on another segment of society. Political power should not be fought over as to who can control other people's religious and moral convictions and the actions stemming therefrom. That is the fundamental question in this whole fight.

After decades of chipping away at the right to an abortion, States now realize that the new conservative majority on the Supreme Court presents an opportunity either to overturn Roe completely or to so radically undermine the right to an abortion as to render it essentially meaningless. But the need for a safe, legal abortion will never be meaningless. The right to have an abortion is fundamental to women's equality, autonomy, and personal liberty. Making decisions about when and how to start a family is essential women's lives and is their decisions, not Congress', not some state legislatures.

As the Supreme Court put it 27 years ago when it upheld Roe after nearly 2 decades of challenges, "The ability of women to participate equally in the economic and social life of the Nation has been facilitated by their ability to control their reproductive lives." We will not go backward. If women cannot make decisions about their reproductive health, they cannot make decisions about starting a career, going to school, opening a business, and planning their lives. When you restrict access to abortion, you strip women of the fundamental freedom to live life on their own terms.

The last few weeks have seen an all-out frontal attack on the right of every woman in this country to access abortion, but this fight is not new, and these laws have not come out of nowhere. The bans and extreme restrictions and enactments in States like Alabama, Georgia, and Louisiana, as well as in many others, represent some of the most extreme legislation coming from the States. But over the last decade, State legislatures have passed hundreds of bills designed to block women from accessing care and for making their own choices. These laws impose medically unnecessary regulations on doctors and on clinics, right down to the clinics' physical dimensions. Some States have even gone so far as to require women who receive abortions by taking a pill rather than through surgery, to take that pill inside a clinic that must meet the standards of a full surgical facility.

Under the disingenuous claim that these types of laws protect women's health, these States are deliberately attempting to put abortion out of reach, particularly for low-income women and women of color. The result is predictable. Many women will get abortions, illegal abortions, medically unsafe abortions, and the death rate will go up. These laws set arbitrary and unnecessary waiting periods that force women to take extra time off to work and delay care. They require unnecessary tests and biased counseling that do nothing but drive up the cost of abortion care. They set arbitrary regulations for providers that are designed solely to force clinics to close. And, most egregiously, they are designed to intimidate and shame women for making the constitutionally-protected choice to have an abortion.

And this is not only happening in the States. Here in the United States Congress, the Republican-controlled Senate is considered a ban on abortion after 20 weeks, a bill that has no basis in science and is prima facie unconstitutional. Meanwhile, the current Administration has taken every opportunity to undermine the right to access abortion and even contraception.

It seems every other week the Administration nominates a new-anti-choice Federal judge or official, promulgates yet another rule undermining access to birth control or ending unbiased family planning services, and announces yet another new policy to protect those who discriminate against patients seeking an abortion rather than protecting the patients themselves.

Enough is enough. Congress must now stand up with women and men around the country to say we will not turn back the clock on women's constitutional rights and women's autonomy. It is my hope that today's hearing is Congress' first step to shoring up the right to abortion across this country through legislation like Representative Judy Chu's Women's Health Protection Act, which would put an end to States banning or otherwise limiting access to abortion, and Representative Barbara Lee's Each Woman Act, which would end abortion coverage bans, or other legislative initiatives. We must act to ensure that every woman, regardless of State, income, race, or any other factor, retains her constitutional right to make her own choice and to access abortion. Women must have the freedom to make decisions about their lives without anyone questioning their intellect, their morals, or their honesty.

I stand with the members of the committee and millions of women and men around this country ready to fight for their freedom. I yield back my time.

Mr. COHEN. Thank you, Mr. Chair. Mr. Collins is at the end of the table. He is the ranking member of the committee, and he is now recognized for his opening statement.

Mr. COLLINS. Thank you, Mr. Chairman. I do appreciate that. The title of this hearing is "Threats to Reproductive Rights in America." The rights mentioned in the title refer to the Supreme Court's 1973 decision in Roe v. Wade. As members of the Judiciary Committee, it is appropriate to examine why the test of time has exposed Roe as a failure in the viable judicial precedent. As mothers, fathers, sisters, brothers, and friends, it is necessary to consider why Roe is a failure of compassion for both women and children.

While Roe asserts a woman's right to privacy, anchors her right to abortion, abortion destroys the right to life along with liberty, the pursuit of happiness, and all other constitutional rights of the children it kills. It is impossible to imagine the framers intending the right of privacy to eclipse one of the self-evident, unalienable rights that motivated the birth of our Nation.

Contending an unborn child has no life to lose becomes impossible when we reflect, even momentarily, on what an abortion entails, and I am grateful for our witnesses today who are here to look at the lives abortions would have snuffed out. These witnesses are not alone in recognize the humanity of an unborn child. In her dissenting opinion in Gonzales v. Carhart, Justice Ginsburg argued that "Compared to a partial birth abortion, the common dismemberment abortion method could have equally been characterized as brutal, involving, as it does, tearing apart a fetus and ripping off his limbs."

Let us then be honest. Let us not speak of abortion as a victimless crime. At best, abortion is aimed at one person's suffering at the expense of another person's existence. We must cultivate compassion and practical support for women who find themselves pregnant under difficult or oppressive circumstances, and we must protect the most defenseless humans among us, those living in the womb. One person's reproductive right cannot outweigh another person's right to live.

Justice Ginsburg also took issue with Roe on legal grounds. As a law professor, she wrote "Roe, I believe, would have been more acceptable as a judicial decision if it had not gone beyond the ruling of the statute before the Court." Heavy-handed judicial intervention was difficult to justify. Other pro-choice legal experts have also voiced concerns with the foundation of this decision. Edward Lazarus, a former clerk to Justice Blackmun, who wrote the majority opinion in Roe, said, "As a matter of constitutional interpretation and judicial method, Roe borders on the indefensible. I say this as someone who is utterly committed to the right to choose. The problem is that Roe has little connection to the constitutional right it purportedly interpreted. A constitutional right to privacy broad enough to include abortion has no meaningful foundation in the constitutional text, history, or precedent." Mr. Lazarus went on to say, "As a matter of constitutional interpretation, even most liberals, even if you administer truth serum, will tell you it is basically indefensible."

Jeffrey Rosen, formerly of the New Republic and currently the president of the National Constitution Center in Philadelphia, wrote, "Thirty years after Roe, the finest constitutional minds in the country still have not been able to produce a constitutional justification for striking down restrictions on early term abortions that are substantially more convincing than Justice Harry Blackmun's famously artless opinion itself. As a result the pro-choice majority asks nominees to swear allegiance to the decision without being able to identify an intelligible principle to support it." Kermit Roosevelt, a law professor at Penn Law School, said, "It is time to admit in public that, as an example of practice of constitutional opinion writing, Roe is a serious disappointment. As a constitutional argument, Roe is barely coherent. The Court pulled its fundamental right to choose more or less from the Constitution either."

As a result of Roe's lack of legal justification, the Supreme Court has since limited its effect. 1992's Planned Parenthood v. Casey permitted States to regulate abortions in the first trimester or in any State before fetal viability, provided that they do not pose an undue burden on a woman's right to abortion. In 2003, Congress banned partial birth abortions, which none other than Justice Ginsburg had called brutal. In a partial birth abortion, a living baby was delivered feet first, skull crushed before its chin clears the uterus, almost before live birth is complete.

2007, the Supreme Court upheld the Federal ban which applied at any point during pregnancy in Gonzales v. Carhart, ruling the Federal law did not impose an undue burden on a woman's right to an abortion. Justice Kennedy's majority opinion noted the law expresses respect for the dignity of human life and affirmed the government's interest in protecting the medical profession's integrity.

He wrote, "The government may use its voice and its regulatory authority to show its profound respect for the life within the woman." Mr. Chairman, the decade since Roe v. Wade has repeatedly delivered legal decisions making it clear any threat to Roe v. Wade is posed by illogical majority opinion.

Before I finish, however, I will have to take exception with my chairman of the full committee. To call the ranking member of this subcommittee arrogant for expressing his personal beliefs while at the same time sitting hypocritically stating your own beliefs from a belief that would assume comes from a moral or civic background is the height of hypocrisy. At this point in time, we can disagree, but at least if we are going to call it, call the balls and strikes the same way. With that, I yield back.

Mr. COHEN. Thank you, Mr. Collins. We welcome our witnesses and thank them for participating in today's hearing. Please note that your written statement will be entered into the record in its entirety. Accordingly, I ask you to summarize your statement and your testimony in 5 minutes. You have a lighting system in front of you. The green light means you are going, the yellow light means you have 1 minute left, and the red light means over. Stay within that limit. You have got those lights.

Before proceeding, I would remind each of you that all of your written and oral statements made to this subcommittee in connection with this hearing are subject to penalty of perjury pursuant to the U.S.C. 18–1001 that could result in the imposition of fine or imprisonment up to 5 years or both.

Our first witness is Ms. Melissa Murray. She is a professor of law and co-director of the Birnbaum Women's Leadership Network at New York University School of Law, where she teaches con law, family law, criminal law, reproductive rights, and justice, among other courses. Her publications appear or are forthcoming in the California Law Review, the Columbia Law Review, the Harvard Law Review, the Michigan Law Review, the Penn Law Review, and Yale Law Journal, and the Virginia Law Review. I don't see how you have time to teach all those courses.

She is an author of Cases on Reproductive Rights and Justice, the first case book to cover the field of reproductive rights and justice. And prior to joining the NYU faculty, she was on the faculty at the University of California-Berkeley School of Law and served as an interim dean there. Professor Murray received her J.D. from Yale. She is a noted development editor of the Yale Law Journal. After law school she clerked for the Honorable Sonia Sotomayor, then a judge on the U.S. Court of Appeals for the U.S. District Court for the District of Connecticut.

She received her undergraduate degree from the basketball powerhouse, University of Virginia, and she is recognized now for 5 minutes.

STATEMENTS OF MELISSA MURRAY, ESQUIRE, PROFESSOR OF LAW, NEW YORK UNIVERSITY SCHOOL OF LAW, NEW YORK, NEW YORK; BUSY PHILIPPS, ACTOR AND ADVOCATE, OAK PARK, ILLINOIS; OWEN PHILLIPS, MD, FACOG, THE UNIVERSITY OF TENNESSEE HEALTH SCIENCE CENTER, MEMPHIS, TENNESSEE; CHRISTINA BENNETT, COMMUNICATIONS DIRECTOR, FAMILY INSTITUTE OF CONNECTICUT, HARTFORD, CONNECTICUT; MELISSA OHDEN, KANSAS CITY, MISSOURI; JENNIFER DALVEN, DIRECTOR, ACLU REPRODUCTIVE FREEDOM PROJECT, NEW YORK, NEW YORK; YASHICA ROBINSON, MD, MEDICAL DIRECTOR, ALABAMA WOMEN'S CENTER FOR REPRODUCTIVE ALTERNATIVES, HUNTSVILLE, ALABAMA; AND H.K. GRAY, ACTIVIST, YOUTH TESTIFY, DALLAS-FORT WORTH, TEXAS

Statement of Melissa Murray

Ms. MURRAY. Thank you very much for the opportunity to appear before you in these hearings on threats to reproductive rights in United States. I am Melissa Murray, a professor of law at New York University School of Law. I will not recount my credentials as Mr. Cohen is the best PR man that I could have on this subject. [Laughter.]

So let me get right to it. In 1973 in Roe v. Wade, the United States Supreme Court recognized that the Fourteenth Amendment's guarantee of liberty protects a woman's right to determine whether to bear or beget a child. Since then, the United States Supreme Court has consistently affirmed a woman's right to choose an abortion as an essential aspect of the Constitution's guarantees of liberty and equality. In so doing, the Court has held that States may not restrict abortion in ways that are unduly burdensome. More precisely, States may not enact legislation that has the purpose or effect of placing a substantial obstacle in the path of a woman seeking an abortion.

And indeed, as recently as 2016, the Court in Whole Women's Health v. Hellerstedt reiterated this commitment to upholding abortion rights. There, the Court struck down two Texas laws and specifically noted that the undue burden standard was not a permissive endorsement of the State's purported rationales for regulating abortion. Instead, reviewing courts are obliged to review the State's purported justifications and determine independently if the challenged restrictions are appropriate measures to achieve the desired legislative ends.

Still, despite these longstanding precedents, State legislatures have continued to test the Constitution's limits by enacting increasingly restrictive abortion laws. These laws make abortion less accessible and more costly. They purport to promote and protect women's health, but, in fact, these laws are part of a larger effort to legislate abortion out of existence through piecemeal attacks.

Recent changes in the composition of the U.S. Supreme Court and the lower Federal courts have further emboldened those seeking to limit a woman's right to choose an abortion. In the last year, efforts to restrict abortion have taken on a more aggressive and extreme posture, flouting the limits that the Supreme Court has consistently recognized. Those responsible for these laws have made their intentions clear. They are no longer content to chip away at the abortion right through piecemeal legislation, and instead these more recent laws are an obvious provocation designed to relitigate and ultimately to overturn Roe v. Wade.

The prospect of overturning Roe v. Wade is the most obvious threat to reproductive rights, but it is not the only threat, nor is it even the most immediate threat. Even if Roe v. Wade is not overturned, there are a number of cases currently pending in the pipeline to the Supreme Court that concern access to abortion. The law challenges in these cases do not challenge Roe directly, but rather seek to strangle access to abortion, putting this fundamental right out of reach. They are part of this well-worn strategy to dismantle abortion rights through a death by a thousand cuts.

If these laws are upheld, whether by the Supreme Court or the lower Federal courts, their impact will be profound, particularly for our most underserved communities. These communities include individuals struggling to make ends meet, women of color, particularly African-American, Latinx, Asian-American and Pacific Islander and native women, rural women, immigrant women, individuals in the LGBTQ community, parents who already have children, and young people. These constituencies already face enormous barriers to obtaining reproductive care, basic healthcare, and economic security. Threats to abortion access further exacerbate these pressures.

Barriers to healthcare, including reproductive care, go hand-in-hand with economic insecurity. The affordable housing crisis, food insecurity, a lack of clean water, the lack of affordable childcare, the wage gap, which is more pronounced for women of color, the lack of paid family leave, a stagnant minimum wage, all of these issues lead to and compound economic insecurity for underserved communities across this country. These barriers have only increased under this presidential Administration.

For all of these reasons, I urge this subcommittee to keep these urgent threats and these underserved constituencies in mind as you consider ways to support and protect the constitutional right to abortion. Thank you.

[The statement of Ms. Murray follows:]

Testimony of Melissa Murray, Professor of Law, New York University School of Law, before the Subcommittee on the Constitution, Civil Rights, and Civil Liberties, Hearing on Threats to Reproductive Rights in America, June 4, 2019

Thank you very much for the opportunity to appear before you in these hearings on threats to reproductive rights in America. My name is Melissa Murray. I am a Professor of Law at New York University School of Law, where I teach constitutional law, family law, and reproductive rights and justice and serve as a faculty co-director of the Birnbaum Women's Leadership Network. Prior to my appointment at New York University, I was the Alexander F. and May T. Morrison Professor of Law at the University of California, Berkeley, where I taught for twelve years and served as Faculty Director of the Berkeley Center on Reproductive Rights and Justice and as the Interim Dean of the law school.

In 1973's *Roe v. Wade,* the United States Supreme Court recognized that the Fourteenth Amendment's guarantee of liberty protects a woman's right to determine whether to bear or beget a child. Since then, the Supreme Court has consistently affirmed a woman's right to abortion as an essential aspect of the Constitution's guarantees of liberty and equality. In so doing, the Court has held that states may not restrict the abortion right in ways that are unduly burdensome. More precisely, states may not enact legislation that has the purpose or effect of placing a substantial obstacle in the path of a woman seeking an abortion.

Despite these long-standing precedents, state legislatures have continued to test the Constitution's limits by enacting increasingly restrictive abortion laws. These laws make abortion less accessible and more costly. Ostensibly intended to promote and protect women's health, these laws are part of a larger effort to legislate abortion out of existence through piecemeal attacks.

Recent changes in the composition of the Supreme Court and the lower federal courts have further emboldened those seeking to limit a woman's right to abortion. In the last year, efforts to restrict abortion have taken on a more aggressive and extreme posture, flouting the limits that the Supreme Court has consistently recognized. Those responsible for these laws have made their intentions clear. No longer content to chip away at the abortion right through piecemeal legislation, these more recent laws are an obvious provocation designed to relitigate, and ultimately overturn, *Roe v. Wade.*

As we wait for the courts to decide these numerous cases, people are already being harmed. Individuals who already face barriers to health care and economic security, including communities of color, rural families, and LGBTQ individuals, have been and will be particularly impacted. I urge this Committee to keep these communities in mind as you consider ways to support and protect the constitutional right to abortion.

The Constitution's Protection of Personal Liberty, Including Access to Contraception and the Right to Abortion, Is Central to Women's Dignity and Equality and to Other Important Rights

The Fourteenth Amendment guarantees all of us liberty and equality. These guarantees cannot exist without recognition of the dignity afforded every member of society as an autonomous individual. For that reason, the Constitution protects an individual's right to make certain personal decisions about intimacy, marriage, and procreation.

The Supreme Court has specifically recognized that a woman has the right to make her own decision about whether to have an abortion.[1] Indeed, according to the Court "[f]ew decisions are more personal and intimate, more properly private, or more basic to individual dignity and autonomy than a woman's decision ... whether to end her pregnancy."[2] The exercise of this right without undue hindrance from the State is essential to a woman's dignity as an individual and her status as an equal citizen.

A woman's reproductive autonomy is rooted in the deeply personal nature of her decisions about bearing children and expanding her family. However, the decision of "whether to bear or beget a child" has ramifications beyond the home and family. As the Court has recognized, women's ability "to participate equally in the economic and social life of the Nation has been facilitated by their ability to control their reproductive lives."[3]

The Supreme Court's decision in *Roe v. Wade,* recognizing the right to abortion, does not stand on its own; it is part of a long line of cases that recognize the constitutional right to privacy and liberty encompasses personal decisions essential to an individual's dignity and autonomy. These decisions include the right to contraception-first recognized in *Griswold v. Connecticut* (1965)[4] - and the right to procreate-first recognized in *Skinner v. Ok fahoma.*[5] The Court relied on these core precedents in deciding *Roe v. Wade,* and in *Carey v. Population Services,* it relied on *Roe* in turn for its central holding that "the Constitution protects individual decisions in matters of childbearing from unjustified intrusion by the State."[6]

Critically, the right to personal liberty is not limited to reproductive rights. It includes the right to marry, first recognized in *Loving v. Virginia,*[7] and reaffirmed in 2015 in *Obergifell v. Hodges.*[8] It includes the right of parents to direct the upbringing of their children, first recognized in two 1920s cases *Mryer v. Nebraska*[9] and *Pierce*

---

[1] *See* Roe v. Wade, 410 U.S. 113 (1973).
[2] Thornburgh v. Am. College Obstetricians & Gynecologists, 476 U.S. 747, 772 (1986).
[3] Planned Parenthood of Se. Pa. v. Casey, 505 U.S. 833,556 (1992).
[4] 381 U.S. 479 (1965).
[5] 316 U.S. 535 (1942).
[6] Carey v. Population Servs. Int'l, 431 U.S. 678,687 (1977).
[7] 388 U.S. 1, 12 (1967).
[8] 135 S. Ct. 2584, 2604-05 (2015).
[9] 262 U.S. 390 (1923).

v. Society of Sisters.[10] It includes the right to maintain family relationships, including relationships that go beyond the traditional nuclear family.[11] And *Roe* has also influenced the Supreme Court's decision to recognize the right to form intimate relationships,[12] and the right to personal control of medical treatment.[13]

Roe is inextricably bound to this constellation of privacy and personal liberty rights. If *Roe* is dismantled or otherwise eroded, these other rights are threatened too.

The United States Supreme Court Has Consistently Upheld and Protected the Right Recognized in *Roe v. Wade*

For over 45 years-including as recently as 2016-the U.S. Supreme Court has upheld the core principles of *Roe v. Wade,* in case after case. Over that time, a right to abortion has faced numerous threats, and the Court has allowed states to impose some restrictions on the right. But it has never strayed from its core holding that each woman has the right to decide whether to continue a pregnancy before viability.

In *Roe,*[14] the Supreme Court held that the constitutional right to privacy includes a woman's right to decide whether to have an abortion. The Court made clear that the right to privacy is "fundamental," meaning that governmental attempts to interfere with the right are subject to "strict scrutiny."[15] To withstand strict scrutiny, the government must show that its law or policy is necessary to achieve a compelling interest. The law or policy must also be narrowly tailored to achieve the interest and must be the least restrictive means for doing so.

The Court identified those state interests as protecting women's health and protecting the "potentiality" of life.[16] The Court developed a trimester framework to balance the woman's right to abortion against these governmental interests: during the first trimester, the decision must be left completely to the woman and her doctor; during the second trimester, a state could only regulate abortion if necessary to protect a woman's health; in the third trimester, generally after fetal viability, a government could regulate and even ban abortion to further its interest in the potentiality of life, but it must safeguard a woman's life and a woman's health.[17]

---

[10] 268 U.S. 510 (1925).

[11] *See, e.g.,* Moore v. East Cleveland, 431 U.S. 494, 500-06 (1977).

[12] *See, e.g.,* Lawrence v. Texas, 539 U.S. 558, 564 (2003).

[13] *See, e.g.,* Cruzan v. Dir., Mo. Dep't of Health, 497 U.S. 261, 342 (1990) (Stevens,]., dissenting); Planned Parenthood of Cent. Mo. v. Danforth, 428 U.S. 52, 71 (1976) (invalidating a requirement that a married woman obtain her husband's consent for an abortion).

[14] 410 U.S. 113 (1973).

[15] *See id.* at 155.

[16] *Id.* at 162.

[17] A case that accompanied *Roe, Doe v. Bolton,* explained that "health" must be understood "in light of all factors - physical, emotional, psychological, familial, and the woman's age - relevant to the well-being of the patient. All these factors may relate to health." Doe v. Bolton, 410 U.S. 179, 192 (1973).

In the years after *Roe,* the Court struck down most attempts to restrict the right to decide whether to have an abortion,[18] facilitating a woman's ability to control her reproduction, her health, and indeed the course of her life itself.

However, the Court's 1992 ruling in *Planned Parenthood of Southeastern Pennsylvania v. Casry* gave momentum to the strategy of chipping away at the constitutional right to abortion. In *Casry,* the Court was presented with the question of whether to overturn *Roe.* It did not. Instead, the Court expressly reaffirmed *Roe's* "essential holding"[19] that the Due Process Clause's guarantee that no individual shall be deprived of "liberty" applies to the decision of whether or not to have an abortion before viability.[20] Although it retained *Roe's* essential holding, the *Casry* Court announced a new standard of review for abortion restrictions. Instead of "strict scrutiny," the highest standard of review, *post-Casry,* courts must review abortion restrictions under the "undue burden" standard.[21] On this account, states may regulate abortion so long as the regulation does not have the purpose or effect of imposing a substantial obstacle in the path of a woman seeking to terminate a pregnancy. Additionally, the *Casry* Court abandoned the trimester framework, and instead adopted the viability framework and gave more weight to the government's interest in protecting "potential life."

After *Casry,* many state legislatures passed burdensome new restrictions on abortion intended to shame, pressure, and punish women who have decided to have an abortion. The stated intent of these laws was to promote potential life and ensure women's health, but the practical impact was to make it more difficult for women to obtain an abortion.[22]

In 2016, the Court addressed these efforts to make abortion care less accessible, by invalidating some of the most restrictive abortion regulations in *Whole Woman's Health v. Hellerstedt.* In that case, the Court issued a 5-3 ruling holding Texas restrictions that created medically unnecessary, burdensome facility and staffing restrictions to be an unconstitutional undue burden.[23] In concluding that the challenged Texas laws violated the Constitution, the Court emphasized that its

---

[18] *See, e.g.,* Planned Parenthood of Cent. Mo. v. Danforth, 428 U.S. 52 (1976) (invalidating a husband consent requirement, requirement that physicians preserve the life and health of the fetus at every stage of pregnancy, and a prohibition on a particular method of abortion); City of Akron v. Akron Ctr. for Reprod. Health, 462 U.S. 416 (1983) (invalidating a requirement that physicians give women anti-abortion information, a 24-hour mandatory delay requirement, a requirement that all abortions after the first trimester be performed in a hospital, a parental consent requirement, and a requirement related to the disposal of fetal remains).

[19] Planned Parenthood of Se. Pa. v. Casey, 505 U.S. 833,834 (1992).

[20] *Id.* at 846 ("Constitutional protection of the woman's decision to terminate her pregnancy derives from the Due Process Clause of the Fourteenth Amendment... The controlling word in the cases before us is 'liberty.'").

[21] *Id.* at 837.

[22] *See generally* GUTTMACHER INST., AN OVERVIEW OF ABORTION LAWS (May 1, 2019), https://www.guttmacher.org/state-policy/explore/overview-abortion-laws.

[23] *See id.* at 2311-18; *see also* Caitlin Gerdts, Liza Fuentes, Daniel Grossman, Kari White, Brianna Keefe-Oates, Sarah E. Baum, Kristine Hopkins, *Impact of Clinic Closures on Women Obtaining Abortion Services After Implementation of a Restrictive Law in Texas,* 106 AM.J. PUBLIC HEALTH 857, 860-63 (2016), https://ajph.aphapuhlications.org/doi/abs/10.2105/AJPH.2016.303134

finding of an undue burden did not depend on a single finding, but rather from the law's collective impacts. Although only one of the challenged laws had gone into effect in Texas while the litigation was pending, it had the effect of shuttering 54% of Texas facilities-reducing the number of clinics from 41 licensed facilities to 19.[24] A study by the Texas Policy Evaluation Project showed the clinic closures caused the average one-way distance to the nearest abortion provider to increase, and for 44% of this group, the new distance exceeded 50 miles.[25] As the Court noted, the laws posed an undue burden because they had the effect of shuttering clinics, increasing wait times and travel distances, and imperiling women's health.[26]

Further, in invalidating the challenged restrictions, the Supreme Court majority specifically noted that the undue burden standard was not a permissive endorsement of the state's purported rationales. Instead, reviewing courts were obliged to review the state's purported justifications and determine if the challenged restriction were appropriate measures to achieve these legislative ends.[27] In the case of the challenged Texas laws, the Court was emphatically clear that the state had failed to support its supposed "legitimate interest" in promoting women's health with any concrete evidence that the challenged laws served women's health.[28]

In *Whole Woman's Health,* the Supreme Court clarified how *Casrys* undue burden standard should be applied, and reaffirmed the letter and spirit of *Roe.* It once again made clear that the Constitution guarantees each individual the liberty and autonomy to decide whether to continue a pregnancy before viability, and, for that right to have any meaning, women must have access to abortion in practice.

This decisive rejection of medically unnecessary and unduly burdensome abortion laws in *Whole Woman's Health,* however, has not stopped state legislators from enacting such restrictions or lower courts from upholding them. Additionally, since this landmark ruling in 2016, the composition of the Court has once again changed. The addition of Justices Neil Gorsuch and Brett Kavanaugh suggests that the Court may be less willing to adhere to the tenets of *stare decisis* in reviewing abortion restrictions.

The Court's recent action in *June Medical Seroices v. Gee* is instructive on this point. In 2018, just two years after *Whole Woman's Health,* the U.S. Court of Appeals for the Fifth Circuit upheld a Louisiana restriction identical to the Texas admitting privileges law struck down in *Whole Women's Health.*[29] The petitioners, a Louisiana clinic, immediately petitioned the Court for review of the Fifth Circuit's decision. While

---

(discussing survey results from a Texas-resident women assessing travel burdens after the introduction of Texas House Bill 2 in 2013).

[24] Gerdts et al., *supra* note 23, at 857.

[25] *Id.*

[26] *See* Whole Woman's Health v. Hellerstedt, 136 S. Ct. 2292, 2316 (2016) ("At the same time, the record provides adequate evidentiary support for the District Court's conclusion that the surgical-center requirement places a substantial obstacle in the path of women seeking an abortion. The parties stipulated that the requirement would further reduce the number of abortion facilities available to seven or eight facilities, located in Houston, Austin, San Antonio, and Dallas/Fort Worth.").

[27] *Id.* at 2310.

[28] *Id.* at 2311 ("We have found nothing in Texas' record evidence that shows that ... the new law advanced Texas' legitimate interest in protecting women's health.").

the petition for review was pending, five justices of the Supreme Court voted to temporarily block the Louisiana law from going into effect.[30] If the challenged law went into effect, it would reduce the number of abortion providers in the state of Louisiana to just one.[31] Meaningfully, despite *Whole Women's Health* and other directly applicable precedents, the Court's newest members- Justices Kavanaugh and Gorsuch-would have allowed the Louisiana law to take effect, an action that would have eliminated abortion access for thousands of women across Louisiana.[32]

Whether It Is Regulated out of Existence or Overturned Outright, the Right to Abortion Is Imperiled

The changed composition of the Supreme Court, and that of federal courts around the country, have emboldened anti-abortion policymakers across the states to pass increasingly prohibitive, deliberately provocative, bans on abortion in hopes that these laws will be challenged all the way to the Supreme Court, prompting a reappraisal, and eventual overruling, of *Roe v. Wade.*

In recent weeks, anti-abortion lawmakers in several states-including Georgia, Louisiana, Alabama, Mississippi, and Missouri-have passed increasingly radical abortion bans, marking a dramatic escalation in the scope and tenor of abortion restrictions.[33] Whereas earlier abortion restrictions sought to undermine the abortion right by making health care services less accessible and more procedurally cumbersome, these most recent laws are more forthright in their aim to launch a frontal attack on *Roe v. Wade.* Buoyed by their sense that the federal judiciary is more amenable to their cause, the proponents of these laws nakedly announce their true intent-to prompt the Supreme Court to overturn *Roe v. Wade.*

The effort reflects the determination by anti-abortion legislators and advocates that now is the moment they have been building towards for over forty-five years. With two of President Trump's nominees pulling the Court further right, the anti-abortion foes consider that their moment really has come to once and for all overturn *Roe v. Wade.* Indeed, Alabama State Representative Terri Collins, who sponsored the Alabama abortion ban, explained that his "bill is about challenging *Roe v. Wade.*"[34]

---

[29] June Medical Servs. v. Gee, 905 F.3d 787 (5th Cir. 2018).

[30] June Med. Servs., L.L.C. v. Gee, 139 S. Ct. 663 (2019) (granting stay).

[31] June Medical Servs. v. Gee, 905 F.3d 787 (5th Cir. *2018),petition for cert. filed,* No. 18-1323, at 2 (U.S. Apr. 17, 2019).

[32] *See* 139 S. Ct. 663 (2019) (Kavanaugh, J., dissenting).

[33] Adam Liptak, *Path to Nullify* Roe v. Wade *a Little Bit at a Time,* N.Y. TIMES, May 16, 2019, at Al.

[34] Emily Wax-Thibodeaux, *Alabama Senate Passes Nation's Most Restrictive Abortion Ban, Which Makes No Exceptions for Victims of Rape and Incest,* WASH. POST (May 14, 2019), https: //www.washingtonpost.com/national/alabama-senate-passes-nations-most-restrictive-abortion-law-which-makes-no-exceptions-for-victims-of-rape-and-incest/2019/05/14/e3022376-7665-11e9-b3f5-5673edf2d127_story.html?utm_term=.1fd441c61bc9.

Another supporter of the bill, Alabama State Senator Clyde Chambliss, similarly asserted that the goal was "to go directly to the Supreme Court to challenge *Roe v. Wade.*"[35]

If the Court were to overturn *Roe* outright, the practical effects would be staggering. Women could be criminalized and punished in this country for having an abortion.[36] Twenty-two states would be at high risk for quickly making abortion illegal.[37] Access would erode even further in this country, leaving women living in large areas in the South and Midwest with potentially no legal access at all-a burden that would weigh most heavily on women of color, women struggling to make ends meet, immigrant women, and rural women in these states.

The fact that women would have to flee to other jurisdictions in order to access abortion highlights the degree to which overturning *Roe* would render women reproductive refugees who have been stripped of their dignity and equality as citizens. This would deprive many women of their dignity and autonomy.

Yet even if the Supreme Court did not overturn *Roe* as a formal matter, it could nonetheless uphold restrictive legislation, eviscerating abortion rights *sub rosa* and effectively rendering *Roe's* protections toothless. This would be the continuation of what we have seen over the last thirty years-abortion opponents' decades-long effort to gut *Roe* by an incremental "death by a thousand cuts."

Since 2011, politicians have passed over 400 new abortion restrictions in 33 states across the country.[38] These restrictions aimed to shut down abortion clinics and restrictions that shame, pressure, and punish women who have decided to have an abortion. Many of these laws restrict access to abortion by making the procedure more difficult or expensive to obtain, including requirements that a woman undergo a medically unnecessary ultrasound before obtaining an abortion,[39] requirements that a woman wait a significant amount of time before obtaining an abortion,[40] prohibitions on purchasing a comprehensive health insurance plan that includes coverage of abortion,[41] and medically unnecessary and burdensome facility and staffing requirements imposed on abortion clinics.[42]

---

[35] Daniel Trotta, *Alabama Senate Bans Nearly All Abortions, Including Rape Cases,* REUTERS (May 14, 2019), https://www.reuters.com/article/us-usa-abrtion-alabama/alabama-senate-bans-nearly-all-abortions-including-rape-cases-idUSKCN1SK13E.

[36] *See* SIA LEGAL TEAM, ROE'S UNFINISHED PROMISE: DECRIMINALIZING ABORTION ONCE AND FOR ALL 1-2 (2018), https://www.sialegalteam.org/roes-unfinished-promise.

[37] *See* CTR. REPROD. RTs., WHAT IF ROE FELL?, https://www.reproductiverights.org/what-if-roe-fell (last updated Feb. 21, 2019) (providing a state-by-state comparison of state laws threatening abortion rights).

[38] Elizabeth Nash et al., Policy Trends in the States, 2017, GUTTMACHER INST. (Jan. 2, 2018), https://www.guttmmacher.org/article/2018/01/policy-trends-states-2017.

[39] Eleven states now require women to undergo a medically unnecessary ultrasound before obtaining an abortion. GUTTMACHER INST., *Requirements for Ultrasound* (May 1, 2019), https://www.guttmacher.org/state-policy/explore/requirements-ultrasound.

[40] Twenty-seven states require that a woman wait at least 24 hours between receiving state-mandated counseling and obtaining an abortion. GUTTMACHER INST., *Counseling and Waiting Periods far Abortion* (May 1, 2019), https://www.guttmacher.org/state-policy/explore/counseling-and-waiting-periods-abortion.

[41] Eleven states now prohibit women from buying an insurance plan that includes abortion coverage, except in limited circumstances, in all private insurance plans written in the state. Twenty-six states

As we have seen over the last twenty years, this slow and steady strategy is incredibly effective. If the Texas restrictions challenged in *Whole Women's Health v. Hellerstedt* had been upheld, more than 75 percent of abortion clinics in Texas would have closed.[43] And even during the time in which one of the restrictions was in effect, several clinics were forced to close-and most have never reopened. The closure of these clinics has meant that the average one-way distance to the nearest abortion provider has increased four-fold.[44] In this regard, although they were eventually invalidated, the Texas restrictions nevertheless had devastating and irreversible effects on access to abortion and other essential health care.

Texas is not alone in this regard. Over the last ten years, the number of abortion providers and clinics has steadily decreased across the country, in part due to restrictive legislation, aggressive clinic protests, and unnecessary licensing requirements.[45] Currently, six states have only one abortion clinic within its borders.[46]

Critically, these laws go beyond undermining abortion to restrict access to other critical health care services, as clinics providing abortion care also typically provide a range of necessary reproductive health care services. As importantly, these clinics often provide care to underserved communities that are the least likely to have access to other health care providers.[47]

---

restrict coverage in the insurance exchanges. GUTTMACHER INST., *Restricting Insurance Coverage of Abortion* (May 1, 2019), https://www.guttmacher.org/state-policy/explore/restricting-insrance-coverage-abortion.

[42] Twenty-four states have laws that contain medically unnecessary facility and/or staffing requirements for abortion providers. GUTTMACHER INST., *Targeted Regulation of Abortion Providers* (May 1, 2019), https://www.guttmacher.org/state-policy/explore/targeted-regulation-abortion-providers.

[43] CTR. REPROD. R.Ts.., *Women's Health Care Providers Ask U.S. Supreme Court to Take On Texas Clinic Shutdown Law* (Sept. 03, 2015), https://reproductiverighrs.org/press-room/womens-health-care-providers-ask-us-supreme-court-to-take-on-texasclinic-shutdown-law.

[44] Gerdts et al., *supra* note 23, at 857.

[45] *See generally* Rachel K. Jones & Jenna Jerman, *Abortion Incidence and Service Availability In the United States, 2014,* 49 PERSPECTIVES SEXUAL & REPRODUCTIVE HEALTH 17 (2017), https://www.guttmacher.org/sites/default/files/article_files/abortion-incidence-us.pdf (examining the relationship between TRAP laws and decreased abortion service availability nationwide); Rachana Preadhan, Renuka Rayasam, & Mohana Ravindranath, *Even if Roe is Upheld, Abortion Opponents are Winning,* POLITICO (May 30, 2019), https://www.politico.com/story/2019/05/30/ abortion-opponents-winning-roe.-vs-wade-1488818 (last updated May 31, 2019) (describing the "piecemeal state laws" that have decreased abortion service availability).

[46] Preadhan, Rayasam, & Revindranath, *supra* note 45 ("Six states - Kentucky, Missouri, Mississippi, North Dakota, South Dakota and West Virginia - have only one clinic left that performs abortions[.]").

[47] Women of color have long experienced stark health disparities in areas like cervical and breast cancer, unintended pregnancy, pregnancy-related complications, and burdens to accessing safe abortion. Marcela Howell & Ann Starrs, *For Women of Color, Access to Vital Health Services Is Threatened,* HILL'S CONGRESS BLOG (July 27, 2017), https://www.guttmacher.org/artricle/2017/07/women-color-access-vital-health-services-threatened.

Restrictions on Legal Abortion Will Disproportionally Impact Communities That Already Face Barriers to Health Care, Economic Security, and Social and Political Equality

State laws that restrict abortion access disproportionately impact individuals struggling to make ends meet, women of color (particularly Black, Latinx/Latina, Asian American and Pacific Islander (AAPI), and Native people), rural women, immigrant women, individuals in the LGBTQ community, parents who already have children, and young people. However, the impact of restrictions on abortion on underserved communities cannot be understood in a vacuum. These communities already face multiple barriers to economic opportunity, health care and reproductive health care in particular. Thus, restrictions on abortion-and associated costs that such restrictions impose-make it difficult, and sometimes impossible, for a person in such communities to obtain an abortion. These restrictions jeopardize an individual's long-term economic security and have a negative impact on a person's equal participation in social and economic life by threatening financial well-being, job security, workforce participation, and educational attainment. In practice, these types of restrictions mean that *Roe* is merely an empty promise, not a reality for many living in these underserved communities.

For these most impacted communities, the consequences of being denied an abortion can be dire. Those who are denied access to abortion care have been found to suffer adverse physical and mental health consequences. For example, women denied abortion care are more likely to experience serious medical complications during the end of pregnancy.[48] They are also more likely to remain in relationships where interpersonal violence is present and are more likely to suffer anxiety.[49] Further, studies show that a woman who wants to get an abortion but is denied is more likely to fall into poverty than one who is able to obtain an abortion.[50] Therefore, the brutal irony is that those who face the biggest hurdles to health care and income security are the very individuals who will be most harmed by the state laws that restrict or even ban abortion access. And the impact of being denied such care further exacerbates the health and economic insecurity threats they face.

---

[48] Women of color have long experienced stark health disparities in areas like cervical and breast cancer, unintended pregnancy, pregnancy-related complications, and burdens to accessing safe abortion. Marcela Howell & Ann Starrs, *For Women of Color, Access to Vital Health Services Is Threatened,* Hill's Congress Blog (July 27, 2017), https://www.guttmacher.org/artricle/2017/07/women-color-access-vital-health-services-threatened.

[49] *See* Nat'l Women's L. CTR., Moving Women & Families Forward: A State Roadmap to Economic Justice 13-14, 53 (2015), https://nwlc.org/wp-content/uploads/2015/02/final_nwlc_2016_State Roadmapv2.pdf.

[50] *See* NAT'L LATINA INST. REPRODUCTIVE HEALTH, ¡SIN SEGURO, No MAS! WITHOUT COVERAGE, No MORE: LATINXS ACCESS TO ABORTION UNDER HYDE 2 (Oct. 2018), https://latinainstitute.org/sites/default/files/NLIRH_Hyde%20Amendment18_Eng_R3.pdf ("Research shows that one in four low-income women on Medicaid who seek abortion care is unable to afford to pay out-of-pocket cost and is forced to carry the pregnancy to term. A woman who wants to get an abortion but is denied is more likely to fall into poverty than one who can get an abortion."); *see also* TURNAWAY STUDY, *supra* note 48.

Taken together, the impact of these barriers results in a range of negative health outcomes. Take, for example, the crisis of preventable maternal mortality and morbidity that disproportionately affects Black and Native women. Black women in the United States die from pregnancy-related complications at a rate more than 3 times greater than that for white women, and American Indian and Alaskan Native women die at a rate of 2.5 times greater than that for white women.[51] There is a strong correlation between these negative health outcomes and state support for reproductive rights.[52] Many of the same states that have recently enacted extreme restrictions on abortion, including Louisiana, Georgia, Missouri, and Arkansas, have some of the highest maternal mortality ratios in the United States. Eliminating health care options for pregnant persons in these states will only exacerbate this crisis.

Barriers to health care and reproductive care go hand in hand with economic insecurity. The affordable housing crisis, food insecurity, the lack of clean water, the lack of affordable child care, the wage gap (a gap that widens significantly for women of color), the lack of paid family leave, a stagnant minimum wage, all of these issues lead to and compound economic insecurity for underserved communities across the country. And these barriers have only increased under President Trump, as his administration has engaged in a series of executive actions to undermine income security supports, including food security, housing, and Medicaid. The administration has also specifically targeted low- income immigrants by threatening to jeopardize their immigration status if they seek basic care and public benefits.

Only with a fuller picture of these multiple, intersectional, and compounding barriers to health and economic security can one fully understand the impact of these abortion restrictions on people of color. An individual seeking abortion care in states that have enacted restrictive abortion laws must navigate a state-created obstacle course. Last weekend, the *New York Times* reported on a recent study that found that over 11.3 million women of reproductive age live over an hour from an abortion clinic.[53] That's over two hours round trip. And in many places the travel time is even greater. What if you have kids and cannot get child care at a moment's notice? What if you cannot get the time off work? What if you do not have a car? This is what people are forced to manage, just to exercise their fundamental right to basic health care.

These obstacles are further compounded by the impact of health care insecurity and economic insecurity. Take for example, a woman who works a minimum wage

---

[51] Patti Neighmond, *Why Racial Gaps in Maternal Mortality Persist,* NAT'L PUB. RADIO (May 10, 2019), https://www.npr.org/sections/health-shorts/2019/05/10/722143121/why-racial-gaps-in-maternal-mortality-persist.

[52] CTR. Reprod. RTS. & IBIS Reprod. Health, Evaluating Priorities: Measuring Women's and Children's Health and Well-Being against Abortion Restrictions in the States 2017 Research Report 3, 16, 25 (2017), https://reprodnctiverights.org/sites/defaul/files/documents/USPA-lbis-Evaluating-Priorities-v2.pdf.

[53] K.K. Rebecca Lai & Jugal K. Patel, *For Millions of American Women, Abortion Access Is Out of &ach,* N.Y TIMES (May 31, 2019), https://www.nytimes.com/interactive/2019/05/31/us/abortion-clin.ics-map.html?action=click&module=Top%20Stories&pgtype=Homepage (discussing research from the Advancing New Standards in Reproductive Health project at the University of California, San Francisco).

job that provides neither paid leave nor health care. To seek an abortion in a state with a legislatively-imposed waiting period and only one clinic, she must take multiple days off from work at her own expense, identify child care for her children, and pay out of pocket for the abortion and associated travel costs to access a provider. Not surprisingly, these kinds of pressures are a strong deterrent to those seeking abortion care. For undocumented persons, many of whom cannot travel for fear of detention and deportation, there are even fewer options. Similarly, young people may be forced to go through judicial bypass procedures, forcing them to take additional time to appear in front of a judge before being allowed to access abortion care services-or they may be denied access altogether if a judge does not approve the decision to terminate a pregnancy.

These dire scenarios all show that these structural barriers to health care and economic security heighten the pressures that restrictive abortion laws impose on underserved communities. Indeed, in moving to restrict abortion, anti-abortion legislators make clear that they have no intention of addressing the structural barriers that impair the autonomy, dignity, and equality of these vulnerable communities. Instead, they have pursued a legislative agenda that makes these hardships more grave.

Conclusion

Reproductive rights are imperiled in the United States. Anti-abortion forces have set their sights on overturning *Roe v. Wade* with renewed vigor, confident that they will find a receptive audience in the Supreme Court. But even if the Court declines this invitation to overrule *Roe v. Wade,* unduly burdensome abortion restrictions continue to stymie and strangle access to abortion care. These issues are compounded for our most vulnerable communities.

Women, especially those in underrepresented communities, require government action-not to restrict the constitutional rights to which they are entitled, but to protect this fundamental right and those who seek to exercise it. If state legislators will not abandon their efforts to undermine and overrule *Roe v. Wade,* then Congress must act to secure the right to abortion for all.

Mr. COHEN. Thank you, Professor. Our next witness is Ms. Busy Philipps. She is a best-selling author, an actress, a writer, and a host of a late-night talk show. She has appeared in a number of movies and television shows. Last month she revealed in her talk show that she had had an abortion when she was a teenager. She has been a vocal advocate for abortion rights, a brave lady, and we recognize her for 5 minutes.

STATEMENT OF BUSY PHILIPPS

Ms. PHILIPPS. Chairman Cohen, Ranking Member Johnson, members of the subcommittee, thank you for having this important conversation and for inviting me to be a part of it. My name is Busy Philipps. I am many things. I am a mother of two wonderful girls, age 10 and 5. I am a professional actor for over 20 years. I am a New York Times best-selling author. I am a wife. I am a daughter. I am a talk show host and a volunteer for various children's charities and my kids' schools. I am a sister, and I am a best friend. I am also the 1 in 4 women in this country who have an abortion.

After the governor of Georgia signed Bill H.B. 481, which would ban abortion at 6 weeks, before most women know they are pregnant, I felt compelled to share my own story on my televisions and online. I had an abortion when I was 15 years old in my home State of Arizona in 1994. It was not a decision that I made lightly, but I have never for one moment doubted that it was the right decision for me. But so much has changed in Arizona and many other States since then. If I were that same 15-year-old in Arizona today, legally I would have to get parental consent. I would be forced to undergo a medically unnecessary ultrasound, go to a State-mandated in-person counseling session designed solely to shame me into changing my mind, and then take a State-mandated 24-hour timeout to make sure I really know what I wanted. And finally, I would be forced to give the State a reason why. Well, here is mine. It is my body, not the State's.

Women and their doctors are the ones that are in the best position to make informed decisions about what is best for them, no one else. Since I shared my story and I called on others to do so using the hashtag, #YouKnowMe, on social media, the response have been overwhelming. I have heard from thousands with their own stories, women who were raped, people who very much wanted children and had severe, severe fetal anomalies, women who were in an abusive relationship, people whose birth control failed or who simply were not ready. I also heard from many women who had abortions before abortion was legal in 1973, putting themselves in dangerous circumstances.

No bill that criminalizes abortion will stop from making this incredibly painful decision. These bans will not stop abortions from happening, but they will drive women and girls and people into the shadows, which is what this has always been about, shaming and controlling women's bodies. In the week after I shared my story on my show, women were coming up to me in the street, in the supermarket, at my gym, with tears in their eyes thanking me for my bravery. But the word "brave" didn't sit right with me. Why is it brave to speak to an experience that millions of people around the world throughout history have gone through? And then I realized it is considered brave because as women, we have been taught to feel shame about our bodies since birth. In my life, I have had many medical procedures, but no one has ever called me brave for talking about them. Abortion is healthcare and should not be treated as different from any other healthcare.

I am so sad that we have to sit here in front of a row of politicians and give deeply personal statements because the why doesn't matter. It should not matter. I am a human being that deserves autonomy in this country that calls itself free, and choices that a human being makes about their own bodies should not be legislated by strangers who can't possibly know or understand each individual's circumstances or beliefs. I am here today because I stand by the decision that I made when I was 15 years old. I am here today because my platform has allowed me to connect with thousands and thousands of people around the country that you represent, who have made the same choice I have made, but who will not all get the same chance to talk to you directly.

I am here today to help de-stigmatize a legitimate medical procedure and continue to encourage women not to allow themselves to be shamed for their choices. And finally, I am here today for my two little girls, Birdie and Cricket. My dream for them is that they will live in a world in which women are truly equal with complete control over their own reproductive health. That is the dream I hold for all people, regardless of their privilege or parents or what State they live in.

That dream is slipping further and further from reality with every ban passed. I hope that you, our elected leaders, can help us reverse the tide. Thank you. I look forward to today's discussion.

[The statement of Ms. Philipps follows:]

Chairman Cohen, Ranking Member Johnson, members of the subcommittee, thank you for having this important conversation, and for inviting me to be part of it.

My name is Busy Philipps.

I am many things. I am a mother to two wonderful girls, 10 and 5, I am a professional actor for over twenty years and a *New York Times* bestselling author. I am a wife and a daughter and a talk show host and a volunteer for various children's charities and my kid's schools. I am a sister and I am a best friend.

I am also the one in four women in this country who have had an abortion. After the Governor of Georgia signed bill HB 481, which would ban abortion at six weeks, before most women know they're pregnant, I felt compelled to share my own story on my late night TV show and online.

I had my abortion when I was 15 years old, in my home state of Arizona in 1994. It was not a decision I made lightly. But I have never for a moment doubted that it was the right decision for me.

But so much has changed — in Arizona and other states — since then.

If I were that 15 year old girl in Arizona today, legally I would have to get parental consent. I would be forced to undergo a medically unnecessary ultrasound, to go to a state-mandated in-person counseling, designed solely to shame me into changing my mind, then take a state-mandated 24-hour time out to make sure I really knew what I wanted. And finally, I would be forced to give the state a reason WHY.

Well, here is mine: my body belongs to me, not the state. Women and their doctors are in the best position to make informed decisions about what is best for them. No one else.

Since I shared my story and called on others to do the same using the hashtag #YouKnowMe on social media, the response has been overwhelming.

I have heard from hundreds of thousands with their own stories: women who were raped, women whose very wanted children had severe fetal anomalies, women who were in abusive relationships, women whose birth control failed or who simply weren't ready. I also heard from women who had abortions before abortion was legal in 1973, putting themselves in dangerous circumstances.

No bill that criminalizes abortion will stop anyone from making this incredibly personal decision. These bans will not stop abortion from happening. But they will drive women and girls into the shadows. Which is what this has always been about. Shaming and controlling women's bodies.

In the week after I shared my story on my show, women were coming up to me on the street, in the supermarket and at the gym with tears in their eyes, thanking me for my bravery. But the word bravery didn't sit right with me. Why is it brave to speak to an experience millions of people in the world throughout history have gone through? And then I realized. It is considered brave because as women we have been taught to feel shame about our bodies from birth.

In my life I have had many medical procedures. But no one has ever called me "brave" for talking about them. Abortion is health care, and should not be treated as different from any other health care.

I am sad that we have to come before a row of politicians and give these deeply personal statements. Because the WHY doesn't matter, it should not matter. I am a human being that deserves autonomy in this country that calls itself free. And choices that a human being makes about their own bodies should not be legislated by strangers who can't possibly know or understand each individual's circumstances or beliefs.

I am here today because I stand by the decision I made when I was 15. I am here today because my platform has allowed me to connect with thousands and thousands of people around the country who have made the same choice I made, but who will not all get the chance to come speak to you directly. I am here today to help destigmatize a legitimate medical procedure and continue to encourage women to not allow themselves to be shamed for their choices.

And finally, I am here today for my two little girls, Birdie and Cricket. My dream for them is that they will live in a world in which women are truly equal, with complete control over their own reproductive health. That is the dream I have for all women, regardless of their privilege or parents or what state they live in.

That dream is slipping further and further from reality, with every ban passed.

I hope that you, our elected leaders, can help us reverse the tide. Thank you, and I look forward to today's discussion.

Mr. COHEN. Thank you very much. Our next witness is Dr. Owen Phillips, a friend from Memphis, Tennessee, who has come to visit me on many occasions about these issues and others. She is a professor at the University of Tennessee Health Science Center in Memphis. She has held that position since 2002. She is a fellow in the American College of Obstetricians and Gynecologist and Board certified by the American Board of Obstetrics and Gynecology and the American Board for Medical Genetics.

She received her M.D. from the University of Mississippi School of Medicine in 1980. She did her residency in obstetrics and gynecology at the University of Mississippi Medical School, and her fellowship in reproductive genetics at the University of Tennessee in Memphis. She has also received a master's in public health degree, summa cum laude from the University of Memphis. She received her B.S. in chemistry from Millsaps.

Welcome. You are recognized for 5 minutes.

STATEMENT OF OWEN PHILLIPS, MD, FACOG

Dr. PHILLIPS. Thank you, Chairman Cohen. Chairman Nadler, Ranking Member Johnson, and members of the committee, thank you again for inviting me to speak with this subcommittee today. My name is Owen Phillips. I am an obstetrician/gynecologist from Memphis, Tennessee. I was asked to testify as to the barriers to care my patients experience because of existing restrictive abortion laws, and to predict what further challenges might arise if even more restrictive abortion regulations become law.

The first I can easily attest to. Tennessee has several laws that were passed under the guise of making abortion safer. None were backed by scientific evidence and all have fulfilled their real purpose: making a safe and legal procedure harder to obtain. The 48-hour wait period requires many women to travel long distances twice to the clinics for face-to-face consenting, adversely affecting their job and childcare. The requirement that physicians provide abortion care have hospital privileges has prevented many experienced doctors from caring for their patients.

My own hospital has bowed to perceived political pressure and severely limits the indication for abortions. None of these restrictions will likely prevent women from attaining the abortion they seek. They just make it harder for women to receive timely, efficient, and equitable abortion services.

To answer the second question, what effects would more restrictive laws have, is harder to answer. I have been practicing since the 1980s. I am not old enough to have personally witnessed the tragedies my physician teacher recalled prior to the Roe decision. No one knows what the consequences will be because almost all doctors practicing now have assumed that safe and legal abortion would always be an option for their patients.

Nevertheless, we physicians are fearful. Commonly a diagnosis of preeclampsia is made in our unit. By definition, this diagnosis is made after 20 weeks. This is a life-threatening condition for which the treatment is delivery. Abortion is often recommended, and the timing of which is made by the doctor with the patient. No politician's opinion should be a part of that medical and personal decision making, but this is where we seem to be headed. And I agree with the vice president of health policy at ACOG, who has opined that one contributing factor to the increasing rates of maternal mortality has been the favoring of fetal wellbeing over that of the patient.

Also typical of my experience is having the heartbreaking conversation with a couple that their pregnancy has a lethal condition, meaning the baby will die within the first few hours or days of life. The couple, after much anguish, may decide to have an abortion or may not, but who among us feels they have the right to make that decision for them? Not me, but I assume people sitting in some State legislatures or maybe even some of you feel that you do.

And it is not just OBGYNs who interface with the issue. The oncologist's decision to treat with cancer-curing drugs is affected by a woman's pregnancy. The cardiologists have to advise women that if they continue their pregnancy, they may or will die from their condition. It is a hard decision, but the woman may look at the young children she has and ask what is the right thing for them. I would never deem myself so arrogant to make this decision for a woman, yet politicians all over this country have decided that they have the right to do just that.

Is this a religious cause? You know, I understand religious conviction. I was raised a Southern Baptist. Was taught to live by the Bible's teaching, "love your neighbor as yourself" and "judge not lest ye be judged." But these laws are not about love and certainly not about refraining from judging others. Where is the ethical and moral high ground in risking a woman's life or wellbeing because she cannot make decisions about her own body, her family, and her wellbeing, whether or not to have a baby, or safely terminate her pregnancy?

Now, most of my patients may have medical conditions for pregnancy termination, but in my experience, every woman who makes this decision has a reason. Abortion is a part of healthcare and should remain safe, accessible, and legal without political interference. I agree with ACOG's recommendation that existing restrictive abortion laws should "be immediately repealed." These laws do not seek to make abortion safer. They instead seek to punish the healthcare systems and doctors who provide abortion care, and, above all, to punish the women who seek abortion services.

The decision to have an abortion should be a woman's decision in consultation with her doctor, period. Thank you.

[The statement of Dr. Phillips follows:]

June 4, 2019

Testimony from Dr. Owen Phillips to the Subcommittee on the Constitution, Civil Rights and Civil Liberties on Threats to Reproductive Rights in America

Thank you, Chairman Cohen and Ranking member Collins for inviting me to speak with the subcommittee today.

I am an obstetrician-gynecologist in Memphis Tennessee. I was asked to testify as to the barriers to care my patients experience because of existing restrictive abortion laws and to predict what further challenges might arise if even more restrictive abortion regulations become law.

The first, I can easily attest to. Tennessee has several laws that were passed under the guise of making abortion safer. None were backed by scientific evidence and all have fulfilled their real purpose-making a legal and safe procedure harder to obtain. The 48-hour wait period requires many women to travel long distances twice to the clinics for face to face consenting, adversely affecting their job and child care. The requirement that physicians providing abortion care have hospital privileges has prevented many experienced doctors from caring for patients. My own hospital has bowed to perceived political pressure and severely limits the indications for abortions. None of these restrictions will likely prevent women from obtaining the abortion they seek. They just make it harder for women to receive timely, efficient, and equitable abortion services.

To answer the second question, what affects would more restrictive laws have, is harder to answer.

I have been practicing since the 1980's. I am not old enough to have personally witnessed the tragedies that my physician teachers recalled prior to the Roe decision. No one knows what the consequences will be, because almost all doctors practicing now have assumed that safe and legal abortion would be an option for their patients.

Nevertheless, we physicians are fearful. Commonly, a diagnosis of preeclampsia is made in our unit; by definition this diagnosis is made after 20 weeks. This is a life-threatening condition for which the treatment is delivery. Abortion is often recommended and the timing of which is made by the doctor with the patient. No politician's opinion should be a part of the medical and personal decision-making. But this is where we seem to be headed. And, I agree with Dr. Barbara Levy, vice president of health policy at the American College of Obstetricians and Gynecologists who opined that one contributing factor to the increasing rates of maternal mortality has been the favoring of fetal well-being over that of the mother. Also, typical of my experience is having the heart-breaking conversation with a couple that their pregnancy has a lethal condition, meaning the baby will die within the first few hours or days of life. The couple, after much anguish, may decide to have an abortion. Or may not. But who among us feels they have the right to make that decision for them. Not me. But I assume people sitting in some state legislatures or maybe even some of you feel you do.

And, it is not just Ob-Gyns who interface with the issue. The oncologist's decision to treat with cancer-curing drugs is affected by a woman's pregnancy. The cardiologists have to advise women that if they continue their pregnancy, they may or will die from their condition. It is a hard decision. But that woman may look at the young children she has and ask what is the right thing for them, as any mother would. I would never deem myself so arrogant to make this decision for a woman. Yet, politicians all over this country have decided that they have the right to do just that.

Is this a religious cause? You know, I understand religious conviction. I was raised a Southern Baptist. I was taught to live by the Bible's teachings: love your neighbor as yourself and judge not lest ye be judged. But these laws are not about love and certainly not about refraining from judging others. Where is the moral high ground in risking a woman's life or well-being because she cannot make decisions about her own body, family and well-being, whether or not to have a baby or safely terminate her pregnancy?

Most of my patients may have medical indications for pregnancy termination, but in my experience every woman who makes this decision has a reason. Abortion is a part of healthcare and should remain safe, accessible and legal and without political interference. I agree with the American College of Obstetricians and Gynecologists recommendation that existing restrictive abortion laws "should be immediately repealed." These laws do not seek to make abortion safer. They instead seek to punish the health care systems and doctors who provide abortion care and above all to punish the women who seek abortion services. The decision to have an abortion should be the woman's decision in consultation with her doctor period.

Thank you.

Mr. COHEN. Thank you very much, Dr. Phillips. Our next witness is Christina Bennett. She is the communications director of the Family Institute of Connecticut. She has been active in the pro-life movement for 15 years. She is a licensed Christian minister and has served on prayer missions in a number of locations, including Washington, Atlanta, and several overseas countries. She has a B.S. in communications from Southern Connecticut State University.

Ms. Bennett, you are recognized for 5 minutes.

STATEMENT OF CHRISTINA BENNETT

Ms. BENNETT. Thank you, Chairman Nadler, Chairman Cohen, Ranking Member Johnson, and members of the committee. I am grateful for the opportunity to share my story with you today.

In 1981, my mother scheduled to abort me at Mount Sinai Hospital in Hartford, Connecticut. She was pressured by my father to abort and rejected by a mentor in her church who told her she wasn't welcome anymore because she was pregnant out of wedlock. She met with a counselor at the hospital who assured her she was making the right decision, but didn't offer counseling on available alternatives. A black elderly janitor approached my mother after seeing her crying in the hospital hallway. She asked her if she wanted to have her baby. My mother said yes. She told her that God would give her the strength to have me.

When she went to leave, my mother was called into the doctor's office, and she saw that he hadn't cleaned up the blood from the last abortion. She was disgusted and told him she wanted to keep me. He insisted that she go through with the abortion and said, "You have already paid for this. You are just nervous." She repeated, "I want my baby," and he yelled at her saying, "Do not leave this room." She felt his anger came from fear of losing her business and those that could possibly follow her, yet with courage she walked out.

Children conceived less than a decade prior to my birth never experienced the threat of death through legalized abortion. It is easy for people to say, "Well, I am glad your mother had a choice," but a statement like that devalues my existence and the reality of what that choice would have done to me. Human life should not be weighed in the balance of whether or not they are wanted or measured in terms of circumstances or convenience. I deserved legal protection and a right to life.

My mother's experience is similar to the experiences I have heard from women throughout this country, women who faced the same rejection, pressure, lack of counseling, lack of support, and disgusting facility conditions. My desire to assist women and children led me to work for years at a nonprofit pregnancy resource center, and there I witnessed the power of hope and the ways in which love and practical support can strengthen women and their families.

Two years ago I had a profound experience while visiting the National Museum of African-American History. I was reminded of the ways black Americans were denied the right to equal protection and due process, treated as property, and dehumanized because of the color of our skin. The museum memorialized the many ways black Americans have been unjustly targeted and killed for centuries. And while I rejoice over the progress that we have made as people of color, an ache remains in my heart because of the denial of equal protection and due process to another class of people: the baby in the womb.

The sacrifices my ancestors suffered to achieve the civil rights I enjoy today are not able to protect future generations because of legalized abortion. I am burdened that the Fourteenth Amendment, which gave us liberty, was unjustly used to invent a supposed right to destroy a human life. Sojourner Truth in her day said, "Am I not a woman?," and in mine I say, "Am I not a person?" Abortion is not a victimless act. We just can't hear the voices of those who have been silenced and discarded.

Roe v. Wade rendered 60 million lives unworthy of legal protection and had led to the deaths of 20 million black babies since 1973. In the dark history of Planned Parenthood, founder Margaret Sanger's philosophy of eugenics was recently documented by Supreme Court Justice Thomas in his concurring opinion about Fox v. Planned Parenthood. And today, an increasing number of black Americans recognize this eugenic population control philosophy that is having a genocidal impact.

Seventy-eight percent of Planned Parenthood surgical facilities are located in black and Latino neighborhoods, and black women, such as Cree Erwin, Lakisha Wilson, and Tonya Reaves, have lost their lives at the hand of an abortion industry that offered them substandard medical care. Others have left by ambulance, suffered botched procedures, and been left with physical and emotional scars. And we are tired of the targeting and the lies that abortion is an answer to our challenges.

As a pro-life feminist, I support body autonomy, but abortion impacts two bodies. I am a unique individual, and just as my heart is beating today, it was beating inside of my mother's body. I was not just a part of her body. And liberation never comes through oppressing other human beings. Roe v. Wade was built on lies that Norma Mccorvey spent her entire life trying to correct. We can love both women and children and strive for a society that treats us all with the dignity we deserve, and this is true empowerment.

[The statement of Ms. Bennett follows:]

Christina Bennett
Director of Communications
Family Institute of Connecticut
June 4, 2019
Threats to Reproductive Rights in America

Dear Chairman Nadler, Chairman Cohen, Ranking Member Johnson and members of the committee:

My name is Christina Bennett and I'm submitting this testimony in hopes that my personal story will shed light on the issue of abortion in America. In 1981 my mother scheduled to abort me at Mount Sinai Hospital in Hartford, CT. She was pressured by my father to abort and rejected by a mentor in her church who told her she wasn't welcome anymore because she was pregnant out of wedlock. She met with a counselor at the hospital who only assured her she was making the right decision and did not offer counsel on available alternatives.

A black elderly janitor approached my mother after seeing her crying in the hospital hallway. She asked her if she wanted to have her baby and when she said yes, she told her God would give her the strength to have me. When she went to leave my mother was called into the doctor's office where she could see he hadn't cleaned up the blood from the last abortion which disgusted her. He insisted she stay and when she said she wanted to keep me he said, "You've already paid for this. You're just nervous." She repeated her desire to keep me and he yelled at her screaming "Don't leave this room," but she walked out. My mother's experience in that hospital is being repeated every day that abortion is performed in this nation. Women are facing the same coercion, the same shunning, the same lack of counseling and disgusting facility conditions.

Unfortunately, many women lack a compassionate advocate to offer them the support and resources they need. This is why I spent four years working at a non-profit pregnancy resource center, practically serving hundreds of women and their children.

Two years ago, I had a profound experience while visiting the National Museum of African-American History. I was reminded of the ways Black Americans were denied the right to equal protection and due process, treated as property and dehumanized because of the color of our skin. The museum memorialized the many ways Black Americans have been unjustly targeted and killed for centuries. While they showcased examples of the progress Black Americans have made, an ache remains in my heart because of the denial of equal protection and due process to another class of people – the baby in the womb. The sacrifices my ancestors suffered to achieve the freedom and civil rights I enjoy today are not able to protect future generations from a decision made just 8 years before my birth. The Roe v

Wade decision rendered 60,000,000 lives unworthy of legal protection and has led to the deaths of over 20 million Black babies since 1973.[54]

Babies conceived just a decade prior did not experience the threat of death through legalized abortion. Their lives were not weighed in the balance of whether or not they were wanted. The value of their lives was not measured in terms of their parents' challenging circumstances or convenience.

The dark history of Planned Parenthood founder Margaret Sanger's philosophy on Eugenics and population control was documented by Supreme Court Justice Clarence Thomas' concurring opinion in Box v. Planned Parenthood in Indiana and Kentucky. Today, an increasing number of Black Americans recognize this eugenic and population control philosophy that is having a genocidal impact.

Recently close to a hundred black women of influence-gathered in Charlotte, NC to protest the stealth opening of a Planned Parenthood in the city's oldest Black neighborhood. Along with my testimony I've attached a statement from Lesley Monet, International Director of The Church of God in Christ's Family Life Campaign. Lesley explains the largest Black denomination with over 6 million members' opposition to the abortion industry's targeting of Black babies and the Church's program to protest abortion and encourage adoption.

Many of us are tired of the targeting. 78% of Planned Parenthood's surgical facilities are located in Black and Latino neighborhoods.[55] Black women such as Cree Erwin, Lakisha Wilson, and Tonya Reaves have lost their lives at the hands of an abortion industry that offers substandard medical care as increasingly women are leaving abortion centers by ambulance.[56]

Taking the lives of our children through abortion doesn't empower or strengthen our communities. Abortion has left behind countless wounded women and men as it silenced millions of children who otherwise would have had a voice and lived out the purpose for their life.

Mr. COHEN. Thank you, Ms. Bennett. Ms. BENNETT. You are welcome.

Mr. COHEN. Ms. Melissa Ohden is an anti-abortion activist. In 2012, she founded the Abortion Survivors Network and has previously testified before the U.S. House of Representatives and the U.S. Senate. She has worked as a speaker for Feminists for Life. You are recognized for 5 minutes.

STATEMENT OF MELISSA OHDEN

Ms. OHDEN. Chairman Cohen, Chairman Nadler, Ranking Member Johnson, members of the committee, I just want to thank you for inviting me to this hearing.

As a now famous saying goes, "Women's rights are human rights." I am here today to give a face and a voice to women whose rights are not just being

---

[54] Centers for Disease Control and Prevention, Abortion Surveillance-United States, 2011, available at: http://www.cdc.gov/mmwr/preview/mmwrhtml/ss6311a1.htm?s_cid=ss6311a1_w.

[55] https://www.protectingblacklife.org/pp_targets/index.html.

threatened, but have been under attack for the past 46 years in our country, and are clearly being even more heavily threatened as abortions throughout all 9 months of pregnancy with no restriction are being introduced and celebrated in States like New York, Illinois, and now Nevada.

Today you have heard countless stories already about how abortion is a difficult, yet necessary, decision, how every woman has the fundamental right to abortion. Every story is important. Every experience deserves to be heard. However, when we hear the stories about abortion, this narrative is woefully one-sided. Our culture has been inundated with messaging in which abortion controls the narrative, yet largely ignored in this abortion narrative that is woven so skillfully throughout our culture, behind even the words in the title of this hearing, "Reproductive Rights," are stories buried beneath the narrative of abortion that has been sewn since Roe v. Wade.

Is there space for stories like mine, women who are alive today after surviving failed abortion procedures? For stories like my biological mother's, who have been coerced or forced into an abortion? Do we ever create space for the stories of women who regret their abortions? The most important stories, though, are those that you will likely never hear, the stories of the little girls who will never live outside of the womb. In all of this discussion about women's rights, some lose sight of the fact that without the right to life, there are no other rights. This is the greatest human rights issue we are facing as a country.

And I am here to tell you that in August of 1977, that is when the attack on my human rights began. My biological mother as a 19-year-old college student had a saline infusion abortion forced upon her by her own mother, a prominent nurse in their community, with the help of her friend and colleague, the local abortionist, Dr. Kelberg. That abortion procedure involved injecting a toxic salt solution into the amniotic fluid surrounding me in the womb. It was meant to poison and scald me to death. I soaked in that toxic salt solution over a 5-day period as they tried time and time again to induce my birth mother's labor with me.

When I was finally expelled from the womb on that 5th day of the abortion procedure, my arrival into this world was not so much as a birth, but an accident, a live birth after a saline infusion abortion. My medical records actually state a saline infusion for an abortion was done, but was unsuccessful. This record is available to you to review along with some other records that talk about how a complication of my birth mother's pregnancy was a saline infusion.

Despite the arguments being made that people like me don't exist or that children aren't left to die after failed abortions, I need you to listen to the words of a nurse who have been connected with who was there that day. I was initially laid aside after my grandmother instructed the nurses to leave me to die, and arguments ensued about whether would be provided medical care. In the words of Nurse Jan, who received me in the NICU that day, a tall, blonde nurse courageously rushed me off, shouting out, "She just kept gasping for breath. And so I couldn't just leave her there to die."

---

[56] https://www.sba-list.org/negligence.

My medical records state that when I was delivered alive in that abortion procedure, I suffered from severe respiratory problems, jaundice, seizures. I weighed a little less than 3 pounds. I was 2 pounds, 14 ounces, which led a neonatologist to remark in my records that I was approximately 31 weeks gestation as opposed to the 18 to 20 weeks that the abortionist had written on my medical records. It is easy to talk about women's reproductive rights until you recognize that without first the right to life, there are no other rights. How do you reconcile my rights as a woman, who survived a failed abortion, with what is being discussed here today?

The abortion industry talks in abstract and gray when it comes to the science of when life begins and what abortion does, but the reality is much clearer. I am alive today because someone else's reproductive right failed to end my life, as are the 287 abortion survivors I have connected with through my work in the Abortion Survivors Network. One hundred and eighty-four of them are female. There is something wrong when someone's right results in another person's death. There is something deeply disturbing about the reality in our world that I have a right to an abortion, but I had never the simple right to live.

As you examine the so-called threat to women's reproductive rights, I would ask you to look behind the language and see stories like mine that are hidden, that might seem inconvenient or rare, and consider there is more to this discussion. And there is more to be done to protect our most vulnerable constituents and meet the needs of women and families in our communities in a way that supports life at all stages of development and in all circumstances, not ends it.

[The statement of Ms. Ohden follows:]

Melissa Ohden

MSW, Founder & Director, The Abortion Survivors Network

June 4, 2019

House Judiciary, Subcommittee on the Constitution, Civil Rights and Civil Liberties

Chairman, Representative Steve Cohen

Representative Cohen and Members of the Subcommittee, thank you for inviting me to this hearing titled "Threats to Reproductive Rights in America."

As the now-famous saying goes, "women's rights are human rights."

I'm here today to give a face and a voice to women whose rights are not just being threatened, but have been under attack for the past forty-six years in our country. And, are clearly being even more heavily threatened as abortion throughout all nine months of pregnancy, with no restriction, are being introduced and celebrated in states like New York, Illinois and now, Nevada.

Today, you will hear countless stories, I suspect, about how abortion is a difficult, yet necessary decision; how every woman has the fundamental right to abortion.

Every story is important. Every experience deserves to be heard.

However, when we hear stories about abortion, the narrative is woefully one-sided. Our culture has been inundated with messaging in which abortion controls the narrative.

Yet, largely ignored in the abortion narrative that is woven so skillfully throughout our culture, behind even the words in the title of this hearing, "reproductive rights," are stories buried beneath the narrative of abortion that has been sewn since Roe v. Wade.

Is there space for stories like mine, women who are alive today after surviving failed abortion procedures; for stories like my biological mother's, women who have been coerced or forced into an abortion? Do we ever create space for the stories of women who regret their abortions?

The most important stories, though, are likely the ones that you'll never hear. The stories of the little girls who will never live outside of the womb. In all of the discussion about women's rights, some lose sight of the fact that without the right to life, there are no other rights. This is the greatest human rights issue we are facing as a country.

In August of 1977, the attack on my human rights began. My biological mother, as a nineteen-year-old college student, had a saline infusion abortion forced upon by her mother, a prominent nurse in their community, with the help of her colleague, the local abortionist, Dr. Kelberg.

This abortion procedure involved injecting a toxic salt solution into the amniotic fluid, that was meant to poison and scald me to death. I soaked in that toxic solution over a five day period as they tried time and time again to induce my birthmother's labor with me.

When I was finally expelled from the womb on that fifth day of the abortion procedure, my arrival into this world was not so much as a birth, but an accident, a "live birth" after a saline infusion abortion. My medical records actually state, "a saline infusion for an abortion was done, but was unsuccessful." I've included this record for you to review, along with another that identifies a complication of my birthmother's pregnancy as a saline infusion.

Despite the arguments being made that people like me don't exist or that children aren't left to die after failed abortions, listen to the words of a nurse who I've been connected with who was there that day. I was initially "laid aside," after my grandmother instructed nurses to leave me to die, and arguments about whether I would be provided medical care, ensued.

In the words of Nurse Jan, who received me in the NICU that day, "a tall blond nurse," courageously rushed me off to the NICU, shouting out, "she just kept gasping for breath, and so I couldn't just leave her there to die!"

My medical records state that the doctors initially suspected I had a fatal heart defect due to the high level of distress I presented with. I suffered from severe respiratory problems, jaundice, and seizures. I weighed in at 2 pounds, 14 ounces, which is what led a neonatologist to remark in my medical records that I was approximately 31 weeks gestation, as opposed to the 18-20 weeks that the abortionist had indicated.

It's easy to talk about women's reproductive rights until you recognize that without first the right to life, there are no other rights. How do you reconcile my rights as a woman who survived a failed abortion with what's being discussed here today?

The abortion industry talks in abstract and gray when it comes to the science of when life begins and what abortion does, but the reality is much clearer.

I'm alive today because someone else's "reproductive right" failed to end my life, as are the 287 abortion survivors I've connected with through my work with The Abortion Survivors Network, 184 of whom are female.

There's something wrong when one person's right results in another person's death. There's something deeply disturbing about the reality in our world that I have a right to an abortion but I never had the simple right to live.

The 14th Amendment says that "nor shall any State deprive any person of life, liberty, or property, without due process of law; nor deny to any person within its jurisdiction the equal protection of the laws." But with states passing laws that state a "fertilized egg, embryo or fetus does not have independent rights," aren't states participating in the deprivation of life? Are states providing equal protection to all children? I don't think so. Each of you as a legislator has sworn to provide equal protection to your constituents under the law.

As you examine the so-called "threat to women's reproductive rights," I would ask for you to look behind the language and see the stories that are so often hidden, the stories that may seem inconvenient or even rare to you, and consider that there's more to this discussion.

And there's more to be done to protect your most vulnerable constituents and meet the needs of women and families in our communities in a way that supports lives at all stages of development and in all circumstances, not ends it.

Mr. COHEN. Thank you. Ms. Jennifer Dalven is the director of the American Civil Liberties Union Reproductive Freedom Project. In that role, she oversees and directs the ACLU's litigation, State advocacy, and communications work on issues affecting access to reproductive health services. Prior to that she was on the staff with the ACLU for more than 10 years and then in private practice. She graduated magna cum laude from the NYU School of Law and served as law clerk for the Honorable Pierre Leval of the U.S. Court of Appeals for the Second Circuit.

You are recognized for 5 minutes.

STATEMENT OF JENNIFER DALVEN

Ms. DALVEN. Chairman Cohen, Chairman Nadler, Ranking Member Johnson, and members of the subcommittee, thank you for inviting me to testify today. My name is Jennifer Dalven, and I am the director of the ACLU's Reproductive Freedom Project.

I have been litigating abortion cases for more than 2 decades, and I am here to tell you that today we are facing a crisis. Since March, seven States have passed laws banning abortion, and make no mistake about it. This has happened because President Trump was able to put two new justices on the Supreme Court, and abortion opponents believe that this new Court will take an extraordinary step of actually taking away one of our constitutional rights.

That is a very real and very frightening possibility, but here is the thing. The Court doesn't have to overturn Roe v. Wade in order for States to push abortion entirely out of reach. That is because these bans are just the culmination of a decades-long strategy, a strategy to pile restriction on top of restriction in order to make it near impossible for a person to get an abortion if they need one.

Congress started by passing the Hyde Amendment, which bans coverage for people insured through Medicaid. Representative Hyde openly admitted what his goal was, that it was to prevent people with low incomes from being able to get abortion care they needed. State legislatures followed suit, and since the 2010 elections, States have quietly passed 479 medically unnecessary restrictions on abortion care.

Lawyers at the ACLU, Planned Parenthood, and the Center for Reproductive Rights are challenging dozens of these restrictions in court. And while litigation is a powerful tool, it alone cannot stop the avalanche of restrictions. The unfortunate truth is that these restrictions have severely eroded access to care, so much so that for many today in our country, abortion is already more theoretical than real. This is particularly true for people with low incomes, people of color, immigrants, young people, and LGBTQ people.

Kentucky is a good example of what is happening around the country. In the 1970s, there were 17 places in Kentucky where a person could get an abortion if they needed one. Today because of hostile State action, there is only one, and Kentucky isn't alone. Six States have only a single abortion provider, and several more have only two or three. And yet there are efforts in Kentucky, Missouri, and other places to shut down even those last clinics. Like many others, Kentucky's governor, Governor Bevin, has been trying to use bogus health regulations to end abortion care in his State, and he would have been successful, but the sole clinic, EMW Women's Surgical Center, refused to abandon its patients. Instead, the ACLU and EMW rushed to court to get an emergency order stopping the governor from shutting down the clinic. After trial, the Court found that the governor's regulations "resulted in no benefit to patients." All they would do is make it impossible for a person to get an abortion in the State. But unfortunately, the State appealed, and so the clinic's ability to keep caring for patients remains in jeopardy.

Now, this was a prime strategy used before 2019, using phony health regulations to prevent people from getting abortions. But since Justice Kavanaugh's confirmation, States are increasingly dropping the pretense. Now they are making a claim to what their goal has been along, which is to ban abortion entirely. Now, of course these laws have never been motivated by a concern for women or families. If they were, Georgia wouldn't have one of the highest maternal mortality rates in the country, a rate that is 3 times higher for black women than it is for white women. If they were concerned about women and children, two-third of Alabama counties would not lack a hospital that provides obstetrical care. If they were concerned about children, Alabama wouldn't have one of the highest infant death rates in the country. But instead of addressing these problems, these States are passing blatantly unconstitutional abortion bans.

Now, we must fight those bans and we are, but at the same time, States are also continuing to quietly regulate away abortion access. It is happening in Missouri, which is on the verge of forcing the last clinic in the State to stop providing abortion care. It is happening in Louisiana where, unless the Supreme Court steps in, there will be only a single doctor left in the entire State eligible to provide abortion care. And it is happening in Alabama where but for lawsuits brought by the ACLU on behalf of doctors, like Dr. Robinson, every single clinic in the State would have been forced to close. That is why Congress must pass the Women's Health Protection Act. That bill would safeguard against not only outright bans, but also clinic shutdown laws and other restrictions that prevent people from getting care.

As the mother of two fabulous children, I know that the decision about whether to become a parent is one of the most important ones we make in our lives. It is the job of our government to ensure that we can actually make real decisions, whether that is to continue a pregnancy or to end it, in a way that is best for ourselves and our families. Thank you.

[The statement of Ms. Dalven follows:]

STATEMENT OF JENNIFER DALVEN, DIRECTOR, REPRODUCTIVE FREEDOM PROJECT, AMERICAN CIVIL LIBERTIES UNION, FOR A HEARING ON THREATS TO REPRODUCTIVE RIGHTS IN AMERICA, BEFORE HOUSE JUDICIARY COMMITTEE, SUBCOMMITTEE ON THE CONSTITUTION, CIVIL RIGHTS, AND CIVIL LIBERTIES, JUNE 4, 2019

Chairman Cohen, Ranking Member Johnson, and Members of the Committee,

Thank you for holding this hearing and inviting me to testify. My name is Jennifer Dalven and I am the Director of the Reproductive Freedom Project at the American Civil Liberties Union, where I oversee litigation seeking to protect and expand access to abortion and reproductive health care. We are honored to bring that litigation on behalf of abortion providers and their patients, including Dr. Yashica Robinson, an obstetrician-gynecologist from Alabama who is on the panel today as well. I am proud to testify today on behalf of our nearly three million members, activists and supporters.

I have been litigating abortion rights cases for more than two decades and have argued cases throughout the country, including before the United States Supreme Court.[57] I am here to tell you that we are facing a crisis.

---

[57] *Ayotte v. Planned Parenthood of Northern New England*, 546 U.S. 320 (2006).

In recent months, seven states--Alabama, Georgia, Kentucky, Louisiana, Mississippi, Missouri, and Ohio--have passed extreme laws banning abortion, aimed at prompting the Supreme Court to reverse *Roe v. Wade.*[58] Legislators in these states, emboldened by President Trump's appointment of two new Justices to the Supreme Court, believe that the newly-constituted Court will take the extraordinary step of actually taking away one of our constitutional rights. While it is important to note that today, abortion is still legal in every state, as these bans have been or will soon be challenged in court and have not taken effect,[59] the prospect that *Roe* may be overturned is a very real and very frightening possibility.

However, it's also critical to understand that the Supreme Court doesn't have to overturn *Roe* in order for states to push abortion entirely out of reach. That is because these bans are the culmination of a decades'-long strategy to pile restriction on top of restriction in order to make it nearly impossible for people to get an abortion.

Congress started in on that strategy shortly after *Roe* was decided, when it first attached the Hyde Amendment to an appropriations bill to withhold coverage for abortion for people insured through Medicaid. Representative Henry Hyde openly admitted this was designed to prevent people with low incomes from getting abortions. When he first introduced his amendment in 1976, he said "I certainly would like to prevent, if I could legally, anybody having an abortion, a rich woman, a middle-class woman, or a poor woman. Unfortunately, the only vehicle available is the...Medicaid bill."[60] His plan worked. It is estimated that one in four Medicaid-eligible women seeking an abortion is unable to get one,[61] which can have devastating consequences for themselves and their families.[62]

State legislatures followed suit, passing a variety of medically unnecessary and politically motivated laws designed to make it impossible for people to access care. This trend picked up alarming speed after the 2010 elections. Since then, states

---

[58] 410 U.S. 113, 163-64 (1973). *Roe*'s central holding been applied and reaffirmed repeatedly for over four decades, including in *Planned Parenthood v. Casey*, 505 U.S. 833, 871 (1992), and most recently in *Whole Woman's Health v. Hellerstedt,* 579 US (2016).

[59] The laws in Kentucky and Mississippi have been enjoined in cases brought by the ACLU and the Center for Reproductive Rights, respectively. See Alan Blinder, *Federal Judge Blocks Mississippi Abortion Law*, NY Times (May 24, 2019), https://www.nytimes.com/2019/05/24/us/mississippi-abortion-law.html. Challenges have also been filed in Ohio and Alabama by the ACLU and Planned Parenthood. The ACLU has also announced its intention to challenge Georgia's ban.

[60] Heather Boonstra, A*bortion in the Lives of Women Struggling Financially: Why Insurance Coverage Matter*s, Guttmacher Policy Review (July 14, 2016), https://www.guttmacher.org/gpr/2016/07/abortion-lives-women-struggling-financially-why-insurance-coverage-matters.

[61] Henshaw SK, et al., *Restrictions on Medicaid Funding for Abortions: A Literature Review*, Guttmacher Institute, 2009, http://bit.ly/1IK5XcF; *see also* Board of Governors, Federal Reserve System, *Report on the Economic Well-Being of U.S. Households in 2018* (May 2019) at *21*, https://www.federalreserve.gov/publications/files/2018-report-economic-well-being-us-households-201905.pdf?smid=nytcore-ios-share (finding that nearly 40% of Americans would have difficulty covering an unexpected expense of $400).

[62] Foster DG, Roberts SCM, and Mauldon J, *Socioeconomic consequences of abortion compared to unwanted birth*, 2012, http://bit.ly/1PvNd4w.

have quietly passed 479 abortion restrictions.[63] The ACLU is currently challenging more than 30 such restrictions in 14 states. Planned Parenthood and the Center for Reproductive Rights are challenging dozens more.

The laws pushed by abortion opponents include laws known as Targeted Regulations of Abortion Providers (TRAP) that place burdensome requirements on abortion providers that are not placed on other health care providers, such as requirements that they obtain admitting privileges at local hospitals, or that their clinics meet the same standards as ambulatory surgical centers. As courts around the country have found, these laws do not actually make patients safer, and are intended to and do force providers to shut their doors. Indeed, in June 2016, in *Whole Woman's Health v. Hellerstedt*, the Supreme Court struck down two such Texas requirements noting that although the laws would decimate access to abortion, it "found nothing in Texas' record evidence that shows that ... the new law advanced Texas' legitimate interest in protecting women's health."[64]

Despite this ruling, not even three years later, the United States Court of Appeals for the Fifth Circuit upheld a nearly identical Louisiana law,[65] and a petition for review is currently pending before the Supreme Court in that case brought by the Center for Reproductive Rights.[66] That law was patterned after the Texas law and designed to shut down clinics. Indeed, if that law is allowed to stand there would only be a single doctor left in the entire state eligible to provide abortions.

States have also passed a wide range of other laws that create unnecessary obstacles for patients, such as forced ultrasound laws and requirements that patients make unnecessary additional trips to the clinic at least 24 to 72 hours before an abortion. Because TRAP laws have caused many clinics to shut down, patients are often forced to travel hundreds of miles to get to the closest abortion provider, posing significant financial and logistical hurdles for patients seeking abortion care, 75% of whom are poor or low-income.[67] These requirements mean that a person must attempt to take additional days off work (losing needed income), attempt to arrange and pay for childcare, find and pay for transportation, and, in some cases lodging. It is not uncommon for patients seeking abortion care to have to sleep in their cars overnight near the clinic because they lack the means to stay in a hotel. For many people, these barriers prevent them from obtaining an abortion at all.[68]

In addition, hostile state legislatures have passed laws that would criminalize providers for providing the only generally available method of ending a pregnancy in the second trimester. Like every other court in the country to consider a challenge to

---

[63] Elizabeth Nash, *Unprecedented Wave of Abortion Bans is an Urgent Call to Action*, Guttmacher Policy Review (May 31, 2019) https://www.guttmacher.org/article/2019/05/unprecedented-wave-abortion-bans-urgent-call-action.

[64] 579 US__(2016).

[65] *June Med. Servs. v. Gee*, No. 17-30397 (5th Cir. 2019).

[66] *June Med. Servs. v. Gee*, Dkt. 18-1323.

[67] Jerman J, Jones RK and Onda T, *Characteristics of U.S. Abortion Patients in 2014 and Changes Since 2008,* Guttmacher Institute (May 2016), https://www.guttmacher.org/report/characteristics-us-abortion-patients-2014.

[68] *See, e.g., Planned Parenthood of Indiana and Kentucky* v. *Box*, 896 F.3d 809 (7th Cir. 2018) (cert. pet. pending).

such a law, the United States Court of Appeals for the Eleventh Circuit, in a case brought by the ACLU, held Alabama's law was unconstitutional.[69] However, Alabama has asked the Supreme Court to review that decision.

These are just some examples of the types of laws that state legislatures have passed that make it difficult, and in some cases impossible, for a person who has decided to have an abortion to actually get one. Indeed, these restrictions have so severely eroded access to care that already for many people the right to abortion is more theoretical than real. This is particularly true for people who face multiple barriers to accessing quality health care, including people with low incomes, who are more likely to be people of color, as well as young people and LGBTQ people.[70]

Kentucky is a prime example of how severely access has already been limited by the avalanche of restrictions. Shortly after *Roe was* decided, there were 17 locations in Kentucky where a person could get an abortion.[71] Today, there is only a single clinic left standing.[72] Yet Governor Bevin, like many politicians opposed to abortion rights, has attempted to use bogus health regulations to force even that last clinic, EMW Women's Surgical Center, to close. Although the clinic had a transfer agreement with a local hospital signed by the head of the hospital's ob-gyn department, the state argued that it needed an agreement signed by the CEO of the hospital, which it could not get in part due to political pressure from the Governor's office. Refusing to abandon its patients, EMW rushed to court seeking an emergency order to keep its doors open. In the end, the court struck down Kentucky's requirement, finding that the transfer agreement "resulted in no benefit" to patients.[73] All it would do is make it impossible for a person to get an abortion in the state. That case is now on appeal, leaving the clinic's ability to continue seeing patients in jeopardy.

Before 2019, opponents of abortion frequently tried to pretend that restrictions like Kentucky's were put in place to protect women's health. Of course, that claim has always been a farce. After all, some of the states that have passed the most aggressive abortion restrictions also have the most abysmal records when it comes to maternal and infant health outcomes.[74] Georgia has one of the highest maternal mortality rates in the country,[75] with a rate for Black women three times higher than

---

[69] *West Ala. Women's Ctr. v. Marshall*, 900 F.3d 1310 (11th Cir 2018).

[70] *See, e.g.,* Samantha Artiga et al., *Changes in Health Coverage by Race and Ethnicity since Implementation of the ACA, 2013-2017,* Kaiser Family Foundation (Feb 13, 2019), https://www.kff.org/disparities-policy/issue-brief/changes-in-health-coverage-by-race-and-ethnicity-since-implementation-of-the-aca-2013-2017/.

[71] *EMW Women's Surgical Ctr v. Glisson*, 2018 WL 6444391, *9 (Sept. 28, 2018).

[72] *Id.*

[73] *Id.* at *28.

[74] *See, e.g.,* Erika Edwards, *States pushing abortion bans have higher infant mortality rates*, NBC News (May 24, 2019), https://www.nbcnews.com/health/womens-health/states-pushing-abortion-bans-have-higher-infant-mortality-rates-n1008481.

[75] Joseph P. Williams, *Limiting Access to Abortion Could Cause Maternal Deaths to Rise*, U.S. News and World Report (May 31, 2019), https://www.usnews.com/news/healthiest-communities/articles/2019-05-31/reduced-access-to-abortion-could-lead-to-more-maternal-deaths; *see also Maternal Mortality*, America's Health Rankings, https://www.americashealthrankings.org/explore/health-of-women-and-children/measure/maternal_mortality/state/GA (*last accessed* June 1, 2019).

the rate for white women.[76] In Alabama, two-thirds of the counties do not even have a hospital that provides obstetrical care.[77] Alabama also has one of the highest infant death rates in the country.[78] The politicians in these states, while focused on banning women's medical decisions, have failed in their duty to ensure that people who want to have babies can be pregnant and give birth safely.

Now, with the most recent bans, states like Alabama and Georgia have dropped the pretense about women's health entirely. They are making plain what their goal *has always been*: to ban abortion entirely.

Americans are rightly incensed by the passage of these laws which expressly force people to stay pregnant against their will. We must fight these bans, and we are. But, while the headlines are focused on the bans, its important to keep in mind that states are also continuing to quietly regulate away abortion access in the same manner that they have for years.

In fact, medically unnecessary regulations like the one EMW faced in Kentucky are threatening to close clinics throughout the South and Mid-West. Six states today have only a single provider left—Kentucky, Mississippi, Missouri, North Dakota, South Dakota, and West Virginia.[79] Several others have only a handful. And Missouri is at risk of becoming the first state since *Roe* was decided to be without a health center that provides abortions.[80] In Louisiana, unless the Supreme Court steps in in a case brought by the Center for Reproductive Rights, there will only be a single doctor left *in the entire state* eligible and able to provide abortion care.[81] In Alabama, but for lawsuits brought by the ACLU on behalf of providers, every single clinic in the state would have been forced to close.[82] In Ohio, the state has been slowly going after clinics one by one, using regulation after regulation, to force clinics to shut their doors. And the list goes on.

Although litigation is a powerful tool, we cannot always count on the courts to stop these laws. And, I have seen firsthand the impact on patients. I have seen a clinic have to turn away patients who were sitting in the waiting room when a

---

76 Georgia Maternal Mortality Report 2014, Georgia Department of Public Health (March 2019) https://dph.georgia.gov/sites/dph.georgia.gov/files/related_files/site_page/Maternal%20Mortality%20 BookletGeorgi a.FINAL_.hq_.pdf.

77 Jessica Ravitz, *Alabama says it wants to protect life. How does that claim stack up outside the womb?*, CNN (May 16, 2019), https://www.cnn.com/2019/05/16/health/alabama-treatment-ofliving/index.html; *In Rural Alabama, Limited Access To Obstetrics Care*, NPR (May 31, 2015), https://www.npr.org/2015/05/31/411044409/in-rural-alabama-limited-access-to-obstetrics-care.

78 Michael Hiltzik, *States with the worst anti-abortion laws also have the worst infant mortality rates*, LA Times (May 15, 2019), https://www.latimes.com/business/hiltzik/la-fi-hiltzik-anti-abortion-infant-mortality-20190515-story.html.

79 Sabrina Tavernise, '*The Time Is Now': States Are Rushing to Restrict Abortion, or to Protect It*, NY Times (May 15, 2019), https://www.nytimes.com/2019/05/15/us/abortion-laws-2019.html?module=inline.

80 Reis Thebault, *Judge's order means Missouri hasn't yet become the only state without an abortion clinic*, Washington Post (May 31, 2019), https://www.washingtonpost.com/nation/2019/05/31/missouri-could-become-only-state-without-clinic-perform-abortions-pending-judges-ruling/?utm_term=.481ef653fe51.

81 *June Med. Servs. v. Gee*, Dkt. 18-1323.

82 *West Alabama Women's Ctr. v. Miller*, 299 F. Supp. 3d 1244 (M.D. Ala. 2017); *W. Alabama Women's Ctr. v. Williamson*, 120 F. Supp. 3d 1296, 1317 (M.D. Ala. 2015); *Planned Parenthood Southeast v. Strange*, 33 F. Supp. 3d 1330 (M.D. Ala. 2014).

restriction unexpectedly went into effect. I have seen a clinic unable to care for a patient who had been referred by a hospital in another state because we did not get a court ruling in time. And research tells us that being denied a wanted abortion has serious consequences for people and their families. For example, people who were unable to get a wanted abortion are more likely to experience serious health complications associated with pregnancy,[83] to remain tethered to abusive partners;[84] and to experience increased economic insecurity.[85]

In order to ensure that people have not only the theoretical right to abortion but the actual ability to get the care they need, Congress must act. We urge Congress to pass the Women's Health Protection Act, which would provide a powerful federal safeguard against not only outright bans, but also against clinic shut down laws and other restrictions that prevent people from getting the care they need.[86] In addition, Congress should pass the EACH Woman Act, which would lift the Hyde Amendment and related bans on abortion coverage in government insurance programs, and also put an end to political interference in private insurance markets by prohibiting federal, state, and local politicians from meddling with insurance companies that choose to cover abortion.[87] Together, these bills would both keep clinic doors open and make care more affordable. They would protect and expand access for people throughout the country, no matter where they live, how much they make, or what type of insurance they have.

There is overwhelming public support for abortion access. According to the recent polling, two-thirds of Americans do not want to see *Roe* overturned.[88] And a majority of voters agree that everyone should have health insurance that covers reproductive healthcare, including abortion.[89] They agree that once a person has

---

[83] Gerdts C, Dobkin L, Foster DG and Schwarz EB, *Side Effects, Physical Health Consequences, and Mortality Associated with Abortion and Birth after an Unwanted Pregnancy*. Women's Health Issues 25(1):55-59 (Jan. 2016).

[84] Roberts SCM, Biggs MA, Chibber KS, Gould H, Rocca CH and Foster DG, *Risk of Violence From the Man Involved in the Pregnancy After Receiving or Being Denied an Abortion*, BMC Medicine 12:144 (Sept. 2014).

[85] Foster DG, Biggs MA, Ralph L, Gerdts C, Roberts S and Glymour MM, *Socioeconomic Outcomes of Women Who Receive and Women Who Are Denied Wanted Abortions in the United States*, Am. J. Public Health 108(3):407-413 (Mar. 2018); *See also Socioeconomic outcomes of women who receive and women who are denied wanted abortions,* ANSIRH Issue Brief (Aug. 2018), www.ansirh.org/sites/default/files/publications/files/turnaway_socioeconomic_outcomes_issue_brief_8-20-2018.pdf (For women denied a wanted abortion, there was an almost fourfold increase in odds that their household income was below the Federal Poverty Level compared to those who were able to obtain a wanted abortion).

[86] Women's Health Protection Act, H.R. 2975, 116th Cong. (2019).

[87] EACH Woman Act, H.R. 1692, 116th Cong, (2019).

[88] Jennifer DePinto, *Majority of Americans don't want Roe v. Wade overturned, CBS News poll finds*, CBS News (May 21, 2019), https://www.cbsnews.com/news/majority-of-americans-dont-want-roe-v-wade-overturned-cbs-news-poll-finds/.

[89] *New polling shows voters see the impact of abortion coverage on women's economic opportunities and security*, Hart Research Associates (Oct. 18, 2017), https://allaboveall.org/wp/wp-content/uploads/2017/10/Economic-Opportunity-and-Reproductive-Health-Polling-Memo-October-2017.pdf.

decided to have an abortion, they should be able to get care that is supportive and affordable without additional obstacles.[90]

As the mother of two fabulous children, I know that the decision about whether and when to become a parent is one of the most important ones we make in our lives. It's incumbent upon our government to enable us to make these decisions in a way that is best for ourselves and our families. That is critical to ensuring that people and families thrive and that everyone in our community can participate with freedom, dignity, and equality.

Mr. COHEN. Thank you. Our next witness is Dr. Yashica Robinson, attending physician in the Department of Obstetrics and Gynecology at the Alabama Women's Wellness Center of Huntsville, Alabama, where she has worked since 2005. She is a fellow of the American Congress of Obstetricians and Gynecologists and a National Health Service Corps Scholar from 2000 to 2013. She received her M.D. from Morehouse School of Medicine, a recipient of three scholarships. She has a B.A. in chemistry, magna cum laude, from Talladega College. She did her residency in obstetrics and gynecology at the University of Alabama School of Medicine.

Dr. Robinson, thank you, and you are recognized for five minutes.

STATEMENT OF YASHICA ROBINSON

Dr. ROBINSON. Thank you. Thank you, Chairman Cohen, Ranking Member Johnson, and members of the subcommittee. My name is Dr. Yashica Robinson. I serve on the board of Physicians for Reproductive Health and I am an obstetrician-gynecologist in Alabama. I have a busy obstetrics practice where I provide prenatal care, deliver babies, and treat mothers after they have given birth. I also provide abortion care at Alabama Women's Center.

I provide abortion care because I believe that patients deserve the full spectrum of care. I came to this work because of my passion for young people that is deeply connected to my personal experience as a teen mother. Prior to finishing high school I learned that I was pregnant, and as a result of fear and lack of resources, by the time I confided in my mother and grandmother, I had no choice—I was going to be a mother.

Becoming a mother as a teenager came with many harsh realities. I love my children dearly, but I know that everyone should be able to make that decision for themselves. I have been in the shoes of many of the young people that I see in my clinic, and it is important for them to know that regardless of their decision, that I am here to support them.

Providing abortion care in Alabama is challenging, but it is also deeply satisfying. I am proud to provide compassionate, quality care when patients enter our doors, but

---

[90] *See, e.g., Analysis of Voters' Opinions on Abortion Restrictions and Affirmative Policies*, PerryUndem Research/Communication (Jan. 20, 2016), https://www.nirhealth.org/wp-content/uploads/2016/01/Memo-NIRH-Poll_Final_3.pdf.

I know all too often that getting to our doors comes with many unnecessary obstacles. People have to travel long distances to come to our clinic. They receive outdated state-mandated information, and then they are required to wait an additional 48 hours before I can provide them the care they need.

Low income patients have an exceptionally hard time. These obstacles increase the overall cost of care, including costs related to transportation, lodging, missing work, and child care. I know that patients have slept in their cars overnight because they had no other options.

Alabama also has a 20-week abortion ban, and patients needing care after that point have to travel out of state, which further increases costs. And young people have to navigate an onerous, timeintensive process to have an abortion if they cannot involve a parent. I have cared for a 12-year-old who faced numerous delays before getting the final judicial approval necessary to proceed with the abortion she needed. Though I met her in her first trimester of pregnancy, she was well into the second trimester and nearly at the legal limit for being able to obtain an abortion in the State of Alabama by the time she navigated all of these hurdles.

The near total ban on abortion that recently passed in Alabama, H.B. 314, imposes a 99-year prison sentence for a physician unless it is agreed that the abortion is needed for the necessary for the life or meets an extremely narrow exception for the health of the woman. This ban, should it ever go into effect, would be disastrous for Alabamians. H.B. 314 is blatantly unconstitutional and would force doctors like me to choose between what is ethically, medically appropriate care, and being criminalized. There is no other area of medicine where we have legislation threatening physicians with criminal prosecution for simply doing their jobs.

Alabama is already a state with an unconscionably high maternal and infant mortality rate. Nearly two-thirds of Alabama counties lack hospitals that offer obstetrical care. Moreover, the number of pregnancy-related deaths across the country is steadily increasing, and in Alabama, black women are nearly five times more likely to die of pregnancy-related complications than white women. Without access to safe abortion care, maternal mortality rates will rise even more.

By attempting to criminalize abortion providers we endanger women and we harm communities that are already lacking health care providers. This law will make doctors' often split-second judgment calls potential criminal acts. This lack of autonomy may deter new physicians from coming to areas that already have a shortage of physicians and may cause others to leave.

Alabama legislators made it very clear, their ultimate goal is to outlaw abortion, period. This is dangerous, as the consequences extend far beyond that. It will affect all providers who take care of pregnant women, not just abortion providers. Women and their doctors need to have access to the full spectrum of care as they manage undesired and complicated pregnancies. Regardless of how you feel about abortion, we cannot tie the hands of health care providers.

Though H.B. 314 has not taken effect it is negatively impacting patients already. I wish that you all could hear how worried patients are. One young lady told me of the nightmares that she had prior to coming in to the clinic because she felt that she would be denied services because of these restrictive laws. In addition to legal obstacles, providers and patients face constant harassment. To enter the clinic or my obstetrics practice, patients have to walk through a line of protestors who yell hateful, dehumanizing, sometimes racially charged things. The hostility that we endure is completely unacceptable and has gotten worse in the past few years. Recently, a protestor attempted to run over a volunteer with their vehicle. Needless to say, this harassment is unheard of for my colleagues who work in other fields of medicine.

The bottom line is this: abortion is health care. Alabamians deserve better. I urge elected officials to show empathy for the lived experiences of people who need health care, be it abortion, miscarriage management, or prenatal care, for they are all connected. Health care should remain patient-centered, and all medical decisions should remain between a patient and her physician, without any political interference.

Thank you.

[The statement of Ms. Robinson follows:]

TESTIMONY OF YASHICA ROBINSON, MD, BEFORE THE HOUSE JUDICIARY COMMITTEE SUBCOMMITTEE ON THE CONSTITUTION, CIVIL RIGHTS, AND CIVIL LIBERTIES, JUNE 4, 2019

Good morning Chairman Cohen, Ranking Member Johnson, and members of the Subcommittee. My name is Dr. Yashica Robinson, I serve on the board of directors of Physicians for Reproductive Health. I am very happy to have the opportunity to speak with you today. I'm an obstetrician-gynecologist in Huntsville, Alabama. I have a busy obstetrics practice where I provide prenatal care, deliver babies, and treat mothers after they give birth. I also provide abortion care at Alabama Women's Center in Huntsville. I provide abortion care because I believe patients deserve the full spectrum of care. However, it is extraordinarily difficult for many people in Alabama to access abortion services, and it will only get worse as women's rights and access to abortion care continue to be threatened.

I came to this work because of my passion for young people, one that is deeply connected to my personal experience with teen pregnancy. Prior to finishing high school, I learned I was pregnant. As a result of fear and lack of resources, by the time I confided in my mother and grandmother, I had no choice—I was going to be a mother. Becoming a mother as a teenager came with many harsh realities. I love my children with all my heart, but I know that everyone should be able to make the decision to parent for themselves. I have been in the shoes of many of the young people I see in my clinic, and it's important for them to know that regardless of their decision, that I am here to support them.

Providing abortion care in Alabama is challenging, but also deeply satisfying. I am proud to provide patients with compassionate, quality care when they enter our doors, but I know all too well that getting to our doors comes with too many unnecessary obstacles. Abortion clinics are being forced to close at an alarming rate.

People have to travel long distances to come to our clinic. They receive outdated state mandated information, then they are required to wait an additional 48 hours before I can provide the care they need. Low income patients have an exceptionally hard time. Alabama prohibits public funding for abortion, so people with Medicaid have no coverage for abortion care. State law also restricts private insurance coverage of abortion and allows employers to deny insurance coverage for reproductive health services, making abortion unaffordable for too many people. These politically sanctioned obstacles increase the overall cost for care, which also includes costs relating to transportation, lodging, missing work, and childcare. I know of patients who have slept in their cars because they have no other options.

Alabama also has a ban on abortion after 20 weeks gestation. Patients needing care after that point have to travel out of state, making the care even more expensive. And young people have to navigate an onerous, time-intensive process to have an abortion if they cannot involve a parent. I have cared for a 12yo victim of incest who faced so many obstacles and delays before getting the final judicial approval necessary to proceed with the abortion she needed. Though I met her in her first trimester of pregnancy, she was well into the second trimester and nearly at the legal limit for being able to obtain an abortion in the state of Alabama by the time she navigated all of these hurdles.

The National Academies of Sciences, Engineering and Medicine (NASEM) published a comprehensive study concluding that abortion is extremely safe and finding that the biggest threat to patient safety is the litany of medically unnecessary regulations that raise costs and delay procedures, ultimately putting women's health at risk. They confirmed what we already know: that access to safe abortion care all too often depends on where you live and your socioeconomic status.

Over the years, Alabama Women's Center has been forced to comply with onerous, medically-unnecessary building requirements—similar to those that were held unconstitutional by the Supreme Court in 2016 in the *Whole Women's Health v. Hellerstedt* case. The local anti-abortion group even sued the zoning board to try to force us to close. This same group then drafted legislation making it illegal to operate an abortion clinic within 2,000 feet of a school—another law specifically designed to shut our facility down. A federal district court held that law unconstitutional, as well, recognizing it was nothing more than a thinly veiled attempt to try to push abortion out of reach for patients. And this is just a small sample of the politically-motivated restrictions we have to contend with.

The near total ban on abortion that recently passed in Alabama, HB 314, imposes a 99-year prison sentence for a physician determined to have caused an abortion, unless it is agreed the abortion is necessary for the life or meets an extremely narrow exception for the health of the woman. This ban, should it ever go into effect, would be disastrous for Alabamians. HB 314 is blatantly unconstitutional and would force doctors like me to choose between what is ethical, medically appropriate care, and being criminalized. There is no other area of medicine where we have legislation threatening physicians with criminal prosecution for doing their jobs.

Alabama is already a state with unconscionably high maternal and infant mortality rates. According to the Alabama Department of Public Health (ADPH) nearly two-thirds of Alabama counties lack hospitals that offer obstetrical care. Moreover, the number of pregnancy-related deaths across the country has steadily increased. In Alabama, Black women are nearly five times more likely to die from pregnancy-related causes than white women. There are many pre-existing conditions that can be made worse by pregnancy, and other serious health conditions can be caused by pregnancy. We know that racial disparities in health care are exacerbated by policies that make accessing health care more challenging. Without access to safe abortion, maternal mortality rates will rise even more.

By attempting to criminalize practitioners who provide abortion care, we will have the unintended consequence of endangering women and harming communities that are already suffering from lack of health care providers. This law will make doctor's (often) split second judgment calls potential criminal acts. This law compounds the complex scenarios that obstetricians routinely balance as they try to make the best decisions they can about managing complicated pregnancies. The lack of autonomy that this law imposes on physicians may deter new physicians from coming to areas that have a shortage of physicians and may cause others to leave. Alabama legislators made it very clear, their ultimate goal is to outlaw abortion, PERIOD. This is dangerous, as the consequences extend far beyond that. It will affect ALL providers who take care of pregnant people, not just abortion providers. Abortion care is health care and pregnant people and their doctors need to have access to the full spectrum of options as they manage undesired or complicated pregnancies. Regardless of how you feel about abortion, we cannot tie health care providers' hands because of individuals' objection to a medical procedure for political gain.

Though HB 314 has not taken effect, it is negatively impacting patients. I wish you all could hear how worried patients are. One told me of the nightmares she had prior to coming to the clinic about being turned away and denied services because of these restrictive laws.

In addition to legal obstacles, providers and patients face constant harassment. To enter either Alabama Women's Center or my obstetrics practice, patients have to walk through a line of protestors who yell hateful, dehumanizing, sometimes racially charged things. The hostility and intimidation we endure is unacceptable and has only gotten worse in the past few years. Recently, a protestor attempted to run over a volunteer with their vehicle. Thankfully, the volunteer is okay, but this underscores the security concerns for abortion providers in the South. Needless to say, this harassment is unheard of for my colleagues who work in other fields of medicine.

The bottom line is this: Abortion care is healthcare! Alabamians deserve better. I urge elected officials to stop trying to make it harder for people to access full spectrum health care. Instead, show empathy for the lived experiences of many Alabamians and people in other states who continue to need health care—be it abortion, miscarriage management, or pregnancy care, for they are all connected. All aspects of healthcare should remain patient-centered, and medical decisions should remain between the patient and her physician, without political interference.

Thank you.

Mr. COHEN. You are welcome. I notice several of you seem shocked by the—we are used to it here. It was the ghost of Shirley Chisholm expressing her upset about the need for this hearing. [Laughter.]

Mr. COHEN. Now I would like to recognize H.K. Gray, who is an activist with Youth Testify, a program for the Advocates for Youth and the National Network of Abortion Funds. She wrote an opinion piece in Teen Vogue on abortion rights.

You are recognized for five minutes.

STATEMENT OF H. K. GRAY

Ms. GRAY. Good morning and thank you to the chairman and ranking member for this opportunity to share my story and bring to light the very real ways restrictions to abortion access threaten our ability to make autonomous reproductive health decisions and raise the families we want.

My name is HK Gray. I am 18 years old and I came here today all the way from Fort Worth, Texas. I am an activist with Youth Testify, a leadership program through Advocates for Youth and the National Network of Abortion Funds. It is an honor to be able to speak before you today.

I became pregnant for the first time when I was 15 and had my daughter shortly after I turned 16. Immediately upon finding out I was pregnant, I knew I would continue the pregnancy. Despite a bit of preterm labor, my baby arrived right on time. She is in her terrible twos now and I love her. I am fortunate to have the incredible support of my fiancé, but becoming a parent has also had challenges, like losing my friends and not being able to attend school. I have been on my own for a few years now because my father is homeless and my mother was incarcerated. They weren't in situation to support me legally, financially, or emotionally. I know they love me, but they are unable to parent me the way I need them to, and the State requires.

After having my daughter, I tried to get a Paragard IUD, but I was unable to because in Texas, in order to get birth control, I need my parent's consent, something I couldn't get due to my parents' situations. And although my doctor was sympathetic, she couldn't legally give it to me.

A few months later, I became pregnant again, but I miscarried. Ten months after giving birth to my daughter, I realized I was pregnant for a third time. When I told my fiancé, we both knew what the other was feeling. We couldn't afford a second child, and it was harder when I had to go back to work a week after having my daughter because I didn't have paid parental leave. Adoption wasn't the right decision for us because if I continued the pregnancy I would have wanted to parent, and the WIC, SNAP, and Medicaid programs aren't enough as it is.

When I tried to get an abortion, I didn't realize how hard it would be. Texas requires parental consent for anyone under 18 years old. It is not that my parents would have opposed to my decision, it is that they weren't physically able to give the consent. This was a new concept to me because it is something I didn't have to do when I had my daughter. It seemed weird to me that I didn't need anyone's permission to become a parent, but I needed to prove to the state that, as a parent, I was mature enough to not have another child.

Thankfully, I found Jane's Due Process, an organization that helped me find a clinic and connected me to a lawyer who would walked me through the judicial bypass process. I had to get an ultrasound to take to court and prove how far along I was.

A few weeks later, when I finally went to court, it was a long day and honestly it was very hard on me. The judge said some hurtful things about me being sexually active, being a young parent, and wanting an abortion. I felt shamed no matter which decision I made. The judicial bypass process is a burden and barrier to abortion access.

My actual abortion was pretty straightforward. The providers were kind and treated me like an adult, and I was glad to get back home to care for my daughter. The irony of this whole experience is that I could make medical decisions for my daughter, but not for myself. When I take my daughter to see a doctor, I am treated like an adult, but I couldn't get routine care at the dentist or get birth control without my parents' permission.

I believe we need more support in this country for young women and transgender people who want to be able to access birth control or want to parent, or want an abortion, or like me, needed all of those things at different times in my teenage years.

Government restrictions on abortion hurt those of us who have fewer resources, or people of color or undocumented or living with disabilities or poor or queer. In Texas, the State prohibits all types of health insurance from covering abortion care and we have to pay out of pocket. I couldn't afford my abortion, but thankfully a family member lent me the money.

Like me, most people seeking abortions are already parenting and are balancing paying for child care, food, and rent. In Texas, 96 percent of counties do not have abortion clinics, impacting nearly half of Texas women. We have to figure out how to take time off work or school to travel to get an abortion, find some place to stay, and pay for all. We are forced to listen to government-mandated, medically inaccurate counseling, and wait 24 hours and go to the doctor twice before getting an abortion.

Unlike me, the majority of people who have abortions are people of color, and we must respect their decisions. I wish there was more support for people of color who are impacted by these restriction harder than I am. We need more love and compassion for families and young people like me. I had a child, I had a miscarriage, and I had an abortion.

As we say at the National Network of Abortion Funds, "Everyone loves someone who had an abortion." Thank you for your time. I hope my story helps you remember these laws that you pass impact your constituents, like me, and your loved ones who have had abortions.

[The statement of Ms. Gray follows:]

Testimony Submitted to House Committee on the Judiciary Subcommittee on the Constitution, Civil Rights, and Civil Liberties, June 3, 2019, via Electronic Transmission

Good morning and thank you to Chairman Cohen and Ranking Member Johnson for this opportunity to share my story and bring to light the very real ways restrictions to abortion access threaten our ability to make autonomous reproductive health decisions and raise the families we want.

My name is HK Gray. I am 18 years old and I came here today all the way from Fort Worth, Texas to share my abortion story with you. I am an activist with Youth Testify, a leadership program through Advocates for Youth and the National Network of Abortion Funds. It is an honor to be able to speak before you today.

I became pregnant for the first time when I was 15 and had my daughter shortly after I turned 16. Immediately upon finding out I was pregnant, I knew I would continue the pregnancy. Despite a bit of preterm labor, my baby arrived right on time. She's in her terrible twos now and I love her. I am fortunate to have the incredible support of my fiance but becoming a parent has also had challenges, one of the hardest parts, for me, was losing my friends and not being able to attend school. I've been on my own for a few years now because my father is homeless and my mother was incarcerated. They weren't in a situation to support me legally, financially, or emotionally. I know they love me, but they're unable to parent me the way I need them to, and the state requires.

After having my daughter, I tried to get a Paragard IUD, but I was unable to because in Texas, in order to get birth control, I need my parent's consent - something I couldn't get due to my parents' situations.

And, although my doctor was sympathetic, she couldn't legally give it to me. It was an awkward conversation; here I was a parent, but I needed my own parents in order to get healthcare to prevent an unintended pregnancy. These ridiculous legal barriers made it so my doctor wasn't able to provide me with the birth control best for my situation and, of course, led me to need my abortion.

A few months later, I became pregnant again, but I miscarried. Ten months after giving birth to my daughter, I realized I was pregnant for a third time. When I told my fiancé, we both knew what the other was feeling. We couldn't afford a second child, let alone go through an entire pregnancy. It was hard enough when I had to go back to work a week after having my daughter because I didn't have paid parental leave. Raising a child is a joy, but it's also expensive and challenging. I was just starting to get the hang of raising my daughter, and wasn't ready for another. Adoption wasn't the right decision for us because if I were to continue the pregnancy, I would have wanted to raise my child and I simply couldn't afford it. The WIC, SNAP, and Medicaid programs aren't enough as it is. We decided that an abortion was the right decision for us.

When I tried to get an abortion, I didn't realize how hard it would be. Texas requires parental consent for anyone under 18 years old. It's not that my parents would have opposed to my decision, it's that they weren't physically able to give the consent. This was a new concept to me because it's something I didn't have to do when I had my daughter. It seemed weird to me that I didn't need anyone's permission to become a parent, but I needed to prove to the state that, as a parent, I was mature enough to *not* have another child.

So, I started the process of getting a judge's approval through a judicial bypass which was long and complicated. I found Jane's Due Process an organization that helped me find a clinic and connected me to a lawyer who would walk me through the process. I had to get an ultrasound to take to court and prove that I was pregnant and how far along I was. My lawyer explained the process and we started discussing my story to build my case; we talked about what kind of mom I am, the situation with my parents, and why I needed an abortion.

A few weeks later, when I finally went to court, it was a long day and honestly it was very hard on me. The judge said some hurtful things about me being sexually active, being a young parent, and wanting an abortion. I felt shamed no matter which decision I made.

The whole ordeal took over two hours. It was frustrating that it was weeks after I first tried to get an abortion. Forced parental involvement laws create extra barriers to abortion access and cause delays and increase the costs we pay for an abortion. The judicial bypass process is a burden and barrier to abortion access.

My actual abortion was pretty straightforward. The providers were kind and treated me like an adult, and I was glad to get back home to care for my daughter. The irony of this whole experience is that I could make medical decisions for my daughter, but not for myself. When I take my daughter to see a doctor, I'm treated like an adult, but I couldn't get routine care at the dentist or get birth control without my parents' permission.

I believe we need more support in this country for young women and transgender people who want to be able to access birth control or want to parent or want an abortion, or like me, needed all of those things at different points in my teenage years. We should be respected and trusted no matter what decision we make. Young people deserve to be heard and deserve to be leaders on reproductive health, rights and justice issues. We can tell you about all the barriers in this country, because they hit us hard.

Government restrictions on abortion hurt those of us who have fewer resources. The restrictions are harder on those who are people of color or undocumented or living with disabilities or poor or queer. It makes our abortions more expensive and makes it hard to navigate logistics. In Texas, the state prohibits all types of health insurance from covering abortion care. This means each Texan seeking an abortion must pay out of pocket. I couldn't afford my abortion, but thankfully a family member lent me the money. Like me, most people seeking abortions are already parenting and are balancing paying for child care, nutritious meals for our families, and rent. Texans seeking abortions know all about the logistical and financial challenges that come along with abortion restrictions because some 96% of counties do not have clinics that provide abortions, and nearly half of Texas women live in those counties.

We need to not only figure out how to take time off work or school to travel to get an abortion, arrange that travel, find someplace to stay, and how to pay for all those extra expenses. We are also forced to listen to government-mandated medically inaccurate counseling, and wait 24 hours and go to the doctor twice before getting an abortion. These restrictions harm our ability to make decisions about our families that are right for us. I wish our government would create policies that make it easier for us to raise healthy families in safe communities. I wish there was more support for young parents like me; the laws as it is make it hard to have an abortion, but also make it hard for me to raise my daughter. Unlike me, the majority of people who have abortions are people of color, and we must respect their decisions. I wish there was more support for people of color who are impacted by these restrictions harder than I am.

We need more love and compassion for families and young people like me. I had a child, I had a miscarriage, and I had an abortion. As we say at the National Network of Abortion Funds, "everyone loves someone who had an abortion." Thank you for your time and I hope my story helps you remember these laws that you pass impact your constituents, like me, and your loved ones who have abortions.

Mr. COHEN. Thank you, Ms. Gray.

We will now enter the period of our hearing where each member has five minutes to ask questions, and I will begin by recognizing myself for five minutes.

Dr. Phillips, thank you for traveling here from Memphis, and away from the land of the best barbecue in the world to join us today. You have spoken about how some of Tennessee's laws, such as the 48-hour waiting period, make it difficult for women to obtain an abortion, particularly those who have to travel long distances for multiple visits.

You have also spoken about how your hospital has bowed to local pressure and placed severe limits on access to abortion. What are those limits and how have they affected patients in your care?

Dr. PHILLIPS. Thank you. The hospital that I practice in has relatively arbitrarily limited abortion to the case of rape, incest, and save the life of the mother. The issue is that the medical indication of saving the life of the mother is one that requires a great number of events to happen to actually prove, and to document more than just prove.

So we have delays. Cases have to be referred to the administration to consider. Many times there requires a number of medical opinions to be documented, and in the meantime the pregnancy is advancing and advancing. And even though first and second trimester abortions are safe, certainly safer than having a baby, and certainly under these medical circumstances safer than having a baby, the delays are heart-wrenching for the patient and for their families as they wait. This is one of the big issues that we face all the time.

Mr. COHEN. Ms. Dalven, Dr. Phillips mentioned the three exceptions that are generally in the law—rape, incest, or the life of the mother. In your knowledge of laws in the United States, do most states now see those three exceptions, except for these new wave of laws that do not consider those exceptions?

Ms. DALVEN. You are absolutely right that many of the new State bans lack exceptions for rape and incest. That is certainly true and the public is outraged. The public is outraged by the bans themselves as they affect all women, and that is why we saw people take to the streets in more than 500 cities and towns around the country, in the middle of the week, to express how concerned they were about bans like Alabama's and Ohio's and Kentucky's and Georgia's, where we are seeing politicians increasingly step away from this old argument that they were just trying to protect women's health or just trying to ensure that decisions are informed. Now what we are seeing is people just taking this decision entirely out of the hands of women.

Mr. COHEN. It is interesting that with the exception of Ohio, the states that have been the worst on these laws are the same states that had miscegenation laws, the same states that made it difficult to vote and were suspect states in the Voting Rights Act, and left the country—somewhat unpatriotic of them.

Professor Murray, you have explained in your testimony that the reasoning Roe v. Wade was part of a long line of cases recognizing a right to privacy and a right to make one's own personal decision in certain areas of life, including people's choice of who they might want to marry, same sex, et cetera, and the rights of parents to direct the upbringing of their children. If Roe were overturned, in what ways could those other rights be threatened?

Ms. MURRAY. Chairman Cohen, you are absolutely right that Roe v. Wade proceeds from a long provenance of cases. It was not conjured out of whole clock but rather proceeds from a series of decisions that were enacted in the 1920s, Meyer v. Nebraska, Pierce v. Society of Sisters, all of which held that parents have the right to upbringing of their children and upbringing of their choosing.

From those protections, we get Griswold v. Connecticut, the right to privacy and the right to use contraception. From there we have Roe v. Wade and from there we have Lawrence v. Texas, the right to engage in consensual adult sexual relationships; and then from there, Obergefell v. Hodges in 2015, which affirms the right to marry a person of the same sex, and, of course, as you say, 1967, Loving v. Virginia. All of these are predicated on the same judicial founding, and if Roe falls, all of these other decisions are equally imperiled.

Mr. COHEN. Thank you, Professor Murray. It is scary to think that we could go back to that era, and all those things that we consider rights and advancements would fall, and we would be back in the Dark Ages.

I recognize the ranking member for five minutes. Mr. JOHNSON. Thank you, Mr. Chairman.

We have heard some compelling testimony today. It is heartfelt on both sides, and we expected that, and I appreciate the civil tone of the dialogue. It is important for us, as American people.

Look, there is a gallery full of young people here today, and I just want to say one thing before I get to my questions. I want to encourage all of you to examine the evidence for yourself. I had an eighth-grade teacher one time that told me that what is popular isn't always right and what is right isn't always popular, and you owe it to yourself to do your own homework.

One of the majority witnesses today said something that really struck me. She said, quote, "I am a human being that deserves autonomy in this country that calls itself free." Okay, but review the facts for yourself and you will see that the indisputable scientific evidence now shows us that when a human sperm meets and fertilizes a human egg, at the moment of conception, there becomes an unborn, living, genetically distinct and biologically self-directing human being. The question is, you should ask yourself quietly, why shouldn't each of those human beings deserve autonomy in this country that calls itself free?

Let me get to my questions. Ms. Bennett, thank you for being here. Your testimony is compelling, and I appreciate you including in your statement Supreme Court Justice Clarence Thomas' concurring opinion in the Box case.

I wanted to read a quick excerpt from that opinion. He said, quote, "This case highlights the fact that abortion is an act rife with the potential for eugenic manipulation. From the beginning, birth control and abortion were promoted as a means of effectuating eugenics. Planned Parenthood founder, Margaret Sanger, was particularly open about the fact that birth control could be used for eugenic purposes. These arguments about the eugenic potential for birth control apply with even greater force to abortion which can be used to target specific children with unwanted characteristics.

"Even after World War II, future Planned Parenthood president, Alan Guttmacher, and other abortion advocates endorsed abortion for eugenic reasons and promoted it as a means of controlling the population and improving its quality. A growing body of evidence suggests that eugenic goals are already being realized through abortion."

Then he says this: "Eight decades after Margaret Sanger's 'Negro Project,' abortion in the U.S. is also marked by considerable racial disparity. The reported nationwide abortion ratio, the number of abortions per 1,000 live births among black women is nearly 3.5 times the ratio for white women."

Continuing to quote Justice Thomas, "And there are areas in New York City in which black children are more likely to be aborted than they are to be born alive, and they are up to eight times more likely to be aborted than white children in the same area." The question is, why do you believe the black community is being targeted by the abortion industry?

Ms. BENNETT. Thank you for the question. If you look at the history of the American Birth Control League, which later became Planned Parenthood, you will see that Margaret Sanger had this pseudoscience that she believed in eugenics philosophy, and it wasn't just her. It was also members of her board. One of her board members was named Lothrop Stoddard and he had a book called "The Rising Tide of Color Against White Supremacy", and it was all about how mixed races were growing and that was a threat to white supremacy.

You have to ask yourself, what would a man like that, who wrote a book like that, why would he be interested in the birth control movement, particularly with targeting people of color? It was because they believed that certain people groups should prosper and grow and that would be a betterment to society, and other groups should not. And that was seen clearly in the writings of Margaret Sanger when she talked about people of color like weeds that should be exterminated.

And she also had something called the Negro Project, in which she manipulated, you know, black ministers and people of color to go into their communities and to push birth control. Unfortunately, she also pushed sterilization. There are women today, like an African American friend I have, Elaine Riddick, who was sterilized in North Carolina after having one child. And she was told by doctors, "We don't want you to reproduce after your own kind."

America has a dark history, and it involves racism. And now we see 78 percent of abortion facilities, Planned Parenthoods, are located in lower-income, minority neighborhoods. There is a great resource on protecting black life where they lay out the map of the United States, and you can go to that website and you can see the different areas that are targeted.

And this is why people of color are standing up. The Church of God in Christ is the largest black denomination in America with over six million members, and recently they have started a movement to stand up against the targeting of African American community as well as a movement of adoption, encouraging their members to adopt.

I will also say that African American women, being three times more likely to abort, it is not because we desire to have abortions more than anyone else. It is because we often feel like we don't have the resources, we don't have the support that we need.

And so things do need to change. We do need help and I support in these areas. People should not be pressured like my mom was. People should not feel like they have to choose abortion because they don't have the resources to take care of themselves or to take care of their families. And so a lot has to change in order for us to truly be able to have equality in this country and not be targeted because of our lack of resources and who we are.

Mr. JOHNSON. I greatly regret that I am out of time but I yield back. Thank you.

Mr. COHEN. Thank you, Mr. Johnson.

Mr. Nadler, you are recognized for five minutes.

Mr. NADLER. Thank you. Professor Murray, there has been some suggestion, more than a suggestion, this morning, that efforts to provide abortion care are linked to an agenda based on eugenics and our design to control minority populations. As someone who has studied the history of reproductive rights in this country, what is your response to that argument?

Ms. MURRAY. I am really grateful to have the opportunity to clarify the record. Like Ms. Bennett, I, too, have studied this history, and she is absolutely correct that the history of eugenics of this country is laced with the taint of racism, but it goes in both directions. Not only was eugenics used to promote the use of contraception and sterilization, it was also used to promote abortion, but from the other side.

In the 1800s, when the first laws criminalizing abortion were enacted, it was because of nativist anxieties that native-born white women were not having as many children as their darker-hued immigrant sisters, who were having too many. So the early effort to criminalize abortion is actually part of a vestige to overwhelm immigrant populations with native-born white births.

I will also note, in response to Ms. Bennett's testimony, that adoption is an option but African American children are the ones who are most likely to linger in the child welfare system and in foster care, and are the least likely to be adopted.

Thank you.

Mr. NADLER. And it is true that eugenics is also a motivating factor, is it not, in much of the anti-immigration legislation? We have got to keep out the Jews, the Italians, the Slavs, and other Eastern Europeans in the early 20th century. Is that not the case?

Ms. MURRAY. That is the case. My colleague at Berkeley, Jerome Karabel, documents some of that in his accounts of higher education in the United States.

Mr. NADLER. Thank you. Last November, a Federal judge blocked Mississippi's ban on abortion after 15 weeks, ruling it was unequivocally unconstitutional. The court described that law as closer to the old Mississippi, a Mississippi bent on controlling women and minorities.

You have already spoken about how restrictions on access to abortion fall disproportionately on women of color. Could you describe some ways in which an outright ban on access to abortion would impact women of color and other vulnerable populations, Professor?

Ms. MURRAY. Women of color continue to bear the brunt of the burden of the restrictions on abortion access. They are often the most likely to be victims of economic insecurity and will not have the opportunity to travel, to go to places where they are able to get more liberalized access to abortion. They will also be more likely to have employment insecurity and not be in positions where they can take time off of work. They may also already be mothers to children and will have difficulty obtaining child care in order to comply with the waiting period and things of that nature.

All of this is compounded by African American women's limitations in access to health care, the high rate of maternal morbidity in this country, and the high rate of infant mortality among African American children.

Thank you.

Mr. NADLER. And, Professor, the judge in that case also wrote that "the State's professed interest in women's health care is pure gaslighting," unquote. This judge recognized a pretext for what it is. But now the case is on appeal to the Fifth Circuit, a court that is conservative to begin with, and now has five extreme right-wing judges appointed by President Trump.

What are some of the ways in which judges who want to reach a particular political outcome could twist the facts in cases involving restrictions on access to abortion?

Ms. MURRAY. Well, Chairman Nadler, we have already seen episodes where courts have consistently flouted the extant precedents of the Supreme Court. So in Whole Woman's Health v. Hellerstedt in 2016, this court struck down a Texas admitting privileges law that basically helped close a number of clinics in Texas. It was struck down in that case.

Almost immediately after, the State of Louisiana passed a virtually similar admitting privileges law. Again, as we have heard today, these admitting privileges laws are often unnecessary in the case of abortion because abortion providers don't often have to admit their patients to hospitals because the procedure is so safe. So we have already seen, in that Louisiana case, June Medical Services, which is currently pending on cert before the Supreme Court, an effort by the Fifth Circuit, again, to flout the precedents that this court has articulated.

Mr. NADLER. Thank you. Ms. Dalven, most State legislatures that are imposing extreme restrictions on abortion or outright bans are targeting the doctors for criminal penalties rather than the patients, although President Trump slipped up during the campaign. He said patients should be arrested and jailed. It is apparently no longer acceptable to say you will put women in prison for receiving an abortion. Can you describe why these laws would still end up punishing women who seek abortions?

Ms. DALVEN. It would—it can punish women in multiple ways. First, if there is no constitutional right to abortion, if the Supreme Court were to overturn Roe v. Wade, there would be nothing to stop states from going after women and punishing women. The fact that they are not saying that today doesn't mean that they will not say that tomorrow.

Second, these laws do punish women by preventing them from getting the care that they need. These laws, a ban on abortion, is a punishment for a woman who needs one. And we know, in states like Georgia and Alabama, it is particularly galling. These states have some of the highest maternal mortality rates in the country. These are states that lack appropriate health care. They lack OB– GYNs, they lack obstetrical departments, and Georgia is one of the states in this country who has refused to expand Medicaid coverage to ensure that people can get the health care that they need.

So bans on abortions, forcing people to stay pregnant against their will, is a punishment, aside from the criminal punishment that could befall women if Roe is overturned.

Mr. NADLER. Let me ask one further question. If a court adopted a constitutional analysis that bans an abortion, perfectly okay because majorities don't like them, is there any difference that would prevent, constitutionally, a state from passing a ban on blood transfusions or open heart surgery, for example? Is there any juridical difference?

Ms. DALVEN. That is a question I have not considered but it would certainly be concerning if the State could step in and say that—and take medical practice out of the hands of doctors and ensure that—and prevent patients from getting the care that they need.

Mr. NADLER. Thank you. My time has expired.

Mr. COHEN. Mr. Gohmert, you are recognized for five minutes.

Mr. GOHMERT. Thank you, and I have been very pleased to hear some things made by our full committee chairman in this hearing, like the statement that is made, or the question, because I recall President Obama saying, in the White House town hall meeting, that under his Obamacare program a woman who had gotten a pacemaker that kept her alive for over a decade, the best thing would just give her a pain pill. So am glad to know that he now believes the State should not prevent someone like that from getting the health care they need.

Ms. Ohden, it is good to see you again. I am curious. You shared in your testimony your birth mother's abortion was forced upon her. Have you heard of any other cases where potential birth mothers, or women that are talking about a potential abortion, had to deal with pressure to get an abortion?

Ms. OHDEN. Thank you for your question. It is correct. My biological mother, I now know, was forced to have this abortion. I didn't find that out until about six years ago now. My birth mother is now a huge part of my life. She is a great support to me. But I face the reality every day of the fact that not only was my life supposed to end but this is not something she wanted.

And I know that she is not alone in that. There was a study done recently where 48 of women identified being coerced into their abortion. And again, I just want to thank all of the women for being here today. I know we have differing experiences and different opinions, but I think we are all passionate about wanting to help and serve women. And for me, personally, really one of the hardest things is that I receive emails on a regular basis from women who do exist in the shadows, not just other abortion survivors like me but women who had abortions, regret them, and are living in pain.

I have to respond to the emails of women who say, "Melissa, can you help me obtain my medical records from my abortion? Can you help me find out if my child is living still today?" That is an interesting place for someone like me to be in, but that is what I see in my experiences.

Mr. GOHMERT. Well, thank you, and I appreciate your working through that with other individuals.

Ms. Busy Philipps, because you are sitting beside Dr. Phillips, but would you agree that somebody who has survived an abortion like Melisa Ohden has a right, when she is born, to life, to control over her body, where someone else doesn't take her life?

Ms. PHILIPPS. Well, first of all, I want to thank her for sharing her story. I—you know, it is not—although I played a doctor on television, sir, I am actually not a physician. [Laughter.]

Mr. GOHMERT. Right. No, but you have given very compelling testimony and I appreciate it. You have obviously given these issues a lot of thought.

Ms. PHILIPPS. Correct, sir.

Mr. GOHMERT. That is why I was asking you.

Ms. PHILIPPS. Yeah. I think that it is something that is very important. I don't believe that a politician's place is to decide what is best for a woman, and, you know, it is a choice between a woman and her doctor.

I can't——

Mr. GOHMERT. So what about a baby and the doctor? That is my question.

Ms. PHILIPPS. Yes, sir. Well, I, again, I can't speak to her experience because I was not there, and so I do not want to——

Mr. GOHMERT. Okay. Well, I just wondered how far you are feeling about that, because once she is born, would you agree that she is a person in being?

Ms. PHILIPPS. Yeah. See, I am not speaking about birth, sir. I am speaking about——

Mr. GOHMERT. Okay. Well——

Ms. PHILIPPS [continuing]. Abortion.

Mr. GOHMERT. Well, I appreciate that, but the concern here is we have got 21 states that allow the termination, and we have heard the governor here——

Ms. PHILIPPS. Yes, and——

Mr. GOHMERT [continuing]. Just across the river, in Virginia.

Thank you. I appreciate it.

Ms. PHILIPPS. No. I just wanted to say, Mr. Gohmert, I appreciate that, what you are trying to get at, and I do——

Mr. GOHMERT. Well, I wasn't trying to get at anything.

Ms. PHILIPPS. No, no, no.

Mr. GOHMERT. You have answered my question. You were sure—so my time, I only have a minute and a half.

I would like to ask, Ms. Bennett, you have obviously done a great deal of study. Have you run into others that you have personally talked to that were in situations like Ms. Ohden?

Ms. BENNETT. I have other friends who have survived an abortion. My friend, Claire Culwell, she survived an abortion. Unfortunately, the reason that she survived was because the abortion took the life of her twin brother, and the doctor, the abortion doctor didn't know that there was twins and so he thought that he had done a successful abortion. And then later on her mother realized that she was still pregnant and Claire was inside of her, because there was twins. And she was adopted, but when she was born she had to be put in a—she was in a body cast and her hip was dislocated, and she suffered greatly because of that.

And there are other abortion survivors. Josiah Presley is another one, and he is missing part of his arm because of the abortion procedure. And like Melissa said, there are others that are in the shadows. It takes a lot of courage to come out and share a story like that. And so there are many more that we—we are not privileged to know their stories.

Mr. GOHMERT. Thank you. And I am being very serious. I appreciate all of you being here because I know what it is to come and testify, and I wish there were a better way to make laws than so-called politicians to come together and enforce their will through the laws. But, unfortunately, it happens every day. I wish it would happen a whole lot less. But I appreciate you all being here and your obvious concern about the issue.

I yield back.

Mr. COHEN. Thank you, sir. I recognize the chair.

Mr. NADLER. Thank you, Mr. Chairman. I ask unanimous consent that this statement from the National Partnership for Women and Families be placed in the record.

Mr. COHEN. Without objection.
[The information follows:]

HOUSE COMMITTEE ON THE JUDICIARY, SUBCOMMITTEE ON THE CONSTITUTION, CIVIL RIGHTS, AND CIVIL LIBERTIES, HEARING ON "THREATS TO REPRODUCTIVE RIGHTS IN AMERICA," JUNE 4, 2019

Statement Submitted by National Partnership for Women & Families
Washington, DC 20009

Dear Chairman Cohen, Ranking Member Johnson and Members of the Subcommittee:

The National Partnership for Women & Families is a nonprofit, nonpartisan organization that has fought for decades to advance the rights and well-being of America's women and families, including the right to access abortion care free of shame, stigma or barriers.

Abortion is an essential part of health care and a basic human right. Nearly one in four women in the United States will have an abortion by age 45.[91] Access to abortion care facilitates people's autonomy, dignity and ability to make decisions about their bodies, their lives and their futures. It also enables people to adequately care for themselves and their families, and to fully contribute to American society. In short, abortion is fundamental to women's equality, and all people deserve access to abortion care and to comprehensive reproductive health care.

Yet across the country, access to abortion is under attack with increasing levels of inflammatory rhetoric and disregard for science and medicine or the realities of people's lives. Bans on abortion are moving with alarming speed in state legislatures.[92] For example, just since January 2019, bans on abortion after 6 weeks – before most people even know that they are pregnant – have passed in Louisiana, Ohio, Georgia, Kentucky and Mississippi and have passed one chamber in legislatures in South Carolina and Tennessee. A ban on abortion after 8 weeks has passed in Missouri, and the state is currently attempting to revoke the license to provide abortion care from the last remaining Missouri clinic, meaning the state could be the first without an abortion provider since before *Roe v. Wade.* Alabama has passed a law that criminalizes abortion at any stage in pregnancy. Trigger laws, which would automatically criminalize abortion in the event that *Roe v. Wade* is

---

[91] Guttmacher Institute. (2017, October). *Abortion is a common experience for U.S. women, despite dramatic declines in rates.* [News release]. Retrieved 4 April 2019, from https://www.guttmacher.org/news-release/2017/abortion-common-experience-us-women-despite-dramatic-declines-rates.

[92] Nash, E., Cappello, O., Naide, S., Mohmmed, L., & Ansari-Thomas, Z. (2019, April). *Radical Attempts to Ban Abortion Dominate State Policy Trends in the First* Quarter. Retrieved 4 April 2019 from Guttmacher Institute website: https://www.guttmacher.org/article/2019/04/radical-attempts-ban-abortion-dominate-state-policy-trends-first-quarter-2019.

overturned, have recently passed in Arkansas, Kentucky and Tennessee. And bans on a commonly-used second trimester abortion procedure have passed in Indiana and North Dakota and are moving forward in Michigan.

These bans are compounded by other efforts at both the federal and state levels to limit access to abortion care and family planning services, such as this administration's Title X gag rule, state efforts to prohibit Planned Parenthood from receiving reimbursement under state Medicaid programs, and other efforts to limit who can provide abortion care and other reproductive health services.

All of this federal and state level activity is part of a concerted and explicit effort to ban abortion outright. This hearing is a necessary venue for bringing these unprecedented attacks on access to abortion and reproductive health care to light, and for affirming the right of all people to have access to the care that they need, free of barriers, shame or stigma.

We commend the Chairman for holding today's hearing and urge the House to take seriously the very real, devastating impacts that restrictions or bans on abortion access have on people's health, well-being, and economic security.

People who are denied access to an abortion have been found to suffer adverse physical and mental health consequences. For example, according to a longitudinal study that is frequently cited in peer-reviewed journals, women denied abortion care are more likely to experience eclampsia, death, and other serious medical complications during the end of pregnancy, more likely to remain in relationships where interpersonal violence is present, and more likely to suffer anxiety.[93] Restrictions and bans on abortion care also fall disproportionately on people of color and exacerbate existing health disparities, including maternal health and maternal mortality disparities.

In addition to health impacts, having access to abortion care also benefits the economic security of individuals and families. Research has shown that women who seek but are denied abortion care are worse off financially and significantly more likely to fall into poverty than women who are able to get the care they need.[94] People who have an abortion are already disproportionately poor, and lack of access to care only further entrenches their economic insecurity. Additionally, women who are denied an abortion had more than three times greater odds of being unemployed six months later than women who were able to access an abortion;[95] access to abortion is linked with greater workforce attachment and higher lifetime earnings. In one study, women who were able to have an abortion were six times more likely to

---

[93] See Advancing New Standards in Reproductive Health: University of California San Francisco. (2018). *Turnaway Study*. Retrieved 4 April 2019, from https://www.ansirh.org/research/turnaway-study.

[94] Foster, D., Roberts, S.C., & Mauldon, J. (2012, October). *Socioeconomic consequences of abortion compared to unwanted birth*. Paper session presented at the American Public Health Associations annual meeting, from https://apha.confex.com/apha/140am/webprogram/Paper263858.html.

[95] Advancing New Standards in Reproductive Health: University of California San Francisco. (2018, August). *Issue Brief: Socioeconomic Outcomes of Women Who Receive and Women Who Are Denied Wanted Abortions* (p. 1). Retrieved 4 April 2019, from https://www.ansirh.org/sites/default/files/publications/files/turnaway_socioeconomic_outcomes_issue_brief_8-20-2018.pdf.

have positive life plans – most commonly related to education and employment –and are more likely to achieve them than women denied an abortion.[96]

Access to abortion care also benefits children and families, most directly by allowing people to take on the costs of having children when they are best able or to have the resources necessary to care and provide for the children they already have. Research has found that denying women abortion care has negative developmental and socioeconomic consequences for their existing children.[97]

We urge the House to reject efforts to undermine access to abortion care, and to stand up for the health, security and dignity of America's women and families. Following this hearing, the House should swiftly pass the Women's Health Protection Act (WHPA), which would protect abortion access across the country. The House should also promptly pass the EACH Woman Act, which, as a complement to WHPA, would ensure abortion access for people no matter their income or how they are insured.

If you have questions, please contact Jessi Leigh Swenson, director of outreach and engagement for reproductive health and rights, at jswenson@national partnership.org or 202-986-2600.

Mr. COHEN. I now recognize Professor Raskin for five minutes. Mr. RASKIN. Mr. Chairman, thank you very much. It is hard for me to believe that this is a congressional hearing in 2019. It feels like a scene out of The Handmaid's Tale, what we are witnessing across the country and what we are hearing about today. So, Dr. Robinson, you practice in Alabama; is that right?

Dr. ROBINSON. Yes.

Mr. RASKIN. And Alabama may soon have a law—tell me if I am correct—which would compel a 15-year-old girl who has been raped by her stepfather to bring—to bring the pregnancy to term, and if a doctor honored her wish to have an abortion that doctor would be facing 99 years in prison. Do I understand this law correctly?

Dr. ROBINSON. That is correct. And like I said in my testimony, there is no other of medicine where physicians are being threatened with criminalization like this.

If you were the patient, you would want your physician—you would want to be your physician's number one priority when you are sitting in front of them, and with women this should be the same. We shouldn't have physicians put in a place where they are having to contemplate criminal prosecution versus proceeding doing what is best for their patients.

And if you don't mind, I would like to go back and refer to the question that was asked of Ms. Philipps, because I am a physician.

Mr. RASKIN. Please.

---

[96] Upadhyay, U., Biggs, M., & Foster, D. (2015, October). The effort of abortion on having and achieving aspirational one-year plans (pp. e9-10). *Boston Medical Center Women's Health*, *15*, e1-10, from https://bmcwomenshealth.biomedcentral.com/track/pdf/10.1186/s12905-015-0259-1.

[97] Foster, D., Raifman, S., Gipson, J., Rocca, C., Biggs, M. (2019, February). Effects of carrying an unwanted pregnancy to term on women's existing children (p. 183). *Journal of Pediatrics*, *205*, 183-189.

Dr. ROBINSON. And states already have laws in place to protect neonates, but it is very, very important to understand that the scenario that was described is not the situation that we are seeing in abortion care here. I can't imagine any situation where that would happen, and I think it is really, really important that we understand——

Mr. RASKIN. And if it does happen it should be illegal, right, if there are unsanitary conditions.

Dr. ROBINSON. Exactly.

Mr. RASKIN. If the women are not treated properly that is obviously a violation of every regulation and law, and whoever does that should be dealt with accordingly.

Dr. ROBINSON. Exactly, and it is important to keep in mind that the majority of abortions take place early in the first trimester. We are not seeing women having abortions——

Mr. RASKIN. Let me ask you about that.

Dr. ROBINSON [continuing]. In the third trimester.

Mr. RASKIN. Can I ask you about that? I have got a million questions for you, Dr. Robinson.

Dr. ROBINSON. Okay.

Mr. RASKIN. Your story just seems extraordinary to me.

We have heard from our friends across the aisle, and I appreciate the intellectual honesty today. But I want America to hear this. We have heard now that when a sperm unites with an egg that is a human life, and the logic of that is the Alabama law, which is if it was the product of a rape, it was the product of incest, if the woman is in—or girl is in no condition to start a family, to be a mother—still that girl would be forced to go ahead and to have a baby, even if it is week three, week four, because the moment—as I understand my colleagues, and the gentleman from Louisiana, I think, was very clear about it—when the egg and the sperm unite, that is a life and that is when it kicks in.

Now let me ask you about that. You bring a lot of babies into existence, right? You are in OB–GYN and so you are—what do you think about this claim that it should be a criminal act for someone to terminate a pregnancy at one month, which was clearly protected under Roe v. Wade, it was clearly protected under Planned Parenthood v. Casey, which drew the line at viability outside the womb of the mother?

Dr. ROBINSON. Well, I don't support any legislation that pushes abortion care out of the reach of women. I know, as a physician, that it is a really important that all women have access to the care they need, regardless of the point they are in their pregnancy, and I know that any legislation that takes this out of the hands of physicians and patients puts those women at risk.

Mr. RASKIN. Thank you. Ms. Dalven, let me come to you. So it is very clear that all of this litigation is meant to go up to the Supreme Court, which they have successfully gerrymandered now because of the stonewalling of my constituent, Merrick Garland, who didn't get a Supreme Court confirmation hearing. But they think now they have got the perfect straight flush. They are going to be able to destroy

Roe v. Wade and Planned Parenthood v. Casey, and our colleagues across the aisle are cheering them along. Okay.

Now, let us say this were to happen. I want to go back to this very interesting question about sterilization and compulsory abortion. If the choice is not a woman's to decide what happens with her pregnancy, pre-fetal viability, which is the Casey framework— so let us say Roe v. Wade is overturned, Casey is overturned. Could the 30 governments which had compulsory sterilization laws, just in the last century, not even a century ago, could they go back to having a compulsory sterilization law? Could authoritarian, right-wing governments throughout the country go to compulsory abortion laws for populations that they don't like, because it would not be a woman's right to choose? At that point it would just be up to the government to decide what happens in the woman's womb?

Ms. DALVEN. This is a real concern if the court were to say that people do not have the right to control what happens with their own body. Even that is a very frightening prospect and it could lead to the frightening prospects that you describe. But what we also know is that——

Mr. RASKIN. And that is not a crazy hypothetical, right? The majority of the states in the country had compulsory sterilization laws for populations that were deemed unfit by essentially authoritarian governments, and most of them were a lot of them existing in the very states which today are trying to ban the woman's right to choose.

Ms. DALVEN. It is certainly true that this country has a disgraceful history of those types of laws. We see those kinds of—and we see that kind of thing happening today, even today, with the Administration's policy of separating immigrant children from their families, so that is a real part of our history.

Mr. RASKIN. All right. I yield back. Thank you very much.

Mr. COHEN. Thank you, sir.

Mr. Cline, you are recognized for five minutes, our distinguished, young, first-year star.

Mr. CLINE. Thank you, Mr. Chairman. I appreciate the witnesses for being here today. I especially want to thank Ms. Bennett and Ms. Ohden for being here today as well. It is an amazing story for both of you, and it is remarkable that you are able to be here today.

You know, Virginia, the Commonwealth of Virginia, is ground zero right now in the fight over late-term abortions, and while I appreciate the discussions of the chairman about states endeavoring to pass pro-life measures like Mississippi, we only need to look at his own State of New York to see just how extreme these laws have gotten.

The law recently signed into—the bill recently signed into law by Governor Cuomo allows abortion on demand through the moment of birth; it allows non-doctors to perform abortions; could result in forcing health professionals to participate in abortions, even if they object; removes protections for children born alive during abortion attempts but leaves them at the mercy of the abortionist who just minutes earlier was trying to kill them; completely removes unborn children from the criminal code, meaning even those who are victims of violent crimes against pregnant women are unprotected.

In Virginia, my own state, we recently saw similar legislation introduced, and the testimony by the patron, she summarized that the bill would have allowed abortionists to self-certify the necessity of late-term procedures, eliminate informed consent requirements, repeal health and safety standards for abortion facilities, permit late-term abortions to be performed in outpatient facilities, remove ultrasound requirements, and eliminate Virginia's 24-hour waiting period.

In her testimony at the hearing, when she was given the hypothetical of a woman who was about to give birth, that has physical signs she is in labor, would that be a time when she could request an abortion if she were in the middle of labor and dilated? The delegate said, "Mr. Chairman, that would be a decision that the doctor, the physician, and the woman would make at that point," and that her bill would allow that, yes. When she claimed that her bill would have done nothing to change Virginia's late-term abortion law, Politifact rated that false.

We then heard from our own governor who, when discussing that bill, said, on the radio, quote, "If a mother is in labor I can tell you exactly what would happen. The infant would be delivered. The infant would be kept comfortable. The infant would be resuscitated, if that is what the mother and the family desired, and then a discussion would ensue between the physicians and the mother." That is an extreme position.

The 14th Amendment says "nor shall any state deprive a person of life, liberty, or property," to begin, and then it goes on—there is no—the word "abortion" is not found in the 14th Amendment but the word "life" is. And when we talk about protecting life I appreciate the difficult and challenging decisions that were made by the women on the panel, and their testimony is stirring. Two of the women were not talking about the important decisions affecting their lives. They were talking about their lives, the ability to even be here today, and that is significantly different.

So I ask, Ms. Ohden, you have made it your life's work to discuss your story. Could you describe more about your efforts and the impact that your life, which could have been cut short, has had on others?

Ms. OHDEN. Thank you so much for all of your words, and for acknowledging, I think, what the white elephant in this room is, right? All of these people here today had a privilege that I was not given, and that is simply the right to be born, and not be born accidentally. And as you can hear in my voice, I get choked up about it. We see this as a political issue, but I have to live with this every single day.

And like so many of you on this panel, yes, I am a mother. My daughters are 11 and almost 5. My oldest daughter was born at the very same hospital where my life was supposed to end, and trust me, I didn't want to do that. I didn't think I could do that. But my children will grow up knowing that they are only alive because an abortion failed to end their mother's life.

That is why I do the work that I do, because I don't get to run away from this. I don't get to pretend like maybe this happens to someone else, that this maybe is an issue that doesn't affect me. And I truly believe that if each and every one of you in this room ever lived in my shoes, you would feel very differently about this issue.

Mr. CLINE. Thank you.

Mr. COHEN. You are welcome, sir.

Ms. Scanlon, you are recognized for five minutes.

Ms. SCANLON. Thank you, Chairman Cohen, for holding this important hearing, you know, especially in light of recent attempts to limit critical reproductive rights for women across America.

You know, as we are hearing, there are a million reasons why someone might choose to continue or end a pregnancy, reasons including the life or health of the mother; whether a fetus has a fatal illness or a severe anomaly; the circumstances of conception, including rape or incest; the mother's socioeconomic status; religious, philosophical beliefs. We have also heard, very eloquently, from some of our witnesses, of difficult situations that have informed their decisions, including, apparently, criminal acts, in some cases.

As someone who has used Planned Parenthood for family planning services, to plan my own family, and has also held the hand of a young woman who chose to terminate her pregnancy after she was raped by a sexual predator 20 years her senior, I support the right of all women to make those choices based upon their own unique circumstances.

I believe we must protect women's rights to have access to a full range of reproductive health care options and the ability to make those decisions in consultation with their medical providers, based upon their own circumstances and their own religious beliefs, not someone else's religious beliefs. I also want to thank the young people who are here today, particularly the young women who are taking a stand to protect those rights.

Now, I am particularly concerned, based upon experience I have had with my clients in the legal services world, about the fact that a person's ZIP code or their socioeconomic status sometimes determines their ability to access basic medical care. And with that, Ms. Dalven, you have talked about the fact that we shouldn't have a theoretical right to abortions but that women with socioeconomic privilege often have more access to reproductive and abortion health care than others, and women of color or of limited means or in rural America are far more likely to have only a theoretical right to abortion.

Can you speak to that topic and how bills like the Women's Health Protection Act, of which I am a proud co-sponsor, might address that issue of justice with respect to reproductive health care?

Ms. DALVEN. Yes. Thank you for the question. Because of restrictions already in place it is difficult, if not impossible, for many people, particularly low-income people, people of color, immigrants, folks who live in rural America, to get the care they need. And there are—I will just give you an example of three types of laws that contribute to that.

One are laws that prevent insurance coverage from covering abortion care, like the Hyde Amendment, and other State—similar laws. Those laws make it impossible for many people to pay for the care they need. There was a recent study by the Fed that showed that 40 percent of Americans would have real difficulty paying for an unexpected $400 expense. So you can imagine the difficulty of coming up with the money for an abortion.

The second type of laws are clinic shutdown laws that have left 11 million American women more than an hour's drive from a clinic.

And the third are laws that require people to make multiple unnecessary trips to the clinic before they can get the abortion care they need.

So just imagine that you are a person who has a minimum-wage shift job that doesn't allow you any flexibility to take time off of work, doesn't allow you any paid time off, and you are trying to mount these really insurmountable barriers of trying to get to the clinic, not once, not twice, not around the corner but more than 100 miles away, perhaps without a car, often without public transportation systems. It is really near impossible for people to get the care they need.

We heard Dr. Robinson talk about her patients who have to sleep in the car overnight because they lack the means to stay in a hotel and are forced to go to these unnecessary trips.

So I really thank you for the question because it shows that even if the court doesn't overturn Roe, we have tremendous barriers and we need the Women's Health Protection Act and the Each Women Act to ensure that every person who needs an abortion can get it, no matter where they live and no matter how much money they make.

Ms. SCANLON. And, Dr. Robinson, one quick question for you. There has been some arguments made today that providing abortion care harms women of color and minority populations. Do you have a response to the suggestion that by providing the care that you give you are harming minority communities?

Dr. ROBINSON. I am appalled by any insinuation that refers to the painful history that we, as African Americans, have experienced, the oppression that my people have experienced, to use that as a way to restrict abortion access. I know that all women need access to safe abortion care, women from all backgrounds, and it is very important that we focus on what is most important, and utilizing race as a reason or to point out a reason that we should not have this access is unacceptable.

Ms. SCANLON. Thank you. I yield back.

Mr. COHEN. Ms. Garcia from Houston, Texas, is recognized for five minutes.

Ms. GARCIA. Thank you, Mr. Chairman, and thank you for giving us the opportunity to talk about a very important topic, and perhaps prepare for what may be coming later in the Supreme Court.

Before I begin my question I wanted to introduce someone in the audience, Alicia Hutt, who is here with us today, shadowing me. You know, Congresswoman Bass has a shadow program from her Caucus on Foster Youth, and we are really pleased to have her today. I think she is getting a really good, on-the-ground education. She is a social work student in Texas and I would like to welcome her today.

Secondly, you know, I am 1 of 10 children. I am Catholic but I am pro-choice. I know what my church says but I also know that I cannot impose those religious beliefs on others. So I have been an advocate for a woman's right to choose, which simply does mean that it is up to the woman, her physician, and her network—her husband, her family—to make this decision, and it is not something that a politician should set their will on someone else.

So for me it is troubling to hear some of the remarks that have been made by some of my colleagues and some of the witnesses, particularly when it comes to serving vulnerable populations, underserved populations, and women of color. Because I have seen, firsthand, what it does in terms of negative impact when women of color in underserved communities don't have the proper health care that they need.

And I was really struck by the testimony of Dr. Phillips, when you said that the mortality rate is increasing because we are putting more focus on the fetal well-being than on the mother's well-being.

Could you just—I mean, what does that really mean? I mean, how does it impact Latinas like myself? How does it impact African American women, Native American women, if that focus is shifting?

Dr. PHILLIPS. Thank you for this question. There are many avenues by which we are seeing this play out in the medical field. One is perhaps altruistic, in a sense. Physicians are working to promote fetal well-being by postponing deliveries under circumstances where we realize that continuing the pregnancy for even a day or a week may increase that patient's risk of acute issues, including mortality, and now long-term health care risks. They may be doing this because they are hoping for the best and thinking that they can postpone delivery until the fetus is a little bit farther along.

But there are many examples of communities where the doctors themselves have different approaches and are postponing care for the patient, who is in front of them, the person who is front of them with the idea that they are instead promoting fetal well-being. And one way to understand this is to understand the ethical principles that all physicians are guided by. The individual in front of us is our patient, but she is also the person. That is the definition. The fetus is a patient but does not have the personal rights that supersede the woman's. And this plays out all the time care.

Ms. GARCIA. And, in fact, we have one of the highest mortality rates in this country.

Dr. PHILLIPS. Right. Right.

Ms. GARCIA. Higher than some other Third World countries.

Dr. PHILLIPS. Correct, and a lot of research into this, and questioning into this, may very well be that either the health care systems or the doctors themselves or opinions of physicians themselves may be pushing the limits——

Ms. GARCIA. Thank you.

Dr. PHILLIPS [continuing]. Of maternal health and care.

Ms. GARCIA. Thank you. I need to get one more in, and this one is for Ms. Dalven.

You also have had a case that involved the Trump administration's, in my mind, blatant abuse of constitutional law by trying to block abortion access to immigrant woman. What is the status of that case and where might we be going in the future?

Ms. DALVEN. Thank you for your question. This was a case, we call it the Jane Doe case. Jane Doe was a young woman who came to this country without her parents, seeking a better life for herself. She was put into a government-run shelter and found out she was pregnant and requested an abortion, and the Trump administration did everything they could to block her, took every single step they could. They sent her to an anti-abortion counseling center, they told her abusive parents, and then they simply blocked the doors.

So we went to court on her behalf. She was resolute in her decision, and after four weeks of unconstitutional delay Ms. Doe was able to finally get her abortion.

That did not stop the Trump administration. We had to go to court on behalf of young woman, after young woman, after young woman, until we finally got the court to say that we could—that the Administration couldn't enforce this policy against any pregnant person.

The Trump administration did not stop. They have appealed that decision and we are waiting for a decision from the Court of Appeals.

Ms. GARCIA. Thank you. I yield back.

Mr. COHEN. Thank you, Ms. Garcia, and like Ms. Garcia, and like Archie Bell and the Drells, from Houston, Texas, Sheila Jackson Lee.

Ms. JACKSON LEE. Mr. Chairman, thank you, and how important this hearing is to all of the witnesses. Whether agree with your positions or not, this is a crucial human rights question. This is a question of dignity and respect. I take great issue to the fact that anyone who believes in choice, which is far different from flag waivers for abortion, which is how the anti-abortion people try to portray us, and we are not. And I refuse to accept that definition because we are a multi-conglomerate of individuals of faith and other perspectives. We are women and we are men, and we are Americans. And my heart broke with the series of outrageous, despotic legislative acts from pompous, self-righteous men who had the audacity, and it might have been men and women, who had the audacity to take away the liberty of anyone.

Let me say that I believe that in the course of Supreme Court cases and others, the dignity of the unborn is respected. I have been through a lot, partial birth abortion and others, which is not a free-for-all. It is a medical decision being made by a doctor, the faith of the individual and family.

Let me quickly ask these questions so my time does not run out, but I want to be very clear that I take great issue with definitions that are not me. What is a definition of myself is the fact that I lived through the era of coat hangers, brokenhearted lives, and death, bleeding to death, backroom operating tables or back alleys, or young people being in your church and all of a sudden you didn't know where they were. God forbid they had died or they were sent somewhere to have that baby. Is that the life that we want for a free and equal country?

Let me, Ms. Murray, I have great respect for your family, the Hill family, and, of course, Professor Hill. The late Professor Hill himself was a great humanitarian, lost his life shortly after returning from South Africa on the question of climate. What a visionary. Thank you for being here, and thank you for your work. I want you to answer that question of this whole Fourteenth Amendment and the dastardly series of legislative initiatives, and particularly in Alabama, which is absolutely appalling. If you would hold your point, I just want to get all my questions out and be fair to the chairman to make sure that I have all of them.

Let me just say to the ACLU, that case was in our district. We are honored by the fact that you never stopped, that young lady. I may be able to ask you a question, but I am going to just thank you for your work.

Dr. Robinson, you lived it. You are from Huntsville, and I happen to have been on the board of Oakwood College. You are from Huntsville. I couldn't imagine the picture of those who voted for it, but from a health perspective, how devastating is it to women's health? How many lives are we going to lose if we continue in this ridiculous pathway? And let me go to Ms. Dalven, as well. Is it true that States placing such restrictions on reproductive care under the guise of ensuring the health of these constituents is, in fact, deficient of evidence? And you state that in Alabama, two-thirds of the counties do not have a hospital that offer obstetrical care and has the highest infant mortality rate. So for those who love life, how devastating it is to not have this in Alabama, and then look what they do. How outrageous.

So three people I have given a question. Professor Murray, thank you. Welcome.

Ms. MURRAY. Thank you, Representative Lee. Thank you for remembering my father-in-law, Dr. Hill, who was indeed a great man, a greater Houstonian. Let me first start with your point about the Fourteenth Amendment. You are absolutely right that the recent laws enacted in Alabama and Georgia flagrantly flout the precedents of this Court. They are patently unconstitutional. We only need the Supreme Court to follow exigent precedent to discover that.

I also wanted to point out that Representative Cline noted that the right to abortion is not included in the Constitution. I will only note that there are other rights that are not included explicitly in the Constitution, like the right to marry, the right to raise children in the manner of your choosing, the right to travel, and, more recently, the concept of executive privilege that we have heard quite a bit about. None of these are explicitly enumerated in the Constitution. Thank you.

Ms. JACKSON LEE. Thank you. Dr. Robinson? I think that is Dr. Robinson? You heard my question to you?

Dr. ROBINSON. Could you repeat it, please?

Ms. JACKSON LEE. Well, I asked you about the problem, you having experienced it, but the problem of the particular law in Alabama as it impacts on having children or not.

Dr. ROBINSON. Yes, I am experiencing that. I am an obstetrician/gynecologist, and I am already seeing the impacts of people having opposition to abortion care, and like we talked about earlier, focusing more on the fetus and not the mother. As an obstetrician, I have two scenarios that I can explain to you very quickly just so you understand how this impacts patients.

One young lady with severe preeclampsia, which, if she was not delivered, she continues to get worse, and it could cause her to die or either severely harm her health over the long term. I had difficulty getting the approvals I needed to deliver that young lady in the hospital. And also with a mother who was pregnant with twins. She delivered very early. She was only 20 weeks, and after one fetus passed, she was bleeding very briskly in the room. However, we did not want to do a Cesarean section because that would be an unnecessary procedure for that mother. I asked a nurse to go ahead and start her Pitocin just to make her start to contract so that the other fetus could pass to decrease her hemorrhaging. And even in that case, after I had left the room and I came back and asked had the orders that I had given, have they been implemented, I was told that they had not because one fetus, the fetus that was still remaining inside, had cardiac activity or still had a heartbeat. Either way it goes, this mother, she was bleeding. She was very pre-term, and that fetus was going to be expelled. The water had already broken.

And I appreciate the scenarios or the situations that these young ladies shared, but I would like you to know that those are criminal acts, and we already have laws against that. So that is not what abortion providers are doing here. Generally when there is a pregnancy that we induce in the third trimester, it is for fetal indications. And in that case, those fetuses are not going to live outside of the womb. They have medical diagnoses that will prevent that. And when you propose a scenario when you have a fetus born live in a clinic, you ask would we render any care, like I said, we have laws that already protect neonates, but this is not happening in abortion clinics in Alabama.

But I would tell you, if it ever did happen, I would say we should transfer those babies, but that does not happen. And for those that are born because of fetal anomalies, they can't live outside of the womb.

Ms. JACKSON LEE. Thank you.

Dr. ROBINSON. So I would be against implementing any heroic measures in transferring to the hospital.

Ms. JACKSON LEE. Thank you.

Dr. ROBINSON. It would be a waste of resources.

Ms. JACKSON LEE. Thank you. May I get Ms. Dalven to—thank you so very much. I am sorry.

Mr. COHEN. Thank you. We are out of time.

Ms. JACKSON LEE. Well, could she just answer the maternal mortality? She was my third person.

Mr. JOHNSON of Louisiana. Mr. Chairman, if we allow that, could I have 1 additional minute, and we could all be fair?

Ms. JACKSON LEE. Well——

Mr. COHEN. That is why we are not going to allow it. [Laughter.]

Ms. JACKSON LEE. If you could give it to me in writing, Ms. Dalven.

Thank you so very much.

Mr. COHEN. Thank you very much. We have had an excellent hearing. I would want to have one more question, and that is, Ms. Gray, you have been an excellent witness. You are the youngest of the panel, and oftentimes the youngest gets overlooked. A long time ago I was the youngest, and I would just like to ask you if you have anything you would like to express to us about your experience, either in this particular area or just about being here in Congress and what you thought of this panel, and what you think we should do better.

Ms. GRAY. Thank you for asking me. I am very happy to be here and seeing all sides of this debate. The thing that I want us to leave with is that the barriers I personally faced and many people face in accessing abortion, it is really just another step to criminalizing poor people. And in doing that, we are making it harder for people to have families. We are making it harder for people to decide that they can't afford to have families. We are making it harder for people like my father to be able to get homes, and people like my mother to be able to be rehabbed and have normal, successful lives.

Another thing that I would like for us to leave with is that whether we all know it, we know someone who has an abortion. We know someone who has been impacted by these laws, and it is unfair for us to pass our judgment, especially when we are passing judgment on people who want and need our support. I want to thank you for having me here, and I want everyone to know that everyone loves someone who has had an abortion. Thank you.

Mr. COHEN. Thank you, and I want to thank you and everybody else on our panel for being here. We have had a great, great panel. Thank you all.

Without objection, all members will have 5 legislative days to submit additional written questions for the witnesses or any additional materials for the record.

With that, the hearing is adjourned.

[Whereupon, at 12:18 p.m., the subcommittee was adjourned.]

Appendix. Black Women's Maternal Health: A Multifaceted Approach to Addressing Persistent and Dire Health Disparities, April 2018

Black women in the United States experience unacceptably poor maternal health outcomes, including disproportionately high rates of death related to pregnancy or childbirth. Both societal and health system factors contribute to high rates of poor health outcomes and maternal mortality for Black women, who are more likely to experience barriers to obtaining quality care and often face racial discrimination throughout their lives.

Due to racism, sexism and other systemic barriers that have contributed to income inequality, Black women are typically paid just 63 cents for every dollar paid to white, non-Hispanic men.

Median wages for Black women in the United States are $36,227 per year, which is $21,698 less than the median wages for white, non-Hispanic men.[98] These lost wages mean Black women and their families have less money to support themselves and their families, and may have to choose between essential resources like housing, childcare, food and health care.

These trade-offs are evident in Black women's health outcomes and use of medical care. Compared to white women, Black women are more likely to be uninsured,[99] face greater financial barriers to care when they need it[100] and are less likely to access prenatal care.[101] Indeed, Black women experience higher rates of many preventable diseases and chronic health conditions including higher rates of diabetes, hypertension and cardiovascular disease.[102] When, or if, Black women choose to become pregnant, these health conditions influence both maternal and infant health outcomes.

> Black women are three to four times more likely to experience a pregnancy-related death than white women.

To improve Black women's maternal health, we need a multi-faceted approach that addresses Black women's health across the lifespan, improves access to quality care, addresses social determinants of health and provides greater economic security.

Background: Black Maternal Health Disparities

Too Many Black Women Are Dying in Pregnancy and Childbirth

Black women in the United States are more likely to die from pregnancy or childbirth than women in any other race group.[103]

---

[98] National Partnership for Women & families. (2017, September). *Quantifying America's Gender Wage Gap by Race,* retrieved 4 April 2018, from http:// www.nationalpartnership.org/research-library/workplace-fairness/fair-pay/quantifying-americas-gender-wage-gap.pdf.

[99] National Partnership for Women & families. (2017, October). *Women's Health Coverage: Sources and Rates of Insurance,* retrieved 4 April 2018, from http://www.nationalpartnership.org/research-library/health-care/womens-health-coverage-sources-and-rates-of-insurance.pdf.

[100] The Commonwealth fund. (2017, february). *Biennial Health Insurance Survey, 2003-2016.* retrieved 4 April 2018, from http://www.commonwealthfund. org/interactives-and-data/surveys/biennial-health-insurance-surveys/2017/biennial-explorer.

[101] Agency for Healthcare research and Quality. (2012, October). *Disparities in Health Care Quality Among Minority Women Selected Findings From the 2011 National Healthcare Quality and Disparities Reports.* U.S. Department of Health and Human Services, retrieved 4 April 2018, from https://archive.ahrq.gov/ research/findings/nhqrdr/nhqrdr11/minority-women.html#maternal.

[102] Office of Minority Health. (2017, May). *Profile: Black/African Americans.* retrieved on October 30, 2017, from https://minorityhealth.hhs.gov/omh/browse. aspx?lvl=4&lvlid=19.

[103] Tucker, M. J., Berg, C. J., Callaghan, W. M., & Hsia, J. (2007). The Black–White disparity in pregnancy-related mortality from 5 conditions: differences in prevalence and case-fatality rates. *American Journal of Public Health, 97*(2), 247-251, retrieved 4 April 2018, from https://www.ncbi.nlm.nih.gov/pubmed/?term=Tucker+MJ%2C+Berg+CJ%2C+Callaghan+WM%2C+Hsia+J.

Black women are three to four times more likely to experience a pregnancy-related death than white women.[104]

Black women are more likely to experience preventable maternal death compared with white women.[105]

Black women's heightened risk of pregnancy-related death spans income and education levels.[106]

Black Women Experience More Maternal Health Complications Than White Women

- Black women are more likely to experience complications throughout the course of their pregnancies than white women.
- Black women are three times more likely to have fibroids (benign tumors that grow in the uterus and can cause postpartum hemorrhaging) than white women, and the fibroids occur at younger ages and grow more quickly for Black women.[107]
- Black women display signs of preeclampsia earlier in pregnancy than white women.
- This condition, which involves high blood pressure during pregnancy, can lead to severe complications including death if improperly treated.[108]
- Black women experience physical "weathering," meaning their bodies age faster than white women's due to exposure to chronic stress linked to socioeconomic disadvantage and discrimination over the life course, thus making pregnancy riskier at an earlier age.[109]

---

[104] Creanga, A.A., Syverson, C., Seek, K., & Callaghan, W.M. (2017). Pregnancy-related Mortality in the United States, 2011-2013. *Obstetrics & Gynecology, 130(*2), 366-373, retrieved 4 April 2018, from https://www.ncbi.nlm.nih.gov/pubmed/28697109.

[105] Louis, J. M., Menard, M. K., & Gee, r. e. (2015), racial and ethnic disparities in maternal morbidity and mortality. *Obstetrics & Gynecology, 125*(3), 690-694.

[106] Black Mamas Matter Alliance & Center for reproductive rights. (2016). *Research Overview of Maternal Mortality and Morbidity in the United States*. Retrieved 2 April 2018, from https://www.reproductiverights.org/sites/crr.civicactions.net/files/documents/USPA_MH_TO_ResearchBrief_Final_5.16.pdf.

[107] Eltoukhi, H. M., Modi, M. N., Weston, M., Armstrong, A. Y., & Stewart, E. A. (2014). The health disparities of uterine fibroid tumors for African American women: a public health issue. *American Journal of Obstetrics & Gynecology, 210*(3), 194-199, retrieved 30 March 2018, from https://www.ncbi.nlm.nih.gov/ pmc/articles/PMC3874080/.

[108] Shahul, S., Tung, A., Minhaj, M., Nizamuddin, J., Wenger, J., Mahmood, e., & Talmor, D. (2015). racial disparities in comorbidities, complications, and maternal and fetal outcomes in women with preeclampsia/eclampsia. *Hypertension in Pregnancy, 34(*4), 506-515, retrieved 30 March 2018, from https:// www.ncbi.nlm.nih.gov/pmc/articles/PMC4782921/.

[109] Geronimus, A. T. (1992). The weathering hypothesis and the health of African-American women and infants: evidence and speculations. *Ethnicity & Disease, 2*(3), 207-221.

Black-Serving Hospitals Provide Lower Quality Maternity Care

Seventy-five percent of Black women give birth at hospitals that serve predominantly Black populations.[110]

- Black-serving hospitals have higher rates of maternal complications than other hospitals. They also perform worse on 12 of 15 birth outcomes, including elective deliveries, non-elective cesarean births and maternal mortality.[111]

Many Black Women Have a Difficult Time Accessing the Reproductive Health Care That Meets Their Needs

- Access to reproductive health care, which helps women plan their families, improves health outcomes for women and children.
- Black women experience higher rates of unintended pregnancies than all other racial groups,[112] in part because of disparities in access to quality contraceptive care and counseling.[113]
- Many Black women lack access to quality contraceptive care and counseling.[114] For example, in a recent analysis of California women enrolled in Medicaid, Black women were less likely than white or Latina women to receive postpartum contraception, and when they did receive it, they were less likely to receive a highly effective method.[115]
- Black women's access to abortion is limited,[116] and they may be more likely to experience the ill effects of abortion restrictions – such as delayed care, increased costs or lack of access to care.[117]

---

[110] Howell, E. A., Egorova, N., Balbierz, A., Zeitlin, J., & Hebert, P. L. (2016). Black-white differences in severe maternal morbidity and site of care. *American Journal of Obstetrics & Gynecology, 214*(1), 122-e1, retrieved 30 March 2018, from https://www.ncbi.nlm.nih.gov/pubmed/26283457.

[111] Creanga, A. A., Bateman, B. T., Mhyre, J. M., Kuklina, e., Shilkrut, A., & Callaghan, W. M. (2014). Performance of racial and ethnic minority-serving hospitals on delivery-related indicators. *American Journal of Obstetrics & Gynecology, 211*(6), 647-e1, retrieved 30 March 2018, from https://www.ncbi.nlm.nih.gov/ pubmed/24909341.

[112] finer, L. B. & Zolna, M. r. (2011). Unintended pregnancy in the United States: incidence and disparities, 2006 (p. 480). *Contraception, 84*, 478–485.

[113] See, e.g., Dehlendorf, C., Park, S. Y., emeremni, C. A., Comer, D., Vincett, K., & Borrero, S. (2014). racial/ethnic disparities in contraceptive use: Variation by age and women's reproductive experiences (p. 526.e1). *American Journal of Obstetrics & Gynecology, 210*(6), 526.e1–526.e9.

[114] ibid.

[115] deBocanegra, H. T., Braughton, M., Bradsberry, M., Howell, M., Logan, J., & Shwarz, e.B. (2017). racial and ethnic disparities in postpartum care and contraception in California's Medicaid program (pp. e3–e4). *American Journal of Obstetrics & Gynecology, 217(*47), e1–e7.

[116] See note 15; see, e.g., Dehlendorf, C., Harris, L. H., & Weitz, T. A. (2013). Disparities in abortion rates: A public health approach. A*merican Journal of Public Health, 103*(10), 1772–1779.

[117] See, e.g., Dehlendorf, C., Harris, L. H., & Weitz, T. A. (2013). Disparities in abortion rates: A public health approach (p. 1776). *American Journal of Public Health, 103*(10), 1772–1779 (describing that "studies have found that restricted access to abortion services can limit women's ability to abort a pregnancy when they wish to do so, and that these effects may be particularly pronounced for Black women and women with lower educational attainment"); Henshaw, S. K., Joyce, T. J., Dennis, A., finer, L. B., & Blanchard, K. (2009). *Restrictions on Medicaid funding for abortions: A literature*

Policymakers, Health Care Professionals and Communities Can Improve Black Women's Maternal Health

Expand and Maintain Access to Health Coverage

Only 87 percent of Black women of reproductive age have health insurance, and many more experience gaps in coverage during their lives. To improve Black women's health outcomes, policies should focus on expanding and maintaining access to care and coverage.

Women need health coverage throughout their lifespan including access to preventive health care, such as birth control, to maintain their health and to choose when and whether to become a parent. For women who choose to become a parent or expand their families, good prenatal and maternity care are critically important for healthy pregnancies and healthy children. Pregnant women who lack insurance coverage often delay or forgo prenatal care in the first trimester,[118] and inadequate prenatal care is associated with higher rates of maternal mortality.[119]

Black women are more likely to live in the South, where women generally experience poorer health outcomes and where many states have chosen not to expand Medicaid coverage,[120] which leaves many Black women in the "coverage gap." Women fall into the coverage gap because they earn too much to qualify for traditional Medicaid, but not enough to purchase insurance on the Affordable Care Act (ACA) marketplace; as a result, they lack access to health coverage. Expanding Medicaid coverage would improve maternal outcomes for Black women by providing better access to care and reducing financial instability.

Provide Patient-Centered Care That Is Responsive to the Needs of Black Women

Black women should receive health care that is respectful, culturally competent, safe and of the highest quality. Unfortunately, research shows that Black women receive a lower quality of care than white women.[121] Much too often, Black women are subject to discrimination in the health care field – 22 percent report discrimination when going to the doctor or clinic.[122]

---

review. Guttmacher institute. retrieved 27 March 2018, from http://citeseerx.ist.psu.edu/viewdoc/download?doi=10.1.1.295.8439&rep=rep1&type=pdf.

118 egerter, S., Braveman, P., & Marchi, K. (2002). Timing of insurance coverage and use of prenatal care among low-income women. *American Journal of Public Health, 92*(3), 423-427, retrieved 27 March 2018, from https://www.ncbi.nlm.nih.gov/pmc/articles/PMC1447093/.

119 U.S. Centers for Disease Control and Prevention. *Prenatal Care,* retrieved 4 April 2018, from https://www.cdc.gov/healthcommunication/toolstemplates/entertainmented/tips/PregnancyPrenatalCare.html.

120 America's Health rankings. (2018). *2018 Health of Women and Children Report,* retrieved 4 April 2018, from https://www.americashealthrankings.org/explore/2018-health-of-women-and-children-report.

121 See note 9.

122 robert Wood Johnson foundation. (2017, December). *Discrimination in America: Experiences and Views of American Women.* retrieved 4 April 2018, from https://www.rwjf.org/content/dam/farm/reports/surveys_and_polls/2017/rwjf441994.

Public policies and medical practice should incentivize providing patient-centered care that focuses on Black women's individualized needs, including non-clinical, social needs. Moreover, policies should endeavor to eradicate cultural biases and discrimination in medical practice and medical education, increase provider diversity in maternity care and hold individual providers and hospital systems accountable if they fail to provide unbiased, high-quality, evidence-based care.

Address the social Determinants of Health

Social determinants of health are the conditions under which people live, work and play. Social determinants have consequential and varying effects on health outcomes across race and ethnicities. For Black women who are affected by structural inequality and discrimination, the chronic stress of poverty and racism has been shown to have a deleterious effect on health outcomes and is linked to their persistent maternal health disparities.[123]

To improve Black maternal health outcomes, social determinants of health must be addressed through policies that raise incomes and build wealth; provide access to clean, safe and affordable housing; improve the quality of education; prioritize reliable public transportation and transport for medical appointments; and increase the availability of healthy, affordable food.

Expand Paid Family and Medical Leave

Black women need paid leave to take care of their own health needs and to have time to care for their children. More than one in four Black workers report that there was a time in the last two years that they needed or wanted to take time away from work for parental, family or medical reasons but could not.[124] Only 30 percent of Black mothers are both eligible for and able to afford to take unpaid leave under the federal Family and Medical Leave Act.[125]

Only 15 percent of all workers have access to paid family leave through their employers. Paid family and medical leave allows workers to earn a portion of their pay while taking time off from work to care for themselves or their families. But current inadequate leave polices mean that Black mothers are more likely to quit and/or be fired from their jobs after giving birth than white women,[126] or return to work before they are healthy enough to do so. Lawmakers should pursue robust,

---

[123] Prather, C., Fuller, T. R., Marshall, K. J., & Jeffries IV, W. L. (2016). The impact of racism on the sexual and reproductive health of African American women. J*ournal of Women's Health, 25*(7), 664-671, retrieved 4 April 2018, from https://www.ncbi.nlm.nih.gov/pmc/articles/PMC4939479/.

[124] Horowitz, J.M., Parker, K., Graf, N., & Livingston, G. (2017, March 23). *Americans Widely Support Paid Family and Medical Leave, but Differ Over Specific Policies.* Pew research Center, retrieved 18 March 2018, from http://www.pewsocialtrends.org/2017/03/23/americans-widely-support-paid-family-and-medical-leave-but-differ-over-specific-policies/.

[125] diversitydatakids.org. (2015). P*olicy Rankings: The Family and Medical Leave Act.* Brandeis University, The Heller School, institute for Child, Youth and family Policy Publication, retrieved 18 March 2018, from http://www.diversitydatakids.org/data/ranking.

[126] Laughlin, L. (2011, October). *Maternity Leave and Employment Patterns of First-Time Mothers: 1961-2008.* U.S. Census Bureau Publication, retrieved 28 March 2018, from http://www.census.gov/prod/2011pubs/p70-128.pdf.

comprehensive paid leave policies that are accessible and affordable for all working people.

Expand Access to Quality, Patient-Centered and Comprehensive Reproductive Health Care

Quality, patient-centered reproductive health care is critical to improving maternal health and addressing the reproductive health disparities that Black women face including higher rates of unintended pregnancies and restricted access to abortion. Researchers attribute these disparities to a number of factors, including disparities in access to high-quality health care generally, and family planning services specifically.[127] Indeed, women with unintended pregnancies are at increased risk for maternal mortality and morbidity, maternal depression, experiencing physical violence during pregnancy,[128] infant mortality, birth defects, low birth weight and preterm birth.[129]

Black women also live with a legacy of reproductive oppression, and continue to experience reproductive coercion, sometimes leading to a distrust of the health care system that further exacerbates disparities. For instance, Black women are more likely to report having been pressured by a clinician to use a contraceptive method.[130] Moreover, some Black women may be forced to continue pregnancies because onerous restrictions and a lack of insurance coverage have pushed abortion out of reach.

This experience falls short of the level of high-quality, patient-centered care that all women should be able to expect. Policymakers must work to ensure that Black women are able to plan their families in the way that feels best for them, which includes access to counseling on the contraception method of their choice, access to abortion care without restrictions and access to prenatal and maternity care from providers they trust.

---

[127] See note 15; see note 20, Henshaw; see, e.g., Dehlendorf, C., Park, S. Y., emeremni, C. A., Comer, D., Vincett, K., & Borrero, S. (2014). racial/ethnic disparities in contraceptive use: Variation by age and women's reproductive experiences (pp. 526.e7). *American Journal of Obstetrics & Gynecology, 210(*6), 526.e1–526.e9 (citations omitted). A number of studies have demonstrated that there is not a significant disparity in knowledge about contraception between Black women and white women. See, e.g., Craig, A. D., Dehlendorf, C., Borrero, S., Harper, C. C., & rocca, C. H. (2014). exploring young adults' contraceptive knowledge and attitudes: Disparities by race/ethnicity and age. *Women's Health Issues, 24*(3), e281–e289; rocca, C. H. & Harper, C. C. (2012). Do racial and ethnic differences in contraceptive attitudes and knowledge explain disparities in method use? Perspectives on Sexual and Reproductive Health, 44(3), 150–158. See also, e.g., Dehlendorf, C., Harris, L. H., & Weitz, T. A. (2013). Disparities in abortion rates: A public health approach (p. 1776). *American Journal of Public Health, 103*(10), 1772–1779.

[128] See, e.g., generally Tsui, A. O., McDonald-Mosley, r., & Burke, A. e. (2010). family planning and the burden of unintended pregnancies. *Epidemiologic Reviews, 32*, 152–174.

[129] See, e.g., generally Conde-Aguedelo, A., rosas-Bermúdez, A, & Kafury-Goeta, A. C. (2006). Birth spacing and risk of adverse perinatal outcomes: A meta-analysis. *JAMA, 295*(15), 1809–1823.

[130] Becker, D. & Tsui, A. O. (2008), reproductive health service preferences and perceptions of quality among low-income women: racial, ethnic and language group differences (p. 208). *Perspectives on Sexual and Reproductive Health, 40*(4), 202–211.

Expand and Protect Access to Trusted Community Providers

Community health care providers play an essential role in providing Black women with basic, reproductive and maternal health care services. Without these vital resources, many Black women would not have information about or access to birth control, annual exams, Pap tests and other essential preventive care.[131] Policymakers should expand funding for trusted, community-based providers including Planned Parenthood. Community-based providers can help Black women get and stay healthy throughout their lifespan, including when, or if, they choose to become a parent.

Expand Protections for Pregnant Workers

Women report pregnancy discrimination across races and ethnicities, but Black women are disproportionately affected. Nearly three in 10 charges of pregnancy discrimination (28.6 percent) were filed by Black women from 2011-2015, yet Black women comprise only 14 percent of women ages 16 to 54 in the workforce.[132] Pregnancy discrimination has serious consequences for women and their families. Women who are demoted, not promoted or discharged because they are, or might become, pregnant can lose critical income.[133] If they are discharged or have their hours cut, they may lose their health insurance and other workplace supports at a time when their families' budgets are already stretched. Because Black women are also at a higher risk for pregnancy-related complications like preterm labor, preeclampsia and hypertensive disorders,[134] the loss of wages and health insurance due to pregnancy discrimination is especially challenging.

Stronger protections for pregnant workers, including federal and state laws that ensure that employers provide reasonable accommodations to pregnant women, robust enforcement of the Pregnancy Discrimination Act and continued education about existing legal rights are critical to combatting and, ultimately, eliminating pregnancy discrimination in this country.

---

[131] See, e.g., Stevenson, A. J., Flores-Vazquez, I. M., Allgeyer, R. L., Schenkkan, P., & Potter, J. E. (2016). Effect of removal of Planned Parenthood from the Texas Women's Health Program. *New England Journal of Medicine, 374*, 853–860 (describing the negative impact of cuts to family-planning services on women's access to contraception), recent studies have also shown that, in Texas, deep funding cuts to family planning services correlated with dramatic increases in the maternal mortality rate. See generally MacDorman, M. f., Declercq, e., & Thoma, M. e. (2018). Trends in Texas maternal mortality by maternal age, race/ethnicity, and cause of death, 2006–2015. *Birth,* 1–9; MacDorman, M. f., Declercq, e., Cabral, H., & Morton, C. (2016), is the United States maternal mortality rate increasing? Disentangling trends from measurement issues. O*bstetrics & Gynecology, 128*(3), 447–455 (describing how the reported maternal mortality rate in Texas doubled within a two-year period); see also Bassett, L. (2016, August 18). Pregnancy-related Deaths Nearly Doubled in Texas After Cuts to Women's Health. *Huffington Post.* Retrieved 27 March 2018, from https://www.huffingtonpost.com/entry/womens-health-texas_us_57b5d949e4b034dc73260bf3.

[132] National Partnership for Women & families. (October 2016.) *By the Numbers: Women Continue to Face Pregnancy Discrimination in the Workplace*. retrieved 6 April 2018 from http://www.nationalpartnership.org/research-library/workplace-fairness/pregnancy-discrimination/by-the-numbers-women-continue-to-face-pregnancy-discrimination-in-the-workplace.pdf.

[133] ibid.

[134] See note 14.

Invest in Health Care Safety and Quality Improvement Initiatives

Maternal mortality is three to four times higher for Black women than it is for white women, and Black women are more likely to experience complications during pregnancy and childbirth. There are existing, proven safety and quality improvement initiatives that need greater uptake to meaningfully improve health care outcomes for Black women.

Maternal mortality review committees increase understanding of the underlying and contributing causes of pregnancy-related deaths and the reasons maternal mortality affects Black women at such a high rate. A structured death review process can provide powerful data and information to facilitate change that improves the health of women before, during and after pregnancy.[135] Review committees should include medical professionals, community stakeholders, health advocates, patients and family members. Together, they should work to identify factors that lead to complications and corresponding strategies to avoid preventable complications as well as provide recommendations aimed at reducing pregnancy-related deaths.

Hospitals and medical practices should be encouraged and supported in participating in quality improvement efforts that are known to improve maternal health. For example, the Alliance for Innovation on Maternal Health (AIM) is a national data-driven maternal safety and quality improvement initiative based on proven implementation approaches to improving maternal safety and outcomes in the United States.[136]

Similarly, the California Maternal Quality Care Collaborative provides a multifaceted, solutions-based approach to quality improvement including toolkits on how to address the leading causes of preventable death and complications for mothers and infants.[137] State-level perinatal quality collaboratives have begun to address severe maternal morbidity and related quality and safety issues and should be encouraged to expand this critical work as they can scale implementation of the AIM resources and toolkits across states.[138]

Many structural and societal issues affect Black women's health. There is extensive research and evidence that point the way to strategies to improve our health care system and ensure that it delivers safe, effective and evidence-based maternal health care to everyone.

---

[135] Association of Maternal & Child Health Programs. (n.d.). *MMR Resource Portal for States: Building Capacity for Maternal Mortality Review*, retrieved 4 April 2018, from http://www.amchp.org/programs andtopics/womens-health/focus%20Areas/MMr/Pages/default.aspx.

[136] Council on Patient Safety in Women's Health Care. (n.d.). *Alliance for Innovation on Maternal Health.* retrieved 5 April 5 2018, from http:// safehealthcareforeverywoman.org/aim-program/.

[137] California Maternal Quality Care Collaborative. (n.d.). *QI Initiatives.* retrieved 4 April 2018, from https://www.cmqcc.org/qi-initiatives.

[138] U.S. Centers for Disease Control and Prevention. (2018, January 25). *Perinatal Quality Collaborative.* retrieved 4 April 2018, from https://www.cdc.gov/reproductivehealth/maternalinfanthealth/ pqc.htm#success.

Conclusion

Black women deserve to have safe and healthy pregnancies and childbirth. To meaningfully improve Black maternal health outcomes, we need systemic change that starts with the health care system, improves access to care and makes the places Black women live and work healthier, more fair and more responsive to their needs. Only when we do that will Black women be able to achieve their optimal health and well-being throughout their lifespan, including if they choose to become parents.

Fighting Back against Lies and Misinformation About Abortion Care, May 2019

Anti-abortion politicians are engaging in a dangerous effort to mislead and confuse the public about abortion care. They are peddling lies about abortion later in pregnancy in order to push their extreme agenda to ban abortion outright. Lawmakers and advocates are standing on solid ground when pushing back on this misinformation. Below are some ways to respond with the facts using an authentic and values-driven voice.

Punch Back with Facts (Adapted from Planned Parenthood's Messaging Guidance)

- These claims about abortion later in pregnancy are not true. This is a manufactured controversy.
- Abortion care later in pregnancy is rare. According to the Center for Disease Control, 99% of abortions occur before 21 weeks.
- An abortion that happens later in pregnancy is because of very challenging circumstances, such as when something in the pregnancy has gone very wrong and a woman's life or health is in danger or the fetus will not survive.
- Women and families in these situations face devastating decisions. They deserve our compassion and support — not our judgment and certainly not politicians telling them what to do.

Put Them on Their Heels

You have strong ground to stand on. You work every day to advance policies that make progress for women and families in real ways, you don't just pay it lip service. Call out their hypocrisy with your dedication to real policies that would make change and allow families to thrive. Express your indignation that anti-abortion politicians oppose the very policies that would enable people to have healthy pregnancies and support their families.

They are using lies to manipulate and mislead the public about abortion care. They are simply paving the way for their real goal — banning abortion outright.

- Across the country, access to abortion is under attack with increasing levels of inflammatory rhetoric and disregard for science, medicine or the realities of people's lives. An outrageous ban on abortion after only 6 weeks — before most people even know they are pregnant — has passed in four states. A bill was just passed by the Alabama Legislature that would criminalize abortion at any stage in pregnancy. A bill in Texas would have made it possible to impose the death penalty for women who seek abortion care.
- These bans are compounded by other efforts to cut off access to abortion care and family planning services, such as this administration's Title X gag rule, efforts to defund Planned Parenthood and the administration's rollback of contraceptive coverage.

If they care about healthy pregnancies and healthy babies then they should work to address the fact that the United States has the highest maternal mortality rate in the developed/westernized world, and that Black women are three to four times more likely to die in childbirth than white women.

- Highlight your support the MOMMA's Act, the MOMS Act, the MOMMIES Act and the Quality Care for Moms and Babies Act. All of these bills are focused on eliminating maternal health disparities and improving maternal health by expanding access to postpartum Medicaid coverage, funding maternal mortality review committees, adopting best practices and developing better quality standards.

The very same people peddling lies and purporting to care about pregnant women are the ones who would strip maternity care from health care coverage by undoing Affordable Care Act (ACA) protections.

- These are the same politicians that want to undo protections for pre-existing conditions and take away copay-free preventive care under the ACA — two key factors in helping women have healthy pregnancies. To support pregnant women, members of Congress should support legislation like the Protecting Pre-Existing Conditions & Making Health Care More Affordable Act, which would protect people living with pre-existing conditions, lower health care costs and reverse the administration's harmful sabotage of the ACA. And, these same people would dismantle our nation's Medicaid program, which covers nearly 50% of all births in our country and is a frontline program for helping women have healthy pregnancy outcomes. For example, Tennessee legislators approved a bill this month that would make the state the first to request approval from the administration for a Medicaid block grant, a move that could potentially cut their Medicaid program and eliminate health coverage for thousands of low-income pregnant women.

They would do nothing to guarantee safe, supportive workplaces for pregnant and parenting people.

- Pregnant workers are often forced out of their jobs because they are denied reasonable accommodations that would enable them to have a healthy pregnancy. They lose the income they need to support their family. Truly supporting pregnant people means supporting legislation like The Pregnant Workers Fairness Act.
- A national paid family and medical leave policy would allow parents to care for new babies while remaining in the workforce. Paid sick days would help pregnant workers get the prenatal care they need. That's why you support the FAMILY Act and the Healthy Families Act.
- Pregnant people also need fair pay. Mothers with full-time, year-round jobs are paid 71 cents for every dollar paid to fathers. Supporting women and families means ensuring that mothers have fair pay so they can support their families.

INDEX

A

B

C

D

E

F

G

H

M

N

O

P

T

U

V

W

Y